Optimal Aging

Also by Jerrold Winter, Ph.D.

True Nutrition, True Fitness

Optimal Aging

A Guide to Your First 100 Years

By

Jerrold Winter, Ph.D.

ISBN: 1505524067
ISBN 13: 9781505524062
Library of Congress Control Number: 2014922297
CreateSpace Independent Publishing Platform
North Charleston, South Carolina

To
Barbara

ACKNOWLEDGMENTS

There are many to whom I owe thanks. Among those who will remain nameless are the staff of the Health Sciences Library of the University at Buffalo. The superb holdings of the HSL have provided me with many pleasurable hours and form the backbone of this book. The conversion of their journal collection to electronic form has saved me many trips to the HSL but has unfortunately diminished my personal contact with the staff. The medical literature is of course entirely the work of countless scientists, physicians, and scholars; some have been named, many more have not. To each I am indebted.

My colleagues in the Department of Pharmacology and Toxicology of the School of Medicine and Biomedical Sciences have helped me in many ways. In particular I thank Margarita Dubocovich, Ph.D., my chairman during the time that this book was in progress, for providing a stimulating environment. Although I must retain responsibility for any and all possible errors of fact or interpretation, I want to thank all those who kindly read and commented upon parts of the manuscript or provided advice. Among those persons are Alan Reynard, Ph.D., Murielle Doat-Meyerhoefer, M.D, Ph.D., Richard Rabin, Ph.D., Jun-Xu Li, M.D., Ph.D., Fraser Sim, Ph.D., Scott Helsley, M.D., Ph.D., and Lucy Mastrandrea, M.D., Ph.D. In addition, critical comments from my children, Jerrold, Jr., Kurt, and Jessica, are deeply appreciated. Special thanks go to Anne, my elder daughter, who read and commented upon the entire manuscript. The book is dedicated to Barbara, my wife of fifty-four years and a constant source of support.

CONTENTS

PREFACE

Do not go gentle into that good night,
Old age should burn and rave at close of day;
Rage, rage against the dying of the light.[1]

B rave as are the words of Dylan Thomas, it is, alas, futile to "rage, at close of day, against the dying of the light." Not one who has lived has failed to die. But, as a preface to dying, all of us will age and in that process all of us are at the mercy of our genes, our luck, and our free will. Only the last of these is under our control. No, we will not beat death but we all can rage against the ignorance, the stupidity, the gluttony, the sloth which moves many of us from the near perfection of early adulthood to premature debility and a too early death.

This book is an attempt to bring order and genuine understanding to the thousands of bits of information which relate to aging: nutrition, exercise, drugs, hormones, cancer, stroke and heart disease, diabetes, obesity, osteoporosis, Alzheimer's disease; the list is daunting. To accomplish this end we must, as Will Durant suggested many years ago, "put aside our fear of inevitable error" and strive to attain "total perspective."[2]

The rise of the internet has made achieving total perspective both easier and more difficult. Easier because an enormous store of information is readily at hand. More difficult because, as Herbert Spencer expressed it, "When a man's knowledge is not in order, the more of it he has, the greater will be his confusion." An example: In 2009 the Nobel Prize for Physiology or Medicine went to three American scientists, Elizabeth Blackburn, Carol Greider, and Jack Szostak, for their discovery of telomeres and how they are controlled.[3] Their work has profound implications for both aging and cancer, because the same mechanisms which may cause our cells to age may also permit the endless and lethal proliferation of cancer cells. The application of these discoveries to human health is still some years, if not decades, away. Never mind, a quick search of the Internet informs me that, among other things, meditation, exercise, diet, and, most remarkable, something called TA-65, will lengthen my telomeres. TA-65 we are told is "a natural molecule derived from the Astragalus plant, a Chinese herb used since ancient times." A nice package deal offers a measurement of the length of my telomeres, vitamin and mineral supplements, a one-time consultation with an "affiliated age management expert doctor" (by phone if I prefer), and a year's supply of TA-65. The price: $21,010. No Medicaid or Medicare patients need apply. What is not mentioned is that the purveyors of this anti-aging elixir can provide no evidence whatsoever that it has beneficial effects. Still more remarkable, The Dietary Supplement Health and Education Act of 1994 permits any "dietary supplement" to be marketed to the general public without evidence of either efficacy or safety. Hence the statement regarding TA-65 as being derived from a Chinese herb. (See chapter 2 for more on the DSEHA of 1994.)

Quite aside from the hucksters, we have another problem to confront. Science in general, medical science in particular, is a wonderful thing. Anesthesia opened the way to a wide range of surgical procedures. Formerly lethal bacterial infections were tamed by the discovery of sulfa drugs, penicillin, and their descendants. The activation of our immune systems by vaccination has led to the potential eradication of diphtheria, measles, polio, and other killers. We can look back and be confident in the value of these great discoveries. However, things are not nearly as clear in the present time as we personally witness the halting progress of medical science. Consider the Women's Health Initiative (WHI).[4] In the last decades of the 20th century, physicians, mostly male, convinced themselves that the use of estrogen replacement therapy in menopause not only ameliorated the troublesome effects of this aspect of female aging but also reduced the incidence of heart disease and osteoporosis. To confirm these beneficial effects, the WHI was begun in 1993 and eventually enrolled more than160,000 women. In one arm of the study, post-menopausal women received either placebo or a combination of estrogen plus progestin. The results of this study reported in 2002 were remarkable but not in the expected way. It was found that drug treatment *increased* the risk of heart attack, of stroke, of blood clots, and of breast cancer. The words of Mark Twain come to mind: "It ain't so much what we know that gets us into trouble. It's what we know that just ain't so." The broader lesson of the WHI is that there is no place in medical science for dogma. What we believe today is only the best current approximation of truth based upon what has come before. We must ever be prepared to alter our approach to aging as Nature's secrets are revealed.

More than two decades ago I wrote a book about nutrition and fitness.[5] The late Thomas Lanigan, my publisher, advised me at that time to be positive and told me that "debunking doesn't sell." It is true that exposure of sham and falseness is a negative exercise. Kent Sepkowitz put it this way: "We want some pixie dust, a little magic, an eccentric genius who can see through…to the core of the problem… dull, steady scientific observation seems only dull and steady."[6] Fortunately, when it comes to aging and the help that you can provide yourself, there is much about which to be positive. Nonetheless, and despite Tom Lanigan's advice, I will on occasion debunk one or another possibly harmful illusion presented to you by the electronic or print media. Almost always I will provide some historical background. Knowledge of where we have been can help us to understand the uncertainties of today and where we may be going in the future.

Jack Weinberg was 24 years old and a leader of the Berkeley Free Speech Movement when he said "Don't trust anyone over 30."[7] In 2014 Jack turned 74. Most of us who are of a certain age can look back and recall fondly how our ideas have changed with the passage of time.

When it comes to aging, few give thought to the subject until about four decades have passed. Then, to most us there comes, unbidden, a revelation: this life is not a dress rehearsal. And it is at about that time that a fortunate few begin to wonder how they might influence the next 60 years or so. I would like to think that this book can be read profitably at any age but, realistically, a certain maturity is required, a recognition that life will come to an end and, most important, the realization that what I do today can alter in very significant ways the course of the years to follow, can influence even the nature of my death. Unfortunately, before that epiphany, many of us will become addicted to cigarettes, contract a sexually transmitted disease, acquire AIDS from a dirty needle, get fat, or suffer any other of the misfortunes of blissfully ignorant youth and middle age. Nonetheless, all of us, guided by what presently is known and unknown, can profoundly influence whatever years are left to us. The earlier one starts, the better.

Optimal Aging is divided into three parts entitled (I) The Chemicals in Our Lives, (II) The Things We Can Control, and (III) The Things We Wish to Avoid. In part I, the reader will learn of how drugs act and the phenomena of physical dependence and addiction. These will be illustrated by the experience of Fervid Trimble, a lively lady of 87 years who finds herself over-medicated in a nursing home, saved only by the advocacy of her daughter. Next the reader will be told of the Dietary Supplement Health and Education Act of 1994 and how it permits virtually unregulated sale of largely untested products. The third chapter of part I is entitled The Aging Brain, The Drug Industry, and The Battered Child of Medicine. Here will be presented the story of drugs used to treat dementia, anxiety, depression, and psychosis together with an account of the pernicious influence of the pharmaceutical industry illustrated by one prominent psychiatrist on its payroll.

The seven chapters of Part II will discuss the training effect and a program of exercise followed by a review, including historical perspective, of macro- and micronutrients. Part II finishes with chapters on obesity, weight control, and enhancement of performance.

The information in parts I and II lay the foundation for part III, The Things We Wish to Avoid. Chapters will discuss the relief of pain and the treatment and possible prevention of Alzheimer's disease, cancer, stroke, heart disease, and osteoporosis. Closing the book is a discussion of the end of life.

There is, I think, a reasonable sequence to each of these parts, but I have with intent made each chapter nearly independent of the others. It is my hope that informative reading can be found wherever the book is opened. For this reason, I would not object if someone with a particular interest in weight loss or cancer were to begin with chapters 8 or 13. Throughout the writing, I have been buoyed by the hope that this book will provide readers of all ages a rationale framework to minimize disease and disability as well as a means to maximize the probability of a long, happy, and healthy life.

PART I

THE CHEMICALS IN OUR LIVES

CHAPTER 1

DRUGS

The Good, the Bad, and the Ugly

In this chapter, I want to lay a foundation for talking about drugs. I introduce the subject early in the book because drugs are all around us, impinge upon virtually every aspect of health, for good and sometimes for evil, and one or more will be mentioned in nearly every chapter to follow. I will begin with a story told to us by Johanna Trimble about her mother-in-law[1]. It well illustrates the perils of drugs, especially as we age.

Eighty-seven years old, Fervid Trimble was admitted to the health center of the senior residence in which she had lived for many years. The immediate reason was that she awakened one morning in her apartment and felt that she couldn't stand without passing out. The only drug she was taking at that time was Vioxx (rofecoxib), an aspirin-like drug often used to treat arthritic conditions. (Vioxx has a long and sordid story of its own involving falsified data, concealed adverse effects, and eventual withdrawal from the market.[2])

Within weeks, Ms. Trimble was receiving nine different drugs which, the staff assured Johanna, were "not very many." Three of the drugs are known to decrease the actions of the brain chemical, acetylcholine, an effect well known to impair memory. For a urinary tract infection, Ms. Trimble received Macrobid (nitrofurantoin), an antibiotic. The World Health Organization discourages the use of Macrobid in the elderly because its adverse effects become much more common and severe as we age[3].

Two different anti-depressants were administered although the family believed that Ms. Trimble was merely upset about leaving her apartment. These were selective serotonin reuptake inhibitors or SSRI's. Prescribed for millions of Americans for depression and anxiety, their trade names are familiar: Prozac, Celexa, Paxil, Zoloft, Lexapro. A possible adverse effect of the SSRI's is called the serotonin syndrome which may include agitation, confusion, and even convulsions. A large number of other drugs are known to increase the risk of the SSRI-induced serotonin syndrome. Among these drugs is Ultram (tramadol), a morphine-like drug used to treat pain. Ms. Trimble was prescribed Ultram. Within weeks, she exhibited signs of the serotonin syndrome which, unfortunately, went unrecognized. A psychiatrist on the staff diagnosed Alzheimer's disease and recommended additional drug treatment.

Fortunately for Ms. Trimble, she had an advocate in the person of Johanna. She, together with her sister-in-law, a former nurse, went to the internet and learned all they could about Ms. Trimble's treatment. They then met with the medical staff and convinced them to stop all the recently prescribed drugs. In the words of Johanna Trimble, "...the *drug holiday* brought our Mom back to the intelligent and aware woman we'd always known (where did that Alzheimer's go!?). Not only did her mental status return to normal, she improved physically (a huge contrast to her original bedridden and delusional state when she was on the new drugs) and was able to participate in activities and exercise...She improved to the point that we could take her out to her favorite seafood restaurant for oysters and white wine when we visited. This gave great joy to all of us... Our Mom died in October 2008 after showering her family in her last weeks with love, gratitude, (and) praise..."

The story told us by Johanna Trimble, however compelling, is merely an anecdote. It is not the basis upon which health policy or medical practice is changed. However, after we talk a bit more about drugs, I will tell of a recent study which fully supports the notion that the elderly are often done more harm than good by the multitude of drugs so freely prescribed for them.

Pharmacology is that branch of medical science that deals with the interaction of chemicals with living systems. The living system that interests us and our physicians is the human body. When the chemicals do us harm we call them poisons or toxins and that branch of pharmacology is given the name toxicology. When the chemicals cure or prevent or ameliorate a disease we call them drugs and that branch of pharmacology is therapeutics or clinical pharmacology. To help make sense of the myriad of drugs we encounter, I will introduce the concept of the drug receptor. We can use Fervid Trimble's prescriptions as an example.

First, a word about drug names: you may have noticed in my listing of Ms. Trimble's drugs that I said Vioxx (rofecoxib), Macrobid (nitrofurantoin), and Ultram (tramadol). The capitalized name is a trade or proprietary name; the second is the generic name. The trade name is the one most often heard by patients, at least until the patent on the drug runs out and a generic form is available. Because the generic form is almost always less expensive, many medical insurance plans, including the one that I have, require that available generic forms be used unless explicitly objected to by the prescriber. A recent example would be Lipitor which has become available as the generic, atorvastatin; my co-pay dropped by 75%. Henceforth I mainly will use generic names, adding a trade name only if the drug has been so widely advertised that I think it familiar to most readers.

Getting back to Ms. Trimble, I will, for sake of illustration, guess at the other drugs she received. We know that there were two SSRI's, let's say fluoxetine and citalopram. The remaining four can be selected from a long list of possibilities. Commonly used in the elderly are alprazolam (Xanax), clozapine, metoprolol, and hydrochlorothiazide. The drug the psychiatrist had in mind for Ms. Trimble's "Alzheimer's disease" was donepezil (Aricept).

Rofecoxib, nitrofurantoin, tramadol, fluoxetine, citalopram, alprazolam, clozapine, metoprolol, hydrochlorothiazide, donepezil: how in the world do these drugs know where to go? We know where we want them to go: nitrofurantoin to her urinary tract, metoprolol to her heart, fluoxetine to her brain, and so forth. But the answer to our question is simple: Drugs don't know where to go. In fact, they go everywhere. With some exceptions, after a drug is swallowed, it is absorbed in the gut, passes through the liver, and enters the blood circulation. Once in the blood it will reach every cell in the body; it will bathe every tissue of the body. And this brings us to the concept of the receptor. A drug produces its desired effects by attaching itself to a structure of the cell called the receptor. Receptors can be very selective, responding only to certain drugs and ignoring the rest. All of Ms. Trimble's drugs go everywhere in her body but a pharmacologic effect results only in those tissues where an appropriate receptor is present.

But if a drug reaches every cell in the body, might it find other receptors unrelated to those we want the drug to occupy? And might these other receptors lead to unwanted drug effects? Yes and yes. Morphine provides an example. Derived from the opium poppy, morphine remains the gold standard for the relief of severe pain. William Osler, who in 1889 was a founder of the Johns Hopkins School of Medicine, called morphine "God's own medicine." Morphine works its wonders by attaching itself to receptors in the brain and spinal cord to reduce even severe pain. However, there also are receptors for morphine in the gastrointestinal tract. When these are acted upon, GI motility is reduced and constipation results. A nice trade you might think, constipation for pain relief, but constipation can be a very real problem, especially in the elderly. After Robin Williams was treated with morphine following surgery, he said that a priest had to be called in to perform a turd exorcism. But let us complete the circle. Might we sometimes wish to induce constipation? Many parents have become acquainted with the use of paregoric to relieve diarrhea in their children. Paregoric is tincture of opium, the natural source of morphine.

The concept of the receptor is fundamental to an understanding of drug action and I will invoke it repeatedly in the chapters to follow. However, in preparing to talk about a variety of drugs to which many of us will be exposed, I wish to provide three additional definitions. These are for drug tolerance, physical dependence, and addiction. Once again, morphine nicely illustrates the phenomena.

Let us imagine that I suffer from metastatic cancer and I am experiencing severe pain. My physician prescribes morphine and the effects are wonderful. But, over time, in order to maintain analgesia, it is necessary to increase the amount of morphine that I receive. It is now said that I have become tolerant to the pain-relieving effects of morphine. But, blessedly, that tolerance can be overcome with increasing doses of the drug. I may, after a few months, receive on a daily basis a quantity of morphine which would have killed me prior to my development of tolerance. Tolerance, in and of itself, is benign.

During the period that I am treated with increasing doses of morphine for my cancer pain, my brain is undergoing adaptive changes in addition to tolerance. Surprisingly, I am totally unaware that these adaptations have taken place. Only upon stopping my morphine are they manifest. Taken together, the constellation of signs and symptoms that results is called the withdrawal syndrome or abstinence syndrome. I am now said to be physically dependent on morphine. Put another way, after physical dependence has developed, the continued present of morphine is required for me to function normally. So long as the drug of dependence is provided, I will not experience withdrawal.

A more general term for what occurs during the chronic use of morphine is physical dependence of the opioid type. This is a reflection of the fact that many other morphine-like drugs whether derived from opium, heroin is an example, or synthetic narcotics such as meperidine (Demerol) and methadone produce a similar form of physical dependence. The opioid withdrawal syndrome has often been portrayed cinematically; films such as *A Hatfull of Rain, The Man with the Golden Arm,* and *Trainspotting* come to mind. In his classic book, *Junky,* William S. Burroughs provides a personal account. The syndrome is characterized by restlessness, anxiety, vomiting and diarrhea, runny nose, muscle twitching, chills, fever, and sweating. A bad case of the flu gives a pretty good imitation. Recall the last time you had the flu. What would you have paid to relieve, in an instant, all of your misery? Physical dependence and the constant threat of the withdrawal syndrome accounts in part for the continued prosperity of drug dealers.

Because the severity of the withdrawal syndrome is directly related to the rate at which the opioid receptors are deprived of the drug, withdrawal with minimal discomfort can be achieved in a medical setting by a gradual reduction of the doses administered.

Tolerance and physical dependence are invariable pharmacological phenomena. They have nothing to do with will power or your moral character. They certainly have nothing to do with the law. Every human, indeed every living animal going far down the evolutionary scale, will develop physical dependence when exposed to an appropriate drug. Addiction is another matter. It has been defined in a variety of ways, none totally satisfactory. A current biologically-based definition is provided by the American Society for Addiction Medicine: addiction is a primary, chronic disease of brain reward, motivation, memory, and related circuitry.[4] This concept of addiction as a chronic disease is antithetical to many who regard addiction as a moral failure, a condition we bring voluntarily upon ourselves. Given these uncertainties, I prefer a purely operational definition such as that provided by Dr. Alan Leshner, a former director of the National Institute on Drug Abuse: addiction is the behavioral state of compulsive, uncontrollable drug craving and seeking.

We have talked of morphine-induced physical dependence. But there are other forms to be considered. Indeed, any drug for which we can agree upon a withdrawal syndrome fits our definition of an agent of physical dependence. Until relatively recently the only types of physical dependence universally accepted were those of the opiate type, which I have described, and of the ethanol/barbiturate type. With respect to the latter, alcoholics are usually physically dependent on alcohol (more properly stated, ethanol, since there are many alcohols) and will undergo an especially severe withdrawal syndrome if denied alcohol or a similar drug. In addition, there is no question that chronic use of alcohol or opiates can end in addiction, i.e., compulsive drug craving and seeking. But let's consider still another form.

Daniel Davies met with his uncle for lunch. He had not seen him for awhile and now Daniel thought that he looked tense, fidgety, haggard, jittery. His uncle quickly explained: "It's the worst withdrawal I've ever suffered" and he went on to say that he couldn't sleep, couldn't concentrate, couldn't think about anything else. It was affecting his work, his marriage, his daily piece of mind. Many of you may recognize this syndrome. Daniel's uncle was a cigarette smoker. His drug of physical dependence: nicotine. What Daniel and his uncle describe is the nicotine withdrawal syndrome.[5]

I have said that physical dependence is not addiction but, once physical dependence is established to nicotine, avoidance of the withdrawal syndrome is a powerful incentive to continue smoking. To paraphrase Thomas Hardy, once you have been tormented by the withdrawal syndrome, mere relief becomes delight. Despite decades of denial by the tobacco industry, smokers are addicts as surely as are heroin users. Indeed, on a statistical basis, a heroin addict has a better chance of getting off his drug than does a smoker.

Forty years ago an international authority stated with confidence that cocaine would never be a major societal problem because its use was not accompanied by physical dependence. Today we know that cocaine, methamphetamine, and other stimulants are remarkably addictive despite having relatively mild withdrawal syndromes. The stimulants present perhaps the clearest example of a discontinuity between a dramatic withdrawal syndrome and addiction.

With the exception of the cigarette smokers among us, few readers of this book have been, are now, or are destined to become drug addicts. Virtually every reader of this book will be exposed to drugs which induce physical dependence of one form or another. I have mentioned morphine and alcohol but must add anti-anxiety drugs, sleeping pills, SSRI's, and caffeine. Yes, caffeine. The hallmark of the caffeine withdrawal syndrome is headache. Many a regular drinker of coffee, tea, or caffeinated soft drinks has awakened from surgery with, in addition to their post-surgical pain, a crashing headache. Having had no recent opportunity to ingest caffeine, they are undergoing caffeine withdrawal. A few enlightened institutions have recognized this uncomfortable complication and now are careful to provide caffeine post-surgically.

Why is it important for the elderly and their families to have a basic understanding of tolerance, physical dependence, and addiction? There are two major reasons. (1) Quite aside from the discomfort of withdrawal, the syndrome, especially in the elderly, can be confused with deterioration of mental functioning and a possible diagnosis of dementia and all that it portends. (2) Some physicians are reluctant to prescribe adequate doses of pain-relieving opiates because of an unwarranted fear that addiction will result. As I already have stated, physical dependence is not addiction. Perfectly appropriate medical treatment of pain may lead to physical dependence. The patient has not become an addict. Tragically, many governments of the world are so concerned about diversion of drugs for non-medical use and addiction that opiates are essentially banned. Countless terminally ill patients die in agony as a result. In India, it is estimated that only one-tenth of the medically indicated amount of morphine is used.[6] Even in the United States, under-treatment of pain, especially as one nears the end of life, is all too common.[7] Pain and its treatment will be discussed more fully in chapter 11.

I began this chapter with the story of Johanna and Fervid Trimble and the harm which may result when the elderly are over-treated with drugs. I will end the chapter by telling you about something called the Feasibility Study of a Systematic Approach for Discontinuation of Multiple Medications in Older Adults. The investigators were Doron Garfinkle and Derelie Mangin. Their results were published in 2010 in the *Archives of Internal Medicine.*[8]

After careful screening to eliminate persons with cancer or those with a life expectancy of less than three months, 70 patients with a mean age of 82.8 years were enrolled. All were living in the community; 26% were classified as independent and ambulatory, 57% as frail and ambulatory, and 17% required some assistance with activities of daily living. As might be expected in a population of this age, a wide variety of medical conditions was represented; one-quarter of the participants were receiving drug treatment for five different conditions, all at the same time. High blood pressure was being treated in 63%, dementia in 57%, depression or anxiety in 43%. Medications for diabetes, high blood lipids, heart disease, and osteoporosis were common.

When the study began, the participants were receiving an average of 8 medications. The investigators then applied what they call The Good Palliative-Geriatric Practice algorithm. This is simply a step-by-step procedure in which the use of every drug is questioned and decisions are made with respect to continuation of the drug, a shift to a better drug, reduction in dosage, or discontinuation entirely.

The results were remarkable, though, having read Ms. Trimble's story, perhaps not surprising to you. More than half (58%) of the drugs were discontinued, only 2% had to be restarted, and only six of the participants failed to have at least one drug discontinued. No significant adverse events resulted. From the patients' perspective, fully 88% felt that their general health had improved, their mood brightened, and their thinking improved. I mentioned that, at the start, 63% of the participants were being treated for high blood pressure; 84% of those drugs were stopped. This was not a novel finding. Earlier investigators had reached the conclusion that overenthusiastic attempts to lower blood pressure in the elderly may increase mortality and morbidity. All aspirin and similar drugs were discontinued. Again, not surprising. In 2009, the United States Preventative Services Task Force found no evidence for recommending aspirin for people older than 80 years.[9]

Deserving special mention are those drugs used to treat disorders of mood and behavior. These conditions range from anxiety to depression to overt psychosis. In the group studied by Drs. Garfinkle and Mangin, 36 patients (51%) were being treated for anxiety, 33 patients (47%) with an SSRI, and 8 patients (11%) with an antipsychotic drug. After application of their algorithm, one-third of the SSRI's were discontinued,

3 patients remained on their antipsychotic drug, and in only 1 of 36 patients was treatment with an anti-anxiety drug continued. I will say more about these drugs in chapter 3 but will note here that the family of anti-anxiety drugs called the benzodiazepines includes many a familiar name: Xanax, Librium, Valium, Rohypnol, Dalmane, Ativan, Serax, Doral, Halcion. I would note also that chronic treatment with benzodiazepines leads to physical dependence. The withdrawal syndrome from benzodiazepines is characterized by insomnia, tremors, and severe anxiety. Physical dependence upon this class of drugs first came to wide public attention in 1979 with the publication of Barbara Gordon's *I'm Dancing as Fast as I Can*, a vivid description of her withdrawal from Valium (diazepam).[10] Nonetheless, benzodiazepines continue to be used frequently in the elderly and, in addition to the possibility of confusion and physical dependence, are a major contributor to fall-related injuries.

It has been said that overtreatment of the elderly with drugs is a disease with serious consequences. But a word of caution: like other diseases, it is best treated by experienced professionals. Drug discontinuation should never be undertaken without consultation between patient, family members, and the prescribing physician.

CHAPTER 2

DIETARY SUPPLEMENTS

Who is watching out for us?

It will come as no surprise to many that the answer to the question posed above is the Food and Drug Administration. Faith in the FDA is widespread. With respect to prescription drugs, a recent survey revealed that four in ten adults believe that the FDA approves only extremely effective drugs and 25% thought approved drugs are without serious side effects. Truth be told, drugs are approved when the FDA believes that the benefit-risk ratio is favorable, i.e., when the anticipated benefits outweigh the expected harms. Approval is often based on a limited number of patients over a short period of time. Intense political and commercial pressure on the FDA to approve new drugs is not uncommon.

If the FDA's approval process for prescription drugs is less rigorous than many imagine, control of dietary supplements, those health-related products for which no physician's prescription is required, is dramatically more fragile. Responsibility for this sorry state of affairs is to be found in the Dietary Supplement Health and Education Act of 1994.[1] I will return to the DSHEA shortly.

Although the origins of the FDA go back more than a century, the agency gained its present name only in 1930. At that time, its powers to regulate were limited to acting against false and fraudulent claims and even this authority was often challenged in the courts. The FDA owes its present form to two therapeutic disasters.

Hildegard Domagk was a lively 6-year-old descending the stairs, embroidery needle in her right hand, seeking her mother's help. Falling, the needle was driven through her palm and up to the level of her wrist bone where it broke off. The place was Germany, the year was 1935, and Hildegard received excellent medical care. Following an X-ray, the needle was surgically removed, the wound was stitched, and she returned to her home. A few days later, her hand became inflamed and a red streak moving up her arm announced a likely streptococcal infection. At that time, amputation of her arm was the only recourse and even that measure would not guarantee her life.

Three years earlier, Gerhard Domagk, Hildegard's father, working in the laboratories of I.G. Farben Industries, had discovered a drug later to be called Prontosil. Unfortunately, it had not yet been tested extensively in patients and was not available to the public. Facing the impending death of his daughter, Dr. Domagk administered the unproven drug. Her life was saved. Prontosil was the first of a new class of drugs, the sulfonamide antibiotics. Domagk's discovery not only spared Hildegard, it later earned him the Nobel Prize for Physiology or Medicine in 1939.[2] (Unfortunately for Dr. Domagk, he was not permitted to accept the prize because of Hitler's displeasure with the earlier award of the Nobel Peace Prize to Carl von Ossietzky, a German pacifist.)

By 1937, dozens of companies around the world were selling one or more drugs of the sulfonamide family. One of the drawbacks of the new drugs was that they were quite insoluble in water and the other media usually used in making syrups and elixirs. The Massingill Company of Bristol, Tennessee, found the answer in diethethylene glycol and marketed an orally-active, sweet-tasting product called Elixir Sulfanilamide. More than one hundred Americans, including a dozen children, died after taking the drug.[3] The culprit was diethylene glycol. Massingill was fined $26,100, all that was allowed by the Food and Drug Law of 1906, on the grounds that the product contained no alcohol as was required in using the term elixir. The Food and Drug Act of 1906 even as amended in 1912 forbade only false and fraudulent claims; it did not forbid the selling of untested drugs.

Legislative reaction to Elixir Sulfonilamide was swift. In 1938, the Federal Food, Drug, and Cosmetic Act gave the FDA the authority, for the first time, to require that a drug be shown to be safe before it can be marketed.[4] The FD&C Act still did not require that a drug be shown to be effective. Legislation on that issue would wait another 24 years and a second therapeutic disaster far more serious than that of Elixir Sulfanilamide.

Morning sickness, the nausea and vomiting of early pregnancy, is known to virtually every mother. Many drugs have been used to treat morning sickness, none with complete success. In 1956, a German pharmaceutical house introduced thalidomide, with the trade name, Contergan, for the treatment of insomnia. Sold without prescription, a reflection of its remarkable safety when taken in overdose, it soon became popular for the relief of morning sickness as well. Use of the drug spread from Germany to other European countries, Canada, and Australia. For marketing in the United States, under the provisions of the Food, Drug, and Cosmetic Act of 1938, it would be necessary to demonstrate that the drug was safe. A simple matter it seemed. A lethal dose of the drug had never been found despite several suicide attempts with it. Kevadon was the name assigned to thalidomide by Richardson-Merrell, Inc., the intended marketer in the United States. The drug was given for evaluation to a new member of the FDA staff, Frances Oldham Kelsey. Much to the annoyance of the executives at Richardson-Merrell, Dr. Kelsey, with a Ph.D. in pharmacology as well as her medical degree, was, as Stanley Scheindlin described her, a nitpicker.[5]

The final issue of the *British Medical Journal* for 1960 carried a letter noting that thalidomide is "generally regarded as being remarkably free of toxic effects." However, the writer, Dr. A. Leslie Florence, went on to say that four of his patients who had been taking the drug exhibited signs of nerve damage.[6] After seeing this letter, Dr. Kelsey, who, as a graduate student had helped to solve the toxic mystery of Elixir Sulfanilamide, continued to delay the approval of thalidomide despite protests to her superiors from Richardson-Merrell. Less than a year later, note was taken in Germany of a sharp increase in infants born with a very rare condition called phocomelia in which the limbs are flipper-like.

In addition, because of internal malformations, four in ten of the babies died before their first birthday. The connection of these events to the use of thalidomide by the mothers was made by Widukind Lenz, a pediatrician.[7] The German government quickly removed the drug from the market. Despite this rapid response, more than 10,000 thalidomide babies would be born. But, thanks to the nitpicking of Frances Kelsey, there were only 17 in the United States. Why were there any in this country? Richardson-Merrill had distributed free samples of the drug to many physicians for use while awaiting approval from the FDA.

On October 10, 1962, John F. Kennedy signed into law the Drug Amendments of 1962, also known as the Kefauver-Harris amendments, which gave the FDA broader authority over the testing of drugs prior to marketing.[8] Included was a requirement that a drug be shown to be efficacious. To this day, disputes continue to occur regularly between drug makers and the FDA regarding the approval process; the most common complaint is a lack of speed on the part of the FDA, speed thankfully lacking in the case of thalidomide. (In March 2012, Senator Orrin Hatch of Utah introduced a bill intended to speed up FDA approvals so that, in his words, "patient care will not be slowed down by government red tape"; more about Senator Hatch later.) But most would agree that the FDA now has the resources and the appropriate legislative tools to protect us from dangerous or ineffective drugs. The same cannot be said for supplements.

Nearly all Americans know Donald Duck and his familiar quack. Fewer may be familiar with the word *quacksalver* or its shortened form *quack* with the meaning of a pretender to medical knowledge, a charlatan, a practitioner of quackery. The fact that this year Americans will spend about $30,000,000,000 (yes, thirty billion) for "dietary supplements" leads me to believe that many of us are unaware that quackery is enshrined in American law. I refer to the Dietary Supplement Health and Education Act of 1994.

A dietary supplement is legally defined in the DSHEA as a vitamin or mineral, an herb or other botanical product, an amino acid, or any combination of these. In contrast with drugs, the FDA cannot require that a supplement as so defined be efficacious, i.e., that it does what it claims to do. In addition, again unlike drugs, sellers of supplements are not required to prove that their products are safe. Instead, the burden is on the FDA to show that a given supplement is *unsafe*. While the FDA budget for 2013 was about $4.5 billion, the resources simply are not available for such tests of safety. Furthermore, the FDA does not have the authority to approve advertisements for dietary supplements before they appear. As one huckster put it, "you can make a lot of money before they catch up to you." Such ads typically talk of a disease, cancer for instance, and then go on to describe "An amazing treatment of Mother Nature"; words such as "safe" and "natural" are used repeatedly. Only then do we detect the presence of the FDA: "Statements made on this advertisement have not been evaluated by the Food and Drug Administration…This product is not intended to diagnose, treat, cure or prevent any disease." In 1994, the year the DSHEA was signed into law, there were about 9,000 dietary supplements on the American market. Today the number exceeds 60,000. The majority are of unproven efficacy and uncertain safety.

We hear much these days about government regulation and how it may infringe upon our freedom as Americans. Indeed, a major facet of the 2012 presidential election was concerned with the proper role of government in society with one side arguing strenuously for less regulation and a diminished role. Should governmental agencies tell me where I can smoke? Are my fries and cheeseburgers of any concern of Washington? Should a bureaucrat tell me I have to carry health insurance? Why should I not be permitted to sell raw, i.e., unpasteurized, milk? In fighting obesity, will the interstate highway system someday have weigh stations for people as well as trucks? None of these questions, and many more like them, is amenable to a simple answer and I will make no attempt to provide one. Nonetheless, with the examples of thalidomide and Elixir Sulfanilamide before us, most would agree that regulation of drugs can save lives. What then is the rationale for the Dietary

Supplement Health and Education Act of 1994? Writing in 2002, Paul Leber called it "an Orwellian 1984-like maneuver by which Congress applied the term dietary supplement to thousands of chemicals which fully meet the definition of a drug." Pieter Cohen in 2009 expressed the view that until the FDA is given the authority to regulate dietary supplements "millions of Americans will continue to be exposed to unacceptable risks in exchange for purported but unproven health benefits."[9]

The roots of the DSHEA are in the State of Utah and the Act is personified by that state's senior senator, Orrin Hatch. Introducing the bill to the Senate on April 7, 1993, Mr. Hatch said that "dietary supplements can promote health and prevent certain diseases." He went on to say that in Utah, healthy life-styles and "common use of dietary supplements, including herbs", have made a difference in terms of the incidence of cancer and heart disease.

It is true that the residents of Utah are a healthy bunch. Their rate of death from heart disease and cancer is among the lowest in the nation. However, before we attribute this fact, as Mr. Hatch does, to dietary supplements, may I suggest his Mormon religion as another possibility. Sixty percent of the state's population belongs to the Church of Jesus Christ of Latter-day Saints.

A central feature of that Church is *The Word of Wisdom* as revealed in 1833 to its founder, Joseph Smith. Based upon this divine revelation, the majority of observant Mormons do not to drink coffee or tea, smoke tobacco, or use alcohol or illegal drugs. Furthermore, they are encouraged to eat fruits and vegetables and grains and to eat meat sparingly. After reading about the DASH and Mediterranean diets in chapter 8, you may be inclined to agree with a Mormon dietician who said that the nutrition guidelines of the United States are coming in line with *The Word of Wisdom*. In Utah, the rate of smoking is the lowest in the country and the incidence of obesity is lower than in all but five other states.

I have no political quarrel with Orrin Hatch. He is a skilled elected official who depends upon the supplement industries in Utah for much of his campaign funding. His son, Scott D. Hatch, is a founder of the

Washington lobbying firm, *Walker, Martin, and Hatch*, and a registered lobbyist for the National Nutritional Foods Association. Mix in appeals to freedom of action, belief in personal responsibility, the merits of free enterprise, the right of consumers to care for themselves, and the creation of jobs in his home state and it is easy to understand why Mr. Hatch might favor a gentle regulatory hand as represented by the DSHEA. He characterized the law as a triumph on behalf of consumer health freedom. Stephanie Mencimer, a Utah native and writer for *Mother Jones* magazine, agrees that the DSHEA fosters freedom, "freedom to serve as guinea pigs for a multi-billion dollar industry, much of which is built on a foundation of fraudulent claims."[10]

My quarrel with Mr. Hatch is about science. How do we know what we know? How do we find truth? For example, how are we to decide whether the relatively good health of the people of Utah is the consequence, as Mr. Hatch suggests, of their use of supplements or if it is due in large measure, as I propose, to the fact that 60% of the population of the state does not smoke, does not drink, and is not obese? The choice is simple. Answers are found in meticulous, unbiased scientific investigation.

Overwhelming evidence from such studies tells us that smoking is the leading cause of death from cancer (chapter 13), alcohol produces extensive medical and societal harm, and obesity dramatically increases our risk of diabetes and heart disease (chapter 7). No remotely comparable evidence exists for health benefits from the use of even the most benign of supplements, the vitamins. And, as next I will illustrate, many of the supplements so freely sold under the rubric of the DSHEA are far from benign.

In mid-2012, I typed the words "dietary supplements" into my Google search engine and got more than 38,000,000 results. I must confess that I have not looked at them all. Instead, I have chosen just two for illustrative purposes. They are vitamin B_{17} and OxyElite Pro. Taken together they demonstrate the fundamental idiocy of the DSHEA as it relates to the health of the American populace.

Cancer will affect all of us, either directly or indirectly, sometime in our lives. Although today's medicine has many tools to treat the disease---surgery, radiation, chemotherapy---cure is often not possible and death, sometimes quick and sometimes lingering, results. In addition, the cost of such treatment is increasingly beyond the financial means of many, insured or not. Into this medical and financial vacuum, come dietary supplements such as laetrile, also known as amygdalin or vitamin B_{17}. (In discussing nutrition in chapter 6, I do not discuss vitamin B_{17}. The reason is that nutritional and medical science does not recognize a vitamin called B_{17}. But, never mind, it has a nice natural sound to it.)

Unlike many other dietary supplements which are without active ingredients and depend solely upon the placebo effect, laetrile is an active toxin. The case of Elizabeth Hankin of Attica, New York, tragically illustrates that fact.[11] Her father was taking a laetrile-containing product for treatment of cancer. Perhaps influenced by the fiction of vitamin B_{17}, he considered the pills to be harmless. Elizabeth was 11-months old when she accidentally ate one or more of the tablets. She rapidly became comatose and three days later she died. Dr. Judith Lehotay, the medical examiner of Erie County, performed the autopsy and listed the cause of Elizabeth's death as cyanide poisoning. It has been known since antiquity that the pits of peaches and apricots contain a substance that can kill. The toxin is hydrogen cyanide, the same substance used in Nazi gas chambers and by Jim Jones to kill the members of his cult in 1978. Those who continue to promote use of laetrile tell us that that cancer cells will be killed selectively. Unfortunately, there exists no evidence to support this claim.

Those with even a casual interest in this area of quackery may have thought that laetrile passed from the scene long ago. Countless law suits were brought against its peddlers and there were many convictions for criminal activity. In 1977, a judge in Wisconsin, in closing down a laetrile factory, said that "the promotion or sale of laetrile for any food or drug use constitutes a fraud on the consuming public."[12] That same year, Donald Kennedy, a distinguished scientist, Commissioner of the FDA, and later president of Stanford University, sent a letter to every physician in the country that said "laetrile is worthless, laetrile is dangerous, laetrile may be contaminated."[13] Dr. Kennedy's statement was based on studies done in thousands of patients treated with the drug.

The medical capstone, what should have been the final stake in the heart of laetrile, came in 1982 in a publication in the *New England Journal of Medicine* entitled A Clinical Trial of Amygdalin (Laetrile) in the Treatment of Human Cancer.[14] The lead author was Charles G. Moertel of the Department of Oncology of the Mayo Clinic. The design of the study was scientifically impeccable. The investigators had given 178 cancer patients laetrile in addition to a program of "metabolic therapy" consisting of diet, enzymes, and vitamins so as to mimic exactly laetrile treatments of the day. The conclusion by Dr. Moertel and his colleagues at the cancer centers of the University of California at Los Angeles and the University of Arizona, Memorial Sloan-Kettering Cancer Center, and the National Cancer Institute was simple: "Amygalin (Laetrile) is a toxic drug that is not effective as a cancer treatment."

In May 2012, thirty years after the publication of Dr. Moertel's study, I read on the Internet an article by Mike Vrentas of the Independent Cancer Research Foundation, Inc., in Lees Summit, Missouri. It begins with these words: "NATURAL CANCER TREATMENTS Information About the Amazing Treatments of Mother Nature!! Laetrile/Vitamin B$_{17}$ for Cancer…This cancer protocol is very effective at getting rid of cancer cells." Accompanying these words is a disclaimer by Mr. Vrentas stating that "The information provided…is for educational purposes only…not intended as medical advice…you must assume risk…products are intended as dietary supplements…products do not make any claim to any specific benefits…we do not attempt to diagnose, treat, cure, or prevent any disease…this information does not carry the approval of organized medicine in the United States, the FDA, the American Cancer Society, or the American Medical Association."

The last disclaimer by Mr. Vrentas is actually a recommendation. In his view, the AMA, the FDA, and the ACS together with what he calls

Big Government comprise a giant cartel designed to "suppress natural treatments" and "to make the people in these organizations very wealthy." Finally, he says that "…it is your God given right and your constitutional right to prescribe treatment for yourself." He might have added, "And facilitated by the Dietary Supplement Health and Education Act of 1994." Directions to Internet sites selling laetrile are provided and, if that is not sufficient, we can, for a fee of $200.00 have a telephone consultation.

The tragedy is two-fold. First, vulnerable cancer patients invest time and money in a worthless and possibly harmful treatment. Second, and more important, proven and potentially highly effective therapy is delayed or ignored entirely. The sickness and death of Steve Jobs, the genius behind Apple computers, illustrates the latter point. In October, 2003, Mr. Jobs had a CAT scan (Computed Axial Tomography) for suspected kidney stones. None were found but a shadow was seen on his pancreas. Soon thereafter he received a diagnosis of pancreatic neuroendocrine tumors. This is a relatively rare condition, constituting less than 2% of all pancreatic cancer. Early surgical removal of these tumors has been found to be curative in the majority of cases. Despite the urging of his family and friends, Mr. Jobs elected to employ alternative treatments including acupuncture, dietary supplements, and juices. Surgery was performed nine months after the original diagnosis and the cancer was found to have spread to his liver. On October 5th, 2011, Mr. Jobs died, age 56. In the words of Walter Isaacson, his biographer, "I think that he kind of felt that if you ignore something, if you don't want something to exist, you can have magical thinking. And it had worked for him in the past." We cannot know if the nine month delay shortened Mr. Jobs' life. We do know that the methods he employed during that period are ineffective however much we might wish otherwise.

With the possible exception of cancer patients, no groups are more susceptible to quackery than those, mostly men, who wish to build their bodies and those, mostly women, who wish to lose weight. (Nutritional supplements for weight loss will be discussed more fully in chapter 8.) You may recall that one definition of a dietary supplement provided by the DSHEA is "an herb or other botanical product." Based on this definition, a favorite tactic of the supplements industry is to combine plant material with a drug. The drugs range from caffeine to chemical relatives of prescription drugs to obscure agents which have escaped regulation. For example, a product for "men's health" (that's supplement-speak for erectile dysfunction) was found to contain an untested analog of sildenafil, the active principle in Viagra. The resulting combinations are of course advertised as "all natural."

A product called OxyElite Pro is but one of fourteen nutritional supplements containing a drug with the chemical name 1,3-dimethylamylamine or DMAA for short. These products are aimed squarely at young body builders with names like Nutrex Hemo-Rage Black and MuscleMeds Code Red. A user quoted by Natasha Singer and Peter Lattman of the *New York Times* said that it "gives you the mad, aggressive desire to lift more weight, pump out more reps, and have crazy lasting energy."[15]

Pharmacologically speaking and as would be predicted from its chemical structure, DMAA closely resembles a family of drugs called the amphetamines (see chapter 9 for more details). Methamphetamine, much in the news lately, is responsible for an epidemic of addiction especially in the American South and Midwest and a favorite commodity of the Mexican drug cartels. Like the amphetamines, DMAA acts on the brain to counter fatigue and induce feelings of energy and strength. An added bonus is that, just as with the amphetamines, appetite for food is suppressed. Indeed, many DMAA-containing products are sold as nutritional supplements for, in the words of one ad, "maximum fat loss." A feature that distinguishes DMAA from the amphetamines is that the latter have been placed in the same category as cocaine and morphine, i.e., drugs having an accepted medical use but a high liability for abuse. In contrast, DMAA is not subject to FDA control though it has been banned by the United States Anti-Doping Agency.

In December 2011, the Department of Defense ordered the removal of DMAA-containing products from the post-exchanges on all military bases.[16] Use of the drug was associated with the death of two soldiers who suffered fatal heart attacks during physical training. A well-recognized effect of the amphetamines, one likely to be shared by DMAA, is the production of unstable heart rhythms especially during strenuous exercise. The makers of OxyElite Pro responded in the expected way. Peter Barton Hutt, a lawyer for the group said that "DMAA is lawfully marketed as a dietary ingredient under Federal law."[17] Mr. Hutt certainly knows the law; he is a former Chief Counsel for the FDA. A company spokesman said that "DMAA is a naturally occurring compound found in an Asian Geranium." This is an important point because, if the DMAA in OxyElite Pro was not of natural origin, the product could not qualify as a supplement under the DSHEA. However, studies conducted in 2013 and 2014, while conceding that minute amounts of DMAA are found in some Geranium extracts, concluded that the amount of the drug in OxyElite Pro could not have been of natural origin.[18, 19]

With the examples of laetrile and OxyElite Pro before us, let us return to the question posed by the title of this chapter. With respect to dietary supplements, "Who is watching out for us?" The answer remains The Food and Drug Administration but I hope that by now you realize the limits put on the FDA by the Dietary Supplement Health and Education Act of 1994 . Indeed, when it comes to dietary supplements, I am inclined to say that the answer is *no one*. You are on our own. *Caveat emptor.*

I do not expect that anything I write will cause a decline in the sale and use of dietary supplements as defined by the DSHEA. Even when adequate evaluations of folk remedies have found them to be ineffective, little has changed. As the chief executive of GNC Corporation, a major seller of supplements, put it, "The thing to do with (these negative studies) is just ride them out. We see no impact on our business."[20] I am reminded of a line from Pat Barker's beautiful novel, *Regeneration:* "The congregation, having renounced rationality, looked rather the happier for it…"[21] Indeed, I am not optimistic that the law will be restored to rationality My only hope is that you will be careful and a bit suspicious and perhaps even a touch cynical when reading advertisements and deciding what to put into your body.

CHAPTER 3

THE AGING BRAIN

The Drug Industry and the Battered Child of Medicine

Anxiety, depression, insomnia, and dementia are common accompaniments of old age. Indeed, among persons living in residential care facilities in the United States, more than half receive a diagnosis of depression[1] and 4 in 10 are demented.[2] To a very significant degree, medicine's answer to these problems has taken the form of drugs acting on the central nervous system, so-called psychotherapeutic agents. For example, a survey of nearly a thousand persons 65 years of age and older newly admitted to nursing homes in Florida revealed that 71% were treated with one or more psychotherapeutic drug; 15% were taking four or more these agents.[3] These drugs are roughly divided into three categories, antipsychotic, antidepressant, and antianxiety agents but there is much overlap between their uses. It is not uncommon for all three types to be used at the same time. These drugs have been relentlessly promoted to the medical profession and directly to the consumer by an industry for which they represent enormous profits. Some good and much harm have been done.

In chapter 1, I introduced you to 87-year-old Fervid Trimble and her unfortunate pharmacological adventures. I want here to expand upon this issue. The first question to be addressed is "When should anxiety, depression, insomnia, or dementia be treated with drugs?" The answer is simple: only when they interfere with the activities of living and only

after other, non-pharmacological means, have been tried. Once instituted, all drug treatment must be monitored regularly and stopped if
found to be harmful or ineffective. As was the case with Ms. Trimble,
the patient often is unable to control or monitor the situation herself and
a strong advocate may be essential.

I am going to begin with antipsychotic drugs. This may seem an odd
place in that psychosis is not generally thought of as being related to old
age. For example, schizophrenia, the most common form of psychosis,
the hallmark of which is episodic departure from reality, usually has its
onset in early adulthood. The reason for our interest here is that antipsychotic drugs are widely used in the aged population particularly among
those suffering from dementia.

William Shakespeare, in commenting on love, provided a neat,
Elizabethan prescription for the treatment of psychosis: "Love is merely
a madness and deserves as well a whip and dark cell as madmen do."
Until the middle of the 20th century, little better was offered.

Henri Laborit was a French military surgeon with a life-long interest in
diminishing the hazards of anesthesiology and surgery.[4] Following his service
in World War II, he developed a three-drug cocktail intended to reduce surgical shock and post-operative illness. The mixture consisted of an antihistamine (a current example familiar to many is Benadryl), a morphine-like drug
(meperidine), and something called RP4560. The RP referred to Rhone-
Poulenc, the French pharmaceutical house that had discovered it.

In reporting his surgical findings to the French medical community
in 1952, Laborit ended with a curious suggestion: RP4560 might have
some uses in psychiatry.[5] And indeed it did. In a span of less than
two years, first in France, then in Canada, and finally in the United
States, RP4560 revolutionized psychiatry and the treatment of psychosis.
RP4560 was to be called Thorazine with the generic name chlorpromazine or simply CPZ. The psychotic wards were silenced, straitjackets
discarded, schizophrenics released to the community, and insane asylums
closed. Thorazine was not a cure for psychosis but, for the first time in
human history, it could effectively be treated.

Fast forward to 2012. In the United States, about 30 percent of all elderly persons in nursing homes receive antipsychotic drugs.[6] However, there is great variation between individual homes. In some, three-quarters of the residents receive these agents. Except in state facilities where cost may be paramount, few any more are treated with generic chlorpromazine. More likely is the use of one of a range of CPZ's descendants. Their intended effect is to reduce the agitation, aggression, and delusions that often accompany advanced old age in general and dementia in particular. Through March 2014, one of these drugs, Abilify (aripiprazole), had sales totaling $6.9 billion, the most of any drug sold in the United States.[7]

Critics argue that antipsychotic drugs are over-prescribed and are used as chemical straitjackets to subdue and tranquilize, some would say zombify, rather than to treat. Many suggest that the beneficial effects of these drugs are minimal. What we do know is that antipsychotics carry with them some very real adverse effects. While the newer drugs are less likely to induce movement disorders, they are more likely to result in obesity and diabetes. Most important, those treated with these drugs are more likely to die. This had been reported earlier in schizophrenics but, beginning in 2005, the Food and Drug Administration issued a series of warnings of a 60-70% increase in the risk of death when these drugs, including Abilify, are given to older patients with dementia particularly those with preexisting heart disease. The FDA's statement in 2008 was unambiguous: Antipsychotics are not indicated for the treatment of dementia-related psychosis.

Writing in the *British Medical Journal* in 2012, Jenny McCleery, Research Director for Dementias at the Oxford Health NHS Foundation Trust, said this: "The use of any antipsychotic in dementia is undesirable given the increased risk of death and the many other adverse effects of these drugs, in addition to their limited efficacy against target behavioral and psychological symptoms…The use of these drugs in this patient population has been much too prevalent in the past and it still is." Together with her colleague, Robin Fox, Dr. McCleery asks "Why then, given their adverse effects, does the use of antipsychotic drugs continue to be so common?" The answers they provide include pressures on physicians to prescribe ("Doctor, just do something.") and a lack of resources to provide non-drug based interventions.[8] I would add a third factor, the pharmaceutical industry itself.

You will recall from chapter 1, that a company can advertise a drug to the medical profession and to the public only for those conditions approved by the Food and Drug Administration. However, once a drug is approved for any condition, e.g., epilepsy, it can be prescribed for any other condition, e.g., dementia. This is called off-label prescribing. However, despite this complete freedom on the part of the physician to prescribe a given drug, it is illegal for a drug manufacturer to promote that drug for off-label uses.

Have drug makers ever violated the law with respect to off-label use of antipsychotic drugs in the elderly? A partial answer is found in the fines levied on some of the largest and most respected pharmaceutical houses in the world for doing just that.

2007 Bristol-Meyers Squibb	Abilify (aripiprazole)	$515,000,000
2009 Pfizer	Geodon (ziprasidone)	$301,000,000
2009 Eli Lilly	Zyprexa (olanzapine)	$1,400,000,000
2011 Johnson & Johnson	Ripserdal (risperidone)	$1,843,000,000
2010 Astra-Zeneca	Seroquel (quetiapine)	$5,200,000
2012 Abbott Laboratories	Depakote (valproic acid)	$1,600,000,000

The size of these fines must be put into the context of sales figures. The 2010 settlement by Astra-Zeneca represents just one tenth of one percent of the 2009 sales of Seroquel ($4.9 billion). Far more important was the blunt warning required by the Food and Drug Administration in all advertisements for the drug: "Elderly patients with dementia-related psychosis treated with this type of medicine are at increased risk of death." In just three years, sales of Seroquel fell to $1.1 billion. But Astra-Zeneca stockholders can take comfort from the fact that in December 2009, the

FDA approved the use of Seroquel as an add-on to antidepressant drugs. Seroquel is now widely promoted for this use in television advertisements and in magazines such as *O The Oprah Magazine*. As they say "Ask your doctor about adding Seroquel."

Those familiar with antipsychotic drugs may wonder about the inclusion of Depakote in our list. It is an old drug usually thought of an anticonvulsant. Its FDA-approved uses are in epilepsy, acute bipolar mania, and migraine headache. However, with a rising tide of objections to the use of antipsychotics in nursing homes, Abbott Laboratories saw an opportunity for their drug. They created a specialized sales force to promote the off-label use of Depakote to control agitation and aggression in patients with dementia.[9] In addition to its illegality, the unscrupulous nature of this sales effort is underscored by the fact that, thirteen years earlier, Abbott terminated a clinical trial of Depacote in patients with dementia because of an increased incidence of adverse effects.

By now one might expect that, with FDA warnings and sizable fines for off-label promotion, the use of these drugs in the elderly would be seriously diminished. Recent surveys suggest otherwise. For example, Lisa Chedekel found that in 2012 in the nursing homes of the State of Connecticut, the overall rate of usage was 26%. Remarkably, rates for individual homes varied between 7% and 68%.[10] For the country as a whole, data for 2009-2010 suggest a rate of 22%. In reporting the latter finding, Becky Briesacher and her colleagues at the University of Massachusetts Medical School said this: "The prescribing of antipsychotic medications persists at high levels in US nursing homes despite extensive data demonstrating marginal clinical benefits and serious adverse effects including death."[11] The fact that the recipients of these drugs are among the most vulnerable among us further saddens the situation.

We are all familiar with periodic variations in our mood. Sometimes we can identify the source: a setback at work, an unhappy relationship, a rebellious teenager, a dream unrealized, the loss of a loved one. Sometimes it's just a gloomy day without sunshine. Hormonal fluctuations are often invoked as causal factors; premenstrual syndrome is a part of our culture. (PMS is now officially called Premenstrual Dysphoric Disorder or PMDD.) For most of us most of the time, these are simple facts of life to be endured and overcome. Over the course of a lifetime, we all will develop tactics to counter a dark mood. These may include a pleasurable book or film, conversation with a trusted friend, escape to a sunnier climate, exposure to the contagious happiness of children. In keeping with a recurrent theme of this book, I would suggest that exercise works for many. Or, as was said in a B movie of the 1930's whose title disappeared from my memory long ago, "There is no problem that won't benefit from scrubbing a few floors."

In contrast with these normal fluctuations in mood and our adaptations to counter it, we have the psychiatric disease of depression and the very common use of drugs to treat it. As I noted earlier, among persons living in residential care facilities in the United States, about half receive a diagnosis of depression. In those over age 65 living independently, the incidence is estimated by the National Alliance on Mental Illness to be 19%; about half of these are prescribed an antidepressant drug. And, just as is the case with antipsychotic drugs, bad things may happen despite the best of intentions.

In the Diagnostic and Statistical Manual (DSM) of the American Psychiatric Association, the diagnosis of depression is based on nine symptoms: (1) depressed mood, (2) diminished interest in activities (Shakespeare was eloquent on this point: "With what I most enjoy, contented least."), (3) significant weight loss or gain or loss of appetite, (4) insomnia or excess sleepiness, (5) psychomotor agitation or retardation, i.e., restlessness or being slowed down, (6) fatigue or loss of energy, (7) feelings of worthlessness or guilt (Shakespeare again: "Yet in these thoughts myself almost despising."), (8) diminished ability to think or concentrate or indecisiveness, and (9) thoughts of death or suicide.

I have told you of the revolution in the treatment psychosis brought about by chlorpromazine in the early 1950's. Whenever a drug such as CPZ is discovered, it sets off a process called the study of structure-activity relationships. Hundreds or even thousands of similar drugs are synthesized with the goal of finding an agent with greater therapeutic efficacy or fewer adverse effects and, in the process, arriving at a new, patentable, profitable drug. Thus, using chloropromazine as their model, medicinal chemists at J. R. Geigy, a Swiss pharmaceutical house, synthesized a compound later to be called imipramine with the trade name Tofranil. Chemically it differed from chlorpromazine only slightly. Therapeutically it would mark a second revolution in psychiatry: successful drug treatment of depression.

The evaluation of Tofranil was placed in the hands of Roland Kuhn, a 38-year-old psychiatrist at the Munsterlingen Asylum in Switzerland.[12] Though trained in psychoanalysis, Dr. Kuhn found himself in 1955 the head of pharmacological initiatives at Munsterlingen. Initially, Tofranil was administered to schizophrenics. Their behavior only worsened. But, when tested in forty depressed patients, the effects were remarkable. The patients, Kuhn said, were "…generally more lively…more communicative…a friendly, contented, and accessible spirit comes to the fore…" Dr. Kuhn reported his findings at the 2nd International Congress of Psychiatry in Zurich in September 1957. Tofranil entered the United States market two years later. A decade after that, 10 million prescriptions a year were being written for Tofranil and its cousins. These were called tricyclic antidepressants. They would dominate the treatment of depression for nearly three decades. And then came Prozac.

It has become popular to say that depression is due to a "chemical imbalance", one that can be corrected with another chemical, a drug. Prominent among the chemicals thought to be imbalanced is serotonin, also known as 5-hydroxytryptamine or 5-HT, a neurotransmitter long believed to be involved in mood. Like many other neurotransmitters, there are active processes by which its actions are regulated. One of these is reuptake of serotonin into the neuron from which it has been released. Block that reuptake and the activity in serotonergic systems will be enhanced. (The whole notion of chemical imbalance in general and a role for serotonin in particular in depression have been called into question most notably by Marcia Angell, former editor in chief of the *New England Journal of Medicine*. But that is another story. What concern us here are the beneficial and harmful consequences of the use of these drugs in depression.)

In the early 1970's, in the laboratories of Eli Lilly and Company, a chemical was synthesized and given the designation LY110140. Soon it was shown by Raymond Fuller, Lilly's senior pharmacologist, that the drug would block the reuptake of serotonin following its release from nerve terminals. By 1979 the drug, now called fluoxetine, was under study for the treatment of depression. It became available for prescription in the United States in January 1988 with the trade name Prozac. The family of drugs of which Prozac is the father now includes Zoloft (sertraline), Paxil (paroxetine), Lexapro (escitalopram), and several others. Collectively, they are referred to as SSRI's, selective serotonin reuptake inhibitors.

The next great commercial, if not therapeutic, success for this class of drugs was the approval in 2004 of duloxetine (Cymbalta). Like Prozac, Cymbalta inhibits the reuptake of serotonin but, in addition, acts to block the reuptake of a second neurotransmitter, norepinephrine. Hence, Cymbalta is called not an SSRI but instead an SNRI. As large as is the market for antidepressants, it pales in comparison with the now approved uses for Cymbalta. In addition to depression, these include neuropathic pain associated with diabetes, generalized anxiety disorder, fibromylalgia, and chronic musculoskeletal pain.

There are two groups of depressed people I want to consider, those suffering from dementia and those of us who are elderly or old; 65 years of age or more is the usual criterion. For both groups, our focus will be on (a) how effective antidepressants are and (b) the adverse consequences which may accompany their use.

I have alluded earlier to the suggestion that antidepressant drugs don't work very well or at least not as well as we would like. Others are of the opinion that they don't work at all. With respect to the latter premise, a study by Sube Banerjee, and his colleagues which appeared in 2011 in the medical journal, *The Lancet*, should give us pause.[13] A total of 326 participants with an average age of 80 years, two-thirds of whom were women, with a diagnosis of depression and Alzheimer's disease, were assigned to one of three treatments. One group received Zoloft (sertraline), an SSRI, a second group Remeron (mirtazapine), a newer antidepressant, and the final third an inactive placebo. Neither the physicians nor the caregivers were aware of what treatments had been given. After thirty-nine weeks, it was found that depression had decreased in all three groups but there was no difference in depression scores for the three treatments nor were there differences in the assessments by caregivers; the drugs were no better than placebo. However, the drugs did differ from placebo with respect to an increased incidence of adverse effects including nausea and sedation. For the depressed demented, the authors suggest a three step approach: (1) watchful waiting, (2) community-based interventions, and, only as a last resort, (3) the trial of an antidepressant drug. (Given the incidence of dementia and the widespread use of antidepressants in the demented, I was most surprised by a fact stated in an accompanying editorial: "…this landmark study (was) the largest trial of antidepressant drugs in dementia ever and almost equaling the combined total from previously published work."[14])

Turning to the elderly depressed who are non-demented, I will take it as a given that antidepressant drugs do have therapeutic value in individual patients and instead will focus on possible adverse effects. In a study published in 2011 in the *British Medical Journal*, Carol Coupland and her colleagues followed 60,746 persons age 65-100 who had received a diagnosis of depression.[15] It was, in the words of the authors "the first systematic assessment of the safety of commonly used antidepressants in older patients across a range of serious adverse outcomes." Reflecting current prescribing patterns, ninety percent received treatment with an antidepressant. The majority of these prescriptions were for either an SSRI such as Prozac (55%) or a tricyclic antidepressant such as Tofranil (32%). An SNRI, venlafaxine, and mirtazapine accounted for the rest. The ten percent of subjects not treated with any drug served as a reference point. Data were collected with respect to death, attempted suicide, heart attack, stroke, falls, and fractures. There were minor differences noted between individual drugs but the overall conclusion was that "All classes of antidepressant drug were associated with statistically significantly increased risk of death, attempted suicide, falls, fractures, and upper gastrointestinal bleeding compared to when these drugs were not being used." In addition, SSRI's were associated with an increased risk of stroke, seizures, and heart attack. In a review of depression in older adults subsequently published in the *British Medical Journal*, Joanne Rodda, and her colleagues "...suggest that a practical approach is to regularly review depressive symptoms, side effects, comorbidity, and current psychosocial stressors and to involve the patient in the decision making process about ongoing drug treatment."[16] Once again, a strong advocate for the patient may be needed.

Let us now pause and ask how we reached the point where, despite clear evidence of harm and sometimes minimal benefit, antipsychotic and antidepressant drugs continue to be so widely prescribed for the elderly whether living independently or in nursing homes? A part of the answer is to be found in "Psychiatry: The Battered Child of Medicine." That was the title of an article which appeared in the *New England Journal of Medicine* in January, 1975.[17] In it, Milton Greenblatt, a Harvard psychiatrist, characterized his specialty this way: "Born in witchcraft and demoniacal possession, feared by the public, often scorned by the family of medical specialists, and dependent for much of its existence upon handouts from public agencies, psychiatry has had a very hard life." I would add that in the nearly four decades since, psychiatrists have not always burnished the reputation of their chosen field and that "handouts from public agencies" have been generously supplemented by handouts from multinational pharmaceutical houses with drugs to sell. Marcia Angell, puts it bluntly: "Psychiatrists are in the pockets of industry."

But why should this matter if the majority of psychoactive drugs are prescribed for the elderly by non-psychiatric physicians? The reason it matters is that prescribing patterns are driven to a substantial degree by what psychiatrists have to say about these drugs both in programs of continuing medical education and in periodic guidelines issued by the American Psychiatric Association. These are called Clinical Practice Guidelines. CPG's are always written by groups of leaders in the field and are very influential in the day-to-day practice of medicine. They are often cited by defense lawyers in malpractice suits as establishing what are regarded as standard practices. However, Lisa Cosgrove and her colleagues of the University of Massachusetts found that 90% of the authors of the APA's guidelines for schizophrenia, bipolar disorder, and major depressive disorder had financial ties to the companies whose drugs were recommended.[18] Des Spence, a Scottish physician, put it this way: "... doctors are open to manipulation...medicine's greatest weakness is its culture—authoritarian, hierarchical, deferential, and therefore easy to control through a few powerful individuals."[19]

Charles B. Nemeroff provides an example of the interplay between psychiatrists and drug house dollars. GlaxoSmithKline (GSK) is a multinational manufacturer of drugs including the antidepressant, Paxil (paroxetine), a selective serotonin reuptake inhibitor. Dr. Nemeroff is one of American's most influential psychiatrists. In 2006, he was chairman of the Department of Psychiatry at Emory University School of Medicine. In that year, Dr. Nemeroff received $960,000 from GSK for, among other things, a series of speeches to groups of doctors in which the virtues of Paxil and other GSK drugs were emphasized.[20] At the same time he led a $3.9 million study sponsored by the National Institute of Mental Health of antidepressant drugs including Paxil.

Under the rules of ethics at Emory University, faculty members are required to report income from outside sources in excess of $10,000. Between 2000 and 2006, Dr. Nemeroff received more than $2.5 million from drug companies including GSK. Because it was found that he reported only a tiny fraction of this, Emory ruled that he could not accept federal grants for a period of two years. In referring to one of Dr. Nemeroff's publications, a University official called it "a piece of paid marketing."[21] In 2008, he stepped down as chairman of psychiatry at Emory.

A year later he was named chairman of the Department of Psychiatry and director of the Center on Aging at the University of Miami's Miller School of Medicine. In 2012, he received the annual achievement award from an organization called CME Outfitters for "his commitment to medical research and improving patient care." According to their Internet site, "CME Outfitters develops and distributes live, recorded and web-based, outcomes- and evidence-based educational activities to thousands of clinicians each year." Also in 2012, GlaxoSmithKline agreed to pay a $3 billion fine in part for the illegal off-label marketing of several of its drugs including Paxil. A sliver of light was seen in February 2013 when the Obama administration issued a rule that requires the makers of prescription drugs to disclose what they pay doctors for consulting or speaking on behalf of the manufacturer.[22]

Whatever the mysteries of psychosis and depression, anxiety is familiar to all. Anxiety is Nature's way of keeping us moving. For many it begins with separation from our mothers and proceeds through every phase of our lives. Most agree that anxiety is a normal reaction to stress and serves a useful purpose in driving us to achieve whatever it is we wish to achieve. But uncontrolled anxiety can be disabling and it is here that we may turn to chemicals for relief. While anxiety and its treatment with drugs may run throughout our lives, the aging brain, and especially the demented brain, is particularly susceptible to the adverse effects of these drugs.

While drug treatment of psychosis and depression is a relatively recent phenomenon, humans have been calming anxiety with drugs for countless millennia. Today's drinkers of alcoholic beverages, smokers of marijuana, and devotees of opium are continuing practices which date back to before written history; 12,000 years ago is a reasonable guess.

As ancient as is man's use of alcohol, it was only late in the 20th century that pharmacology provided a plausible explanation of how it works in our brains. Embedded in the outer covering of our neurons are a variety of channels that control the inward and outward flow of essential chemicals and in turn the excitability of the neuron. One such channel is called GABA$_A$, named for *gamma*-aminobutyric acid, the neurotransmitter that acts upon the channel to suppress activity in the nervous system. Alcohol acts at GABA$_A$ to potentiate this effect. I mention this bit of esoterica because it now appears that the same mechanism accounts for the effects of all drugs used for anxiety and insomnia. Even propofol, the drug implicated in Michael Jackson's death, acts this way. Collectively, these drugs are called depressants. A common mechanism also explains how these drugs can be additive or even more additive in their effects. As one amateur pharmacologist put it: A Xanax and two beers is as good as a six-pack. (More about Xanax in a moment.)

A medically accepted alternative to alcohol for anxiety and insomnia was provided by a family of drugs called the barbiturates. The first of these, barbital, was sold in Germany at the turn of the 20th century under the name Veronal. Worldwide use for the treatment of insomnia and neurosis soon followed for Veronal and its many relatives. (In *Grand Hotel*, a classic film from 1932, Greta Garbo famously says "Not even the Veronal can help me sleep.") But there are drawbacks to the barbiturates. Foremost among these is death from overdose whether accidental or with suicidal intent. In addition, physical dependence may develop accompanied by addiction. Nonetheless, barbiturates were the mainstay of the treatment of anxiety and insomnia well into the 1950's.

Having used the term "neurosis" in the preceding paragraph, I should say a bit about terminology. In American psychiatry, we are no longer labeled as neurotics. Instead we suffer from *anxiety disorders*, a category housing a multitude of conditions including panic attacks, obsessive-compulsive disorder, posttraumatic stress disorder, social phobia, and generalized anxiety.

A new era in the treatment of anxiety and insomnia was ushered in by the discovery and sale in 1955 of meprobamate under the names Miltown and Equanil. For marketing purposes, meprobamate was called a *minor tranquilizer* to distinguish it from *major tranquilizers* such as Thorazine. The attachment to these drugs of a common term, tranquilizer, is unfortunate in that the implication is that these are similar drugs differing only in intensity of effects. Much inappropriate prescribing has resulted including the prescription of antipsychotics for simple anxiety. But, for purposes of advertising, tranquilizer is a wonderful word. Who, after all, would not wish to be tranquil?

The popularity of Miltown was short-lived, lasting only until the discovery of the benzodiazepines. First came Librium (chlordiazepoxide) in 1960 to be followed two years later by Valium (diazepam). The family now includes many other familiar names: Xanax (alprazolam), Dalmane (flurazepam), Ativan (lorazepam), Restoril (temazepam), and Halcion (triazolam) among them. Standing marginally apart is a group of "non-benzodiazepine" drugs used largely for insomnia. Included are Ambien (zolpidem), Sonata (zaleplon), and Lunesta (eszopiclone). I say "standing marginally apart" because, though they chemically are not benzodiazepines, they act, as do alcohol and the benzodiazepines, at $GABA_A$ receptors. Hence we should not expect their benefits and risks to be significantly different. Zolpidem is also marketed as Intermezzo, to be taken by insomniacs who awaken in the middle of the night.

A major virtue of the benzodiazepines and their relatives is that it is much more difficult to kill yourself with an overdose. However, their effects in combination with alcohol and opiates are less certain and there is the suspicion that they may contribute to a fatal outcome. Anecdotal evidence for this possibility comes from public disclosure of autopsy results following the death of celebrities. For example, benzodiazepines were among the multiple drugs found in Heath Ledger, Michael Jackson, Corey Heim, and Whitney Houston.

A primary concern surrounding the use of antianxiety drugs in the elderly in general and the elderly demented in particular is an increased risk of falls, a leading cause of injuries, hospitalization, and death. The evidence is clear that all classes of psychotherapeutic drugs, including benzodiazeptines used to treat anxiety and insomnia, increase risk to the point that some have advised that all such drugs be avoided in those prone to falling. In the United States, more than 20,000 elderly persons die each year from head trauma or hip fracture as a result of falls. A study done by the Veterans Administration found that one in three elderly male veterans who fracture a hip die within one year.[23]

With benzodiazepines and related drugs such as Ambien, the occurrence of what have been called paradoxical effects increases with age, especially in the presence of dementia. These may include a deepening of depression and the emergence of agitation and aggression. Such effects may be interpreted as the worsening of an underlying condition rather than a drug effect thus leading to still further drug treatment with still further unfortunate consequences.

If used for prolonged periods, whether for anxiety or insomnia, these drugs induce physical dependence of a form reminiscent of alcohol dependence. The withdrawal syndrome may include anxiety, agitation, cramps, insomnia, sensitivity to light, and seizures. Once again, particularly in the elderly, these signs can be misinterpreted as a worsening of dementia leading to further inappropriate drug treatment.

Earlier we discussed Prozac, the first of the serotonin reuptake inhibitors, and its approval as an antidepressant in 1988. Even before that time, studies in animals revealed what appeared to be antianxiety effects. These were soon confirmed in human studies and today, SSRI's are regarded by many as the drugs of choice for the treatment of anxiety disorders in old and young alike. Unfortunately, like the benzodiazepines, SSRI's, in addition to their other adverse effects, increase the risk of falls and fractures.

Among the indications for the use of an SSRI is premenstrual dysphoric disorder, not a concern for the elderly but, in forming our impression of the pharmaceutical industry, an interesting story nonetheless. At the time that Eli Lilly's patent on Prozac was about to end, the company created a "new" drug for the treatment of PMDD. In fact it was Prozac with a new color, pink, and a new name, Sarafem, and, most important for Lilly, new patent protection. Lilly promised to make you "more like the woman you are." It was Alicia Rebensdorf who alliteratively called this "The Pimping of Prozac for PMS."[24]

I have mentioned the relative safety of the benzodiazepines in caus-ing death when taken in excess but I have noted as well several epide-miological studies which found a peculiar increase in the risk of death in elderly persons treated with acceptable doses of these drugs. It has been difficult to pinpoint an exact cause for this fact but a report published in 2013 suggests a possible contributor. Eneanya Obiora and his colleagues examined the association between the use of benzodiazepines and the occurrence of pneumonia.[25] Use of benzodiazepines increased the risk of pneumonia by almost 50%. In the nearly five thousand patients studied, the risk of death from the disease was increased by 20 to 30%.

In discussing dietary supplements in chapter 2, I asked "Who is watching out for us?" In light of the Dietary Supplement Health and Education Act of 1994, the answer we arrived at was *No one; you are on your own.* With respect to the drugs we have discussed in this chapter, all of which are available only by prescription, it is the Food and Drug Administration to which we look for protection. However, as is wit-nessed by the examples I have provided you, it is clear that the FDA's ability to watch out for us is seriously limited by the political, financial, and advertising power of the drug industry. Whether our democracy and our devotion to capitalism will permit a reversal of this situation remains to be seen. In the meantime, we must look out for ourselves and for those we love. It is never inappropriate to question your physician as to the rationale for the use of any drug either for yourself or for those under your care. This is especially true for the psychotherapeutic drugs we have discussed.

PART II

THE THINGS WE CAN CONTROL

CHAPTER 4

A TRAINING EFFECT

The Alvin Roy revolution

For most of us, exercise is not a neutral subject. Some seek to avoid it as if it were a lethal disease. Others describe their daily routine as would a monk his prayers. J.V. Durnam, a Scotsman and exercise physiologist, says this about jogging: "...even sensible people pretend they enjoy it. The enjoyment is seldom obvious...I find jogging to be a particularly useless form of activity, with little apparent pleasure to be obtained from it."

I must differ with Professor Durnam. After more than fifty years, I continue to find running an almost always pleasurable experience. The fact that it seems to confer benefits other than the purely hedonistic is a bonus. (Confusion sometimes arises on the distinction between running and jogging. I am a runner; all those few people slower than I are joggers. Feel free to use those definitions.)

It was the 17th century when Rene Descartes compared the human body to a machine but that analogy remains useful today. Our bodies generate energy by oxidizing food and in the process emit carbon dioxide and water and waste products. Our eyes and ears and other sensory tools provide a central computer, our brain, with information that is selectively stored or ignored or acted upon. The machines of action are the muscles and, when properly guided by the brain, can wink an eye or run a marathon or sing a song. However, like machines, our bodies wear out with the passage of time---the process of aging. Then, after a few still usable parts have perhaps been removed for use by others, we are recycled: "Thou art dust, and shalt to dust return" was John Milton's elegant line.

But this notion of wearing out can be misunderstood. Unlike a classic automobile that continues to escape the junkyard because it is coddled and protected, the human machine thrives on hard use and becomes stronger in the process. Put your body to bed for the winter and you will emerge with the spring, not bright and shiny and ready for a road trip, but shriveled and weak. The response of our bodies to exercise is called the training effect.

To understand the training effect, we need to know a little about our muscles and how they translate food into motion. The immediate source of energy for muscular contraction is a chemical found in all cells, adenosine triphosphate, ATP for short. If I am about to be run over by a bus, my brain will send an urgent message to my muscles to get me out of the way. Fortunately, there is enough ATP available to allow immediate, bus-avoiding action. This is done without the need for oxygen, hence my life-saving muscular contraction is called *anaerobic* from the Greek *an* (without), *aer* (air), and *bios* (life).

If, instead of a bus, it is slowly rising flood waters that threaten me and the high ground is ten miles distant and me without a wheeled vehicle, I had better respond in a different fashion. Were I to sprint off, the ATP in my muscles would soon be exhausted and collapse would overtake me just before the flood. Instead I will walk or run at a pace I can maintain for the hour or two it will take me to cover the ten miles.

The large amounts of ATP required by my 10-mile jaunt can only be generated from nutrients and oxygen. Nutrients present no problem because my muscular engines can run on carbohydrate or fat or even protein in a pinch. On the other hand, the increased need for oxygen will cause me to breathe more often and more deeply. This need for air gives this kind of exercise its name, *aerobic*.

The consequences of anaerobic and aerobic exercise are not the same. At the risk of insulting one or other, let's compare the appearance of a weight lifter or body builder with that of a long-distance runner. The lifter, whose exercise is primarily of the anaerobic kind, may have the well-defined muscles of a Mr. Universe contestant or simply be massive. In contrast, our model for an aerobic trainer might be one of those remarkably fast but remarkably thin Kenyan marathoners, men and women capable of running 5-minute miles for a couple of hours.

We can understand these differences in appearance by considering how the runner and the body builder train. I will use the *vastus lateralis*, one of the three major muscles of the thigh as an example. Weightlifters may place a bar loaded with several hundred pounds across their shoulders, lower their bodies into a squat, and return to a standing position. One squat takes about three seconds and will be repeated perhaps four times. If the weight has been chosen with care, the fourth repetition requires maximum effort and a fifth is impossible; there simply isn't enough ATP left in the muscle. Twelve seconds of anaerobic exercise doesn't seem like much but over time remarkable changes will take place. The class of muscle fibers best able to contract anaerobically will increase in size producing a bigger and stronger *vastus lateralis*. After a brief period for recovery, this activity may be repeated and other muscles stressed in a similar maximal way.

Anyone who doubts the reality of the anaerobic training effect needs only compare the weights of football linemen over the past decades. In 1955, I had just graduated from high school and was in an August postseason game with players from in and around my hometown in Western Pennsylvania. I was a lineman and on my right was Jim Schaaf, a high school All-American tackle. Jim went on to Notre Dame where he was shifted to guard. His companion at that position on the 1958 team was Al Ecuyer who would finish the season as a collegiate All-American. Al was listed at 205 pounds, Jim at 195. Contrast those figures with the offensive lineman for the Notre Dame team of 2014; on average, they weighed 309 pounds. In 1964, the University of Alabama team that won the national championship had only one starting lineman who weighed more than two hundred pounds, Cecil Dowdy at 206. Less than 20 years later, in his last season of coaching, Bear Bryant's offensive line averaged

258 pounds. In 2014, the Alabama roster listed a total of 21 offensive linemen with an average weight of 308 pounds. Alvin Roy had changed football forever.

Born in Baton Rouge, Louisiana, Alvin Roy[1] served with distinction during World War II in the European theater under General George Patton. In 1946, while still in the Army, Roy was assigned to the United States weight lifting team for the world championships held in Paris. Later he would be the trainer for the United States team in the 1952 Olympic Games. At that time, conventional wisdom was that weight lifting made an athlete slow and muscle-bound and no football coach permitted it. Based on what he had learned from the weight lifters, Roy was ready to challenge that dogma.

Weight training programs for football players were begun by Roy at his high school alma mater in 1954, at Louisiana State University, his college alma mater, in 1957, and finally with the professional San Diego Chargers in 1963 under their head coach, Sid Gillman. The incentive was that each of these teams had suffered through losing seasons. The results were spectacular. In the first year following the introduction of Roy's strength program, his high school team was undefeated, LSU won its first national championship, and San Diego was the American Football League champion. Today, strength training is an integral part of every football program and is found as well in many other sports. (Sid Gillman and Alvin Roy also have the distinction of bringing the use of steroids to American athletes. Roy had learned of these drugs from the Russian Olympic weight lifters. The training camp of the Chargers in 1963 served Diabinol, an analog of testosterone, at every meal.[2] No sport, amateur or professional had banned the use of steroids at that time. Steroids will be discussed more fully in chapters 9 and 10.)

In contrast with the lifter's brief, intense effort, a single stride of the runner places a much smaller demand on the *vastus lateralis*. However, that small demand may be repeated thousands of times without rest. Unlike the lifter, who borrows ATP from the muscle bank, the runner must pay as she goes. To do that she depends on a second major class of muscle fibers, those best able to provide ATP from oxygen and nutrients; in other words, to contract aerobically. If the *vastus lateralis* is exercised by running for 30 minutes a day for a few weeks, these fibers will increase their capacity to produce ATP. However, they will not increase in size. It's for this reason that women who take up running needn't worry about developing massive leg muscles; aerobic exercise does not produce bulky muscles. We may look again at the Kenyans for proof.

The training effect of aerobic exercise does not end with the muscle fibers. If the muscles are to use more oxygen, the whole system of delivery of oxygen must be improved. A trained muscle fiber is seen to have more capillaries, the smallest of blood vessels, surrounding it. The muscular components of the heart become stronger and more efficient so that more blood can be pumped per minute. Respiratory muscles develop the endurance to maintain deeper and more frequent breathing. The nervous system becomes better able to shunt blood from one area to another. Changes such as these separate us from all things mechanical; we respond to the stress of exercise by improving our ability to exercise; we become more fit.

What shall we be, lifters or marathoners, aerobic trainers or anaerobic trainers, strength versus endurance? What will best get us to and through a long, healthy, happy old age? For a long time, we thought that aerobic fitness was the key; LSD stood not only for a hallucinogenic drug but also for Long Slow Distance running. The change in our thinking did not come quickly, certainly not with the speed of the Alvin Roy revolution in football. But it did come. Loss of muscle mass and strength with aging is now recognized as a major hazard for the frail elderly particularly with respect to life-threatening falls.[3] Clearly what is needed is a program of exercise, tailored to the individual at every age, which includes both aerobic and anaerobic components. I will suggest just such a program in the next chapter.

CHAPTER 5

A PROGRAM OF EXERCISE

The good addiction

I have said elsewhere that there is no place for dogma in medical science. Today we act upon the best approximation of truth that we can find but we are always open to challenges to conventional wisdom. Having said that, I now will be dogmatic: exercise of all kinds is good for us. It is good for our health, it is good for our mental state, and, for the narcissists among us, it is good for our appearance. Scattered throughout this book are examples of how exercise favorably influences a variety of conditions: from osteoporosis, heart disease, high blood pressure, rheumatoid arthritis, and obesity to fibromyalgia, dementia, depression and even cancer. The only questions I will entertain are "What kind of exercise? How much exercise? How are injuries and possible harm to be minimized? How do we decide what is appropriate exercise at any given age?"

First off, is it necessary to see a physician before beginning an exercise program? For many years, the answer to that question was an unequivocal yes. A statement by the American Medical Association in 1958 was typical: "All persons should be shown by medical examination to be organically sound before performing training routines...." By 1981, the National Heart, Lung, and Blood Institute was saying "Most people do not need to see a doctor before they start since a gradual, sensible exercise program will have minimal health risks." In the Physical Activities Guideline for Americans issued in 2008 by the Department of Health and Human Services (HHS) it is stated that "The protective value of a medical consultation for persons with and without chronic diseases who are interested in increasing their physical activity level is not established."[1] My own suggestion is that if the condition of your heart, joints, or other parts is less than good, or if you have no idea of what their condition is, see your doctor. Of course, this implies that you have a personal physician. If you don't, please try to get one whether you think yourself healthy or not. Today's medicine is too complex and too specialized for any of us to get along without an advocate. A good primary care physician can fill that role admirably.

The basis of every fitness program is aerobic exercise. Whether you begin by combining aerobic and anaerobic activities right from the start or add the strength component later is up to you. I will take them up sequentially but practice them together as I will make clear below. Regardless of the form of aerobic exercise we choose, the heart and circulatory system must be worked long enough and hard enough to produce a training effect. But what is hard enough? Does a leisurely stroll around the block have the same consequences as a fast run? Common sense tells us that they do not but we need a way to tell the difference.

The maximum effort during aerobic exercise is accompanied by the greatest possible use of oxygen by the muscles; what the exercise physiologists call maximum oxygen uptake (MOU). The intensity of exercise can be measured in terms of the percentage of MOU---a fast run may need 90% of maximum whereas our stroll may require less than 50%. Such measurements are completely impractical for nearly all of us.

Fortunately, we all can measure the rate of beating of our hearts and, it turns out, heart rate is highest when oxygen uptake is greatest. It is for this reason that heart rate can be used as a guide to the intensity of our aerobic exercise. For many years, an estimate of your maximum heart rate, that which will occur with maximum aerobic effort, was gotten by subtracting your age from 220. However, in 2013, Norwegian investigators, after studying 3,320 men and women age 19 to 89, arrived at a formula of 211 minus 64% of age.[2] For a 20-year-old, it matters little, just a difference of 2 beats per minute. However, as we age, the new formula suggests a significant increase in maximum heart rate. Thus, for me, at age 77, the maximum rate increases by a full 19 beats, from 143 under the old formula to 162 under the new.

Our original question, "What is hard enough?" can now be restated as "What percentage of maximum heart rate must be maintained in order to produce an aerobic training effect?" Estimates vary. In 2008, the U. S. Department of Health and Human Services gave a target zone of 60-75%.[3] Again using me at age 77 as an example: 97-122 beats per minute. Be assured that once you get to know your body a little better it will become unnecessary to measure heart rate. Of course, in this digital age, there are wrist watch-like devices you can strap on that will give you an inconspicuous and continuous reading.

Anyone who has run for a bus or a touchdown or an errant child knows that heart rate increases with exercise. We might then guess that, just as our muscles grow with anaerobic exercise, the maximum rate of beating of our hearts might increase as we become more aerobically fit. In fact, our formula for maximum heart rate changes very little with aerobic conditioning. Instead the heart becomes able to pump more blood with each stroke. It is as if a bigger pump, not a faster one has been installed. The consequence is that fit and unfit people tend to have quite different heart rates when at rest. Put another way, as we become more fit, a decrease in resting heart rate can be expected.

A "normal" adult rate of 72 beats for minute is often quoted. Edward Laskowski of the Mayo Clinic defines normality in a broad range of 60-100. These values probably reflect a poorly conditioned heart; a moderate degree of aerobic training results in rates of 50-60 and an elite marathoner may have a resting heart rate less than 40. However, there are exceptions: Jim Ryan, a former holder of the world record for the mile run, was said to have a rather high resting heart rate. As a practical matter, these numbers are not very important. However, for those about to embark on a program of aerobic exercise, all incentives are welcome. For this reason, a beginner at the start may wish to measure heart rate after sitting quietly for five minutes without conversation or other distractions at a specific time of day. This can then be repeated regularly as the fitness level is improved and a gratifying decrease in resting heart rate observed. In chapter 14, I encourage the home monitoring of blood pressure. Heart rate will be measured at the same time.

Now that we know how fast we want our heart to beat during aerobic exercise, we must consider how long we should maintain an elevated rate. The answer depends upon the intensity of our exercise. An activity that fails to raise the rate to 60% of maximum is unlikely to change aerobic capacity no matter its duration. That is why many who sit in an office and work "long, hard hours" can still be in very poor condition from an aerobic standpoint. On the other hand, a relatively brief exercise of high intensity can quickly produce results. In one early study, a very significant training effect in middle-aged sedentary men was achieved with just 36 minutes of exercise a week but it was all at about 85% of maximum heart rate.

Earlier I mentioned the 2008 Physical Activities Guidelines for Americans issued by the Department of Health and Human Services (HHS). While there is much useful information in the guidelines, they make no mention of heart rate as an index of exercise intensity. Instead, something called the Metabolic Equivalent of a Task (MET) is used. The MET is a comparison of the energy used in a given activity and the resting metabolic rate, the energy expended while sitting quietly. The Guidelines then go on to define moderate-intensity physical activity as anything with a MET value of 3 to 6; any exercise with a MET value greater than 6 is called vigorous-intensity. Values are given for activities ranging from ball room dancing to general gardening. For example, running 10-minute miles has a MET value of 9.8 while brisk walking (3.5 miles per hour) comes in at 4.3. The time spent exercising decreases as the MET increases. Thus, the Guidelines suggest that we engage in 150-300 minutes of moderate intensity or 75-150 minutes of high intensity exercise per week. For those already exercising, that's not a lot, walking for 20 to 40 minutes a day or running for 10 to 20. However, much as MET's are loved by exercise physiologists, I remain attached to using heart rate as an index of exercise intensity.

Ultimately, each of us must establish our own program of activities that we enjoy and which we perform with an intensity and duration that broadly fit the guidelines given above. As the years pass, our program will be modified as our interests and abilities change but there will be one constant: regular aerobic and anaerobic exercise. Jack LaLanne, the founder in 1936 of the gym which would become today's Bally Total Fitness chain, was said to have a daily 2-hour routine which he last performed the day before he died at the age of 96. Few of us have the natural abilities of a Jack LaLanne but all of us can hope to exercise the day before we die. As Frederick Stare put it, "Our goal is to die young as late as possible."[4] Dr. Stare, the founder of the Department of Nutrition at the School of Public Health of Harvard University, passed on at the age of 92. Because running is one of the simplest and most efficient means of training and because it has been so well studied in recent years, I will use it to illustrate a beginning program. First, a bit of history.

A group headed by Dr. Waldo Harris at the University of Oregon published an article in the September 4th, 1967 issue of the *Journal of the American Medical Association* with the simple title "Jogging. An adult exercise program."[5] They defined jogging as "walking and running alternately at a slow to moderate pace." Men ranging in age from 30 to 66 exercised three times a week on a quarter mile track. They began with a total distance of just one mile, equally divided between walking and running. Over a period of twelve weeks they progressed to about two and one-half miles, mostly running. It is interesting that now, nearly a half century later, the end point arrived at, about 75 minutes of running per week, is exactly the low end of the 2008 Guideline recommendation of 75 to 150 minutes of high intensity exercise. About 60% of the participants were judged to be overweight at the start. Although no changes in diet were suggested, these men over the course of the 12 weeks lost an average of 8 pounds and 1and ½ inches of waistline. A co-author of the *JAMA* article was William Bowerman, then the track coach at the University of Oregon, who was later a founder of the Nike Shoe Company.

I am confident that once you have accepted the discipline of regular exercise and have begun to feel and see its value, you will need no further encouragement. Until that time comes, a rather rigidly defined program can lend some support. These are my suggestions for starting.

(1) Choose a quarter of the year when you are most likely to be able to devote 30 minutes on each of three days per week to your renaissance. The first month is the most important.

(2) Commit a specific time of day to exercise. It matters not at all when it is but it should be decided in advance. After a few months, when exercise is established as a part of your routine, you can be less rigid about this. Over the years I have exercised at various times of day but now do so first thing in the morning before going to work. This has the advantage, as someone put it, of getting your body to do something before your mind is fully awake to find excuses.

(3) Decide where your jogging is to take place; try to shun traffic, dogs, and other hazards and distractions. Any fairly smooth surface will do. An old-fashioned cinder running track or a modern cushioned artificial surface is nearly ideal. About two years after coming off active duty with the US Navy, I began to run regularly. I ran outside on concrete and asphalt surfaces all year long in Western New York for about 45 years. I then invested in a treadmill and, except when I am away from home, I now use it exclusively. What is lost in outdoor scenery is compensated for by the very great convenience of treadmill running. An unending supply of films from Netflix pleasantly distracts me from the task at hand: nearly daily aerobic exercise.

(4) Be gentle. Set your own pace. The results of years or decades of neglect will not be reversed in a week. Some will have trouble walking for 30 minutes; a few will be able to run that far right from the start. Gradual progress is what we are after. Use your heart rate to measure effort.

Some people make a big thing of warming up and cooling down. My opinion is that it is more a matter of personal preference than physiological necessity. If you want to do a few gentle stretching exercises before or after running, go ahead, but don't count it as part of your 30 minutes. My practice is to gradually increase my pace over the first 9 or 10 minutes of a run. As to the merits of flexibility exercises, very little convincing research has been done; if you like to stretch or think that it does you some good, do it.

(5) Keep a record of your activities. This can be as elaborate as you like but the minimum is the date and duration of your exercise. Use one week as the basic unit of time and try always to exercise three times in each week. To minimize possible muscle soreness, take a day off after each day of exercise rather than lumping the three days together. If two of your three days of exercise must be on the weekend, make Sunday's workout a little easier than Saturday's. As soon as your routine is well established, consider more frequent exercise.

(6) Focus on aerobic exercise for three months. After aerobic conditioning is well established, the next step is to add an anaerobic or strength component to your routine.

One of the features of aging is that, unless active measures are taken to avoid it, there is a gradual loss of muscle mass. Sarcopenia, the fancy word for this phenomenon, is of little concern for those obliged to do physical labor throughout their lifetimes; think of a farmer or rancher. For the rest of us, perhaps sitting before a computer all day or retired to inactivity, something else is needed to go along with our aerobic conditioning.

For the vast majority of us, whatever our age or physical condition, I have few reservations in suggesting a self-monitored program of jogging as I have outlined above. Strength training is another matter. Unless you have prior exposure to weight training, I suggest a gym, club, or community organization in which you can receive some guidance in the use of free weights or exercise machines. Within a short period of time you will know all that you need to know, will have developed a personal program of strength training, and can feel free to go off on your own perhaps with the help of one of the many books and videos available.

A nice mix of aerobic and anaerobic exercise is provided by calisthenics. The word comes from the Greek *kalos* (beautiful) plus *sthenos* (strength). Calisthenics refers to exercise which requires no or minimal equipment and uses the weight of our bodies for muscle building together with aerobic exercises such as jumping jacks and squat thrusts. Though familiar to members of the Greatest Generation who served in the armed forces of World War II, calisthenics have largely been supplanted by modern equipment. However, for those unwilling to invest in free weights or who often find themselves away from their home gym or a training facility, calisthenics remain a valuable adjunct to other activities. Once again, several books provide useful guidance and practical routines. However, we must keep in mind that it is a balance between aerobic and anaerobic exercise which we wish to achieve. For me, that balance is most easily achieved with jogging and free weights.

A personal note on calisthenics: Several years ago, out of the blue, I developed back pain and sciatica. Without the pain relief provided by opiates, I was unable to work even my sedentary job. In a progression familiar to many, I went from internist to orthopedic surgeon to neurosurgeon with stops for X-rays, magnetic resonance imaging (MRI), and physical therapy. Fortunately, before epidural steroid injections or other invasive procedures were brought to bear, nature began to heal me and the pain disappeared as mysteriously as it had come. The whole episode lasted about a year. A residue of that experience is a set of calisthenics provided me during physical therapy. They take only about five minutes, I do them every morning upon arising, and, stimulated by the memory of my previous pain, I plan to do them every day until I am incapacitated or die, whichever comes first.

In laying out a simple plan of aerobic exercise, I suggested jogging three times a week with later addition of a strength-building component. Substitution of biking or swimming or one of the many dance routines now available is perfectly fine so long as the principles of duration and intensity are followed. Paramount in all of this is the avoidance of injury. This is best accomplished by a gradual progression in duration and intensity. Of late, inspired in part by the heroics of the SEAL teams of the United States Navy, there has been much talk of high intensity exercise. Some clubs in New York City and elsewhere even promote intense exercise, including yoga, in studios kept at artificially high temperatures. This is a recipe for disaster for all but the already fit. The worst thing, short of a fatal heart attack, that can happen to a beginning exerciser is to jump into a routine too advanced, suffer an injury, and be turned off to exercise in the future. Most important of all is to choose activities that appeal to you from the start.

One of the nearly universal experiences of advancing age is a subtle loss of balance and, just as loss of muscle mass can be countered by exercise, there are a number of things we can do to hold our unsteadiness at bay. The reason it is so important to do this is that loss of balance with subsequent falls is a major cause of injury and death for the elderly. Strength training aimed at the legs will help considerably. In addition, a number of studies now suggest that the performance of Tai Chi, Pilates, and yoga can each further contribute to improved balance. One again, of course, the qualifications of your instructor are of primary importance. My personal approach is the daily use of a wobble board. As a bonus, regular wobble board use strengthens the tendons and ligaments of the ankle. Any sporting goods store will carry a variety of devices usually called balance boards or wobble boards. They can readily be bought on line but I suggest trying some out before purchase.

We are now left with the question of where and with whom we will exercise. Some of us are social beings, extroverts if you prefer, who seek companionship, the pleasure of human interaction, and the support that others can give. Extroverts may find the milieu of a club or gym or other group to be very helpful. These organizations can provide the same support that we consider in chapter 8 with respect to weight loss. The rest of us, introverts, find the idea of group exercise to be unattractive. The important thing is to find what works best for you within the broad parameters of time and intensity outlined above. (On any introvert/extrovert continuum, I am definitely with William Manchester who said "I had been, and after the war I would be again, a man who usually prefers his own company, finding contentment in solitude." For some years, when I had a son at home who was interested in competitive running, I trained hard and ran with him in local races but now I exercise alone. My "gym" consists of a treadmill, weight bench, an assortment of free weights, and a wobble board.)

DVD's, health clubs, designer outfits to sweat in, and other forms of the commercialization of fitness sometime obscure the simple beauty of the principles of conditioning. Whatever the point from which you begin, nothing stands between you and increased strength and aerobic capacity but you. Be assured that sometime during your progression the pleasure will begin. If you wish to have a plausible explanation for this phenomenon, you need look no further than your endorphins and endocannabinoids. These are naturally-occurring chemicals in our brains which mimic the effects of opiates and marijuana, respectively. Or to put it in a more natural order, opiates and marihuana mimic the effects of endorphins and endocannabinoids, respectively. Activity in the neural pathways mediated by cannabinoids and opiates is increased during and after exercise. But whatever its origins, the pleasure of aerobic and anaerobic fitness is as varied as the individuals who experience it.

I will close this chapter with the words of Jane Brody, a columnist for the *New York Times*. Her wisdom has always been evident in her writing but, in my view, it has grown with time. I have never met Ms. Brody but in a sense we have aged together; she is four years my junior. To the question "Why do I exercise?", she provided these words.[6]

> ...weight control might be my first answer, followed by a desire to live long and well. But that's not what gets me out of bed before dawn to join friends on a morning walk and then bike to the Y for a swim. It's how these activities make me feel: more energized, less stressed, more productive, more engaged and, yes, happier—better able to smell the roses and cope with the inevitable frustrations of daily life.

CHAPTER 6

NUTRITION

6.1 Introduction

Human nutrition is a remarkably complex subject both scientifically and politically. National food policies and food production are influenced to a significant degree by our politicians who in turn are moved by sellers of fast foods, farmers of all kinds, food processors, and any number of other commercial interests. In terms of science, the principles of nutrition are well established. For example, the metabolism of the components of the diet is understood in intricate detail. The last vitamin was discovered in 1948. What is much less certain is how nutrition impinges on human health. Advice coming from authoritative bodies such as the Department of Agriculture or the National Institutes of Health seems ever in flux. Is sugar a poison or a simple source of energy? Does vitamin E prevent cancer or promote it? Should I stop eating eggs? Is salt in the diet a major cause of high blood pressure? Does more calcium prevent osteoporosis or is it bad for your heart? Do vitamin supplements do us good or simply enrich the companies that sell them? Should we all be quaffing fish oil every day? These and a myriad of other questions have no certain answers at this time but an understanding of the principles of nutrition will allow us to separate the plausible from the implausible, fact from fiction, and quackery from honest endeavor. Nutritional literacy will allow us to make sensible decisions about the foods we eat in our quest for a long, happy, and healthy life.

Every living thing requires energy to sustain life. Food provides that energy in the form of fat, carbohydrate, and protein. These are referred to as the macronutrients. The energy content of food is expressed as calories. For example, I require about 3,500 calories a day to maintain a constant weight. Eat less and weight will be lost; eat more and over time I will become obese. It matters not whether the excess calories are in the form of protein, carbohydrate, or fat because my body can convert carbohydrate and protein into fat. But, important as it is, there is more to nutrition than maintaining an ideal body weight. It is for this reason that the proper balance between the macronutrients will be discussed.

If a source of energy in the form of the macronutrients was the only necessity for life, nutritional science would be a relatively simple matter. However, other factors must be considered as well. These are the micronutrients which include vitamins and minerals. These substances are essential for life but, unlike the macronutrients, are required in modest amounts. A brief history of each of the vitamins and essential minerals will be given. In addition, we will consider the amount of each micronutrient currently deemed suitable and how that amount can be gotten, in nearly all instances, without resort to dietary supplements.

It was Queen Victoria's Privy Council which, in 1860, asked Edward Smith to estimate the human need for protein. The occasion for that request was a severe economic depression in England which threatened the provision of adequate food to the working class. In meeting that request, Dr. Smith provided what Isabella Leitch, a distinguished British nutritionist of the 20th century, called "the first true dietary standard based on scientific principles."[1]

Since the time of Queen Victoria, various governments, often stimulated by war or depression, have provided their citizens with dietary guidance. In the United States, the stimulus was provided by the onset of World War II. In 1941, the Food and Nutrition Board of the National Academy of Sciences established a committee charged with establishing recommendations for nutrient intake to insure optimal health as it related to national defense. Issued in 1943, they were called Recommended Dietary Allowances, RDAs.[2]

As with all other guidelines, the RDAs have been modified over the years and are always a work in progress. In addition, the guidelines have become more complex, new terms have been introduced, and there are multiple acronyms to be deciphered.

Beginning in 1993, efforts were begun to replace RDAs with something to be called the Dietary Reference Intake or DRI. The DRI includes the RDA but adds three other values for each nutrient. These are Estimated Average Requirement (EAR), Adequate Intake (AI), and Tolerable Upper Intake (UL). For each, distinctions are made on the basis of gender, pregnancy, lactation, and, most relevant to our discussions, age.[3]

We must add one more acronym to our portfolio. Indeed, it is the only one which will concern the vast majority of us. It is the RDV, the Recommended Daily Value, often referred to as simply the Daily Value or DV. The reason for its importance is that it provides the basis for the "Nutrition Facts" now carried on the labels of most processed foods.[4] For example, the cereal I eat nearly every morning has a side panel which lists "% daily value" for each of 26 different macro and micro nutrients contained in one cup of the cereal. The RDV is based roughly on the RDA and is expressed on the basis of a diet which provides a total of 2,000 calories.

CHAPTER 6

NUTRITION

6.2 Fat
Lessons from sheep sex

For decades fat was the *bête noire* of American nutrition. From puberty to senility, we were in a war against it whether it was the fat in our blood or in our food or in the subcutaneous fat of our pot bellies, love handles, and thunder thighs. While many of us still rightly abhor the fat of obesity, fat as a component of the diet has lost a bit of its sinister reputation. Carbohydrates are the new black beast. We will come to the carbohydrates shortly.

Virtually all who have had a routine physical examination have had some "blood work" done including a measurement of triglycerides. This is simply an assessment of the amount of fat in our blood. In chemical terms, *triglyceride* perfectly describes all manner of fats, a single molecule of glycerin to which are attached three fatty acids. Depending upon the nature and arrangement of their chemical bonds, the fatty acids are classified as poly-unsaturated, monounsaturated, and saturated. A variety of vegetable and fish oils are poly-unsaturated, the classic example of a monounsaturated oil is olive oil, and saturated fats are found largely in animal products. I give you these details because we will see that the quantity and nature of the fatty acids of the foods we eat are important factors both in our energy intake and in the nutritional quality of our foods.

How was it that we began our war on dietary fat in the first place? To answer that question we need to know a bit about cholesterol, a member of the steroid family. Contrary to its reputation as a villain, cholesterol is essential for human life. It is a structural component of every cell of our body. In addition, the ovaries, testes, and adrenal glands use cholesterol as the first step in synthesizing essential hormones. However, when cholesterol is present in excess it may be deposited in the walls of our arteries thus blocking blood flow. If the vessels supply the heart, the result is a heart attack, in the brain, a stroke. We will talk about this in detail in chapter 14.

Without foods of animal origin, there is no cholesterol in the diet. If cholesterol is essential, how do strict vegetarians (vegans) survive? The answer is simple: vegans and the rest of us are perfectly capable of making our own. This occurs principally in the liver and the cholesterol is then moved around the body attached to lipoproteins, nature's detergents that permit cholesterol to be transported in the blood. The terms LDL and HDL, short for low-density and high-density lipoproteins, are familiar to many. High levels of LDL-cholesterol are associated with an increased risk of heart attack and stroke. Millions of Americans have taken a member of the family of drugs called statins with the intention of lowering LDL-cholesterol.

In 1913, the German-trained Russian pathologist, Nicolai Anitschkow, fed large amounts of cholesterol to rabbits; the rabbits developed atherosclerosis.[1] Thus was born the notion, which soon became medical dogma, that eating cholesterol-rich foods contributes to heart and vascular disease. But this simple idea is complicated by a simple fact: rabbits are not humans. Most of us, in contrast with rabbits, are able to maintain appropriate amounts of cholesterol in blood despite large fluctuations in the quantity of cholesterol in the diet. Our bodies do this by controlling the amount of cholesterol that is absorbed, manufactured, and metabolized. The net result is that our cellular and hormonal needs are met and excess is avoided. It is for this reason that all countries but one placed little emphasis on dietary cholesterol. The exception was the United States. In 2006, the American Heart Association recommended that no more than 300 mg of cholesterol be eaten per day.[2] The fact that two large egg yolks contain a total of about 370 mg of cholesterol gives you some idea of how often that advice was ignored. But, in the immortal words of Roseanne Roseannadanna, "never mind." In 2014, the Heart Association's guidelines said this: There is insufficient evidence to determine whether lowering dietary cholesterol reduces LDL-cholesterol.[3]

But if we are agreed that lowering LDL-cholesterol is a good idea, what does cholesterol have to do with the fat that I eat? In 1952, a letter appeared in the *Journal of Clinical Endocrinology* from Lawrence Kinsell of the Alameda County Hospital in Oakland.[4] It reported a single patient in whom the substitution of vegetable oils for animal fat caused cholesterol levels to fall. Since that time abundant clinical and epidemiological evidence has supported the conclusion that saturated fat, the kind found mostly in animal products, is the single most important environmental factor in determining serum cholesterol. For this reason, the National Institutes of Health since 1984 have recommended that Americans from age 2 to 90 consume no more than 10% of their daily calories as saturated fat. For a person consuming 2,500 calories per day that comes to 28 grams of saturated fat. A single Texas Triple Whopper from Burger King provides 33 grams.

But two details of the previous paragraph deserve further comment. First, why does the NIH specify age 2 for beginning a restriction on fat? The answer lies in the composition of mother's milk. There is universal agreement that the milk provided her baby by a nursing mother is an ideal food yet it provides more than half of its calories in the form of fat and more than 40% of that fat is saturated. Furthermore, human milk contains much more cholesterol than cow's milk. Babies and their brains thrive on this high fat, high cholesterol food and we tinker with Mother Nature's formula at great risk to those babies.

Many years ago, Michael Pugliese of North Shore University Hospital on Long Island, described seven of his patients, 7-22 months of age, who were not growing normally. By imposing a low-fat, low-calorie diet on these infants, the parents thought that they were guarding against obesity, heart disease, and unhealthy eating habits. Dr. Pugliese put it this way: "It appears that society's obsession with being slim and trim and its fear of heart disease and obesity have resulted in another disease of poor growth and delayed development in infancy."[5] Whether such dietary insults in early life are ever fully remedied is uncertain but there is no doubt that a diet beneficial to overweight adults may do harm when uncritically applied to infants. Nearly everyone agrees that high-fat, high-cholesterol mother's milk is best for the first six months of life and some extend that recommendation out to 24 months.

A second item of note in the NIH's advice is the suggestion that no more than 30% of calories come from fat. The validity of that advice is very much dependent on the nature of the fat consumed. For example, in chapter 8 we will consider a Mediterranean diet as a means to maintain a healthy body weight and avoid obesity while taking in 40 to 50% of our calories as fat. However, most of the fat of the Mediterranean diet is in the form of mono-unsaturated olive oil and the poly-unsaturated fats contained in vegetables and fish. Extensive epidemiological evidence indicates that such a high-fat diet is good for our girth, our hearts, and even our brains.

Forgetting for a moment that fat contributes much to the pleasures of eating ice cream or buttery mashed potatoes or a nicely marbled steak, do we really need to consume any fat at all? The answer is "yes we do." The reason is that there are two fatty acids, called linolenic and linoleic, that cannot be synthesized by our bodies and thus must be provided in the diet. However, because of their widespread distribution in animal and plant tissues, deficiency of these essential fatty acids has never been observed in a normal human being. Indeed, the only reason I mention them is the enormous current interest in supplements containing fish oil rich in linolenic acid or two of its derivatives, eicosapentanoic acid and docosahexanoic acid, better known by the acronyms, EPA and DHA. Because their names are so similar it is easy to confuse linoleic and lino-lenic but our bodies have no difficulty in distinguishing them. Both are polyunsaturated fatty acids (PUFA), a reference to the nature of their chemical bonds, but they differ in the arrangement of these bonds. For linoleic acid the arrangement is called *omega*-6 and for linolenic acid, *omega*-3.

The first hint that something in fat might be required for complete nutrition came in 1927 when an American scientist, Herbert Evans, observed that rats fed a diet containing no fat at all failed to grow at a normal rate despite being provided adequate calories in the form of protein and carbohydrates. Evans and George Burr, a Minnesotan then working in Evans' California laboratory, suggested the existence of a previously unrecognized vitamin in fat. The idea of a vitamin F was discarded two years later when Burr and his wife Mildred published a paper with the title "A new deficiency disease produced by the rigid exclusion of fat from the diet."[6] The subjects were rats. Odd as it may sound to us today, the disease was cured by feeding tiny amounts of lard to the animals. The curative factors were assumed to be a variety of fatty acids, including linoleic. For the first time, these fatty acids were called *essential*, at least for rats. Humans would take a while longer.

Experiments by Arild Hansen at the University of Texas Medical Branch at Galveston are of interest to us for two reasons. First, they provided convincing evidence that certain fatty acids are essential for humans as well as for rats. Second, they illustrate an ethical dilemma often encountered by clinical investigators.

Hansen's work began as a general comparison of the constituents of the blood of well-nourished and poorly-nourished children. The two groups had about the same total amount of fatty acids but there was very little linoleic acid in the blood of children who lived in poverty. This suggested to Hansen that linoleic acid might, in his words, "be essential for the well-being of healthy children." He was of course aware that retrospective studies could not prove the essentiality of linoleic acid—there were far too many other things that might account for the lack of well-being in poor children. What was needed was a prospective study, one in which groups of infants would be fed varying amounts of linoleic acid and differences in their health could be demonstrated. Just such a study was reported by Hansen and his colleagues in 1963.[7]

A total of 428 newborn children were fed one of four different formulas. Three of these contained 42% of their calories as fat but their linoleic acid contents were 1.3, 2.8, and 7.3%, respectively. For comparison, human milk provides 4-5% of its calories as linoleic acid. The fourth formula contained no fat at all. It quickly became evident that babies fed the no-fat formula were not growing at a normal rate. Therefore it was modified to contain 42% of calories as fat but with virtually no linoleic acid.

After three months had passed, the essentiality of linoleic acid had been proven. Babies who received either 1.3% or no linoleic acid at all were retarded in their rate of growth. In addition, the linoleic acid-poor formulas caused the babies' skin to become dry and scaly; in the skin folds there was redness, oozing, and peeling.

As important as were these studies in establishing the human need for linoleic acid, today's ethical standards would forbid them. Who were these infant volunteers? Dr. Hansen does not tell us but we may, I think, safely assume that they were not the children of the hospital's professional staff. Instead it is likely that they came from what is euphemistically called a clinic population, i.e., those receiving free medical care. We are told that 70% of the babies were "Negro infants." None could benefit from the study and some were almost certain to be harmed, at least transiently. What then was the motivation of the mothers to enroll their babies? The answer most likely lies in the fact that "milk and solid foods were provided free of charge for the duration of participation in the study." Today, such economic coercion would not be permitted. No investigator, however well-intentioned, has the right to treat humans as he would a group of guinea pigs.

The great French scientist, Louis Pasteur, said that "chance favors the prepared mind." Nowhere is this better illustrated than in the discovery of the essentiality of the *omega*-3 fatty acid, linolenic acid. Ralph Holman, a biochemist, was interested in the role of fatty acids in nutrition throughout his long career at the Hormel Institute of the University of Minnesota but thirty years would pass between his first publication on the subject and his contact with a little girl who had lost much of her small intestine to a gunshot wound. As a result, she was being provided all of her nourishment intravenously in a process called total parenteral nutrition. Five months after she was started on TPN, she experienced periods of numbness, weakness, inability to walk, pain in her legs, and blurring of vision.[8] The prepared mind of Dr. Holman realized that the TPN protocols of the day provided little if any linolenic acid. With its addition to the TPN fluid, all of the girl's symptoms disappeared. (Having mentioned the virtues of human breast milk, I will add that it is a rich source of both of our essential fatty acids.)

Few of us, fortunately, will find ourselves receiving total parenteral nutrition, all nutritionists are now aware that essential fatty acids are indeed essential, and, as I have mentioned, it is nearly impossible to become deficient in them. Why then in the 21st century is there so much interest in these substances? To answer that question, I am going to compress about eighty-five years of medical research into a few paragraphs. Our story begins in 1930 in a laboratory at Columbia University where two gynecologists, Raphael Kurzrok and Charles Lieb, observed that semen from sheep contains a substance which affects the muscle tone of the human uterus. A few years later, Ulf Svant von Euler, a Swedish physiologist and later a winner of the Nobel Prize for Physiology or Medicine, isolated the substance and, thinking its origin was the prostate gland, called it *prostaglandin*.[9] Three decades and World War II then passed before the suggestion was made that essential fatty acids are the precursor substances from which the body manufactures a whole family of prostaglandins. The words of the Swedish scientists, Sune Bergstrom and Bengt Samuelsson, who would share the 1982 Nobel Prize for Physiology or Medicine for their discoveries, were prophetic indeed: "Although our knowledge of their biological effects is still fragmentary, their wide distribution (suggests) that the symptoms of essential fatty acid deficiency at least partly are due to an inadequate biosynthesis of the various members of the prostaglandin...system."[10] With the subsequent discovery of dozens of products formed from the essential fatty acids, the term *eicosanoid* was applied to the whole family. It is derived from the Greek word *eicosa*, meaning 20, the number of carbon atoms in the eicosinoids.

The second part of our story requires a brief digression into pharmacology. The bark of the willow tree when chewed has been known since at least the time of Hippocrates to have pain relieving and anti-inflammatory properties. In the 19th century, the active principle in willow bark was identified and, late in the century, gave rise to a related chemical, acetylsalicylic acid. First synthesized in the German pharmaceutical house, Bayer AG, it was in 1899 given the trade name, Aspirin. (In the United States aspirin, with a small A, is the generic name for the same drug.) In 1971, the late Sir John Vane, a British pharmacologist and co-recipient of the Nobel Prize for Physiology or Medicine with Bergstrom and Samuelsson, proposed that the pain-relieving, anti-fever, and anti-inflammatory effects of aspirin are the result of the inhibition of the synthesis of prostaglandins from arachadonic acid, a substance derived from linoleic acid, one of our essential fatty acids.[11]

What Vane's hypothesis did not explain was the ability of aspirin to inhibit the clotting of blood. No known prostaglandin fit the bill. Sune Bergstrom soon provided the answer with his discovery of another product of arachadonic acid whose formation is blocked by aspirin. He called it thromboxane because of its presence in thrombocytes, an element of the blood involved in the formation of blood clots (thrombi).[12] If my presentation to this point has not been too obscure, it is now clear to you why millions of Americans now take aspirin every day in the hope of avoiding a blood clot-mediated stroke or heart attack. The point is to inhibit the synthesis of thromboxane from linoleic acid.

Current advice with respect to the use of low-dose aspirin is relatively simple. In 2009, the United States Preventative Services Task Force said the following.[13] For men age 45-79, the use of aspirin is recommended when the potential benefit due to a reduction in heart attacks outweighs the potential harm due to bleeding in the stomach. For women age 55-79, the use of aspirin is recommended when the potential benefit of a reduction in strokes outweighs the potential harm of an increase in gastric bleeding. Put another way, if your stomach doesn't mind a little aspirin, aspirin is a good idea over those age ranges. Aspirin is not recommended at earlier ages. No recommendation is made for age 80 and beyond. At present, I take 81 mg of aspirin each day. Unless new evidence emerges, I will stop doing so at age 80. (That last sentence reminds me of a Woody Allen line: "If you want to make God laugh, tell him about your plans.")

If aspirin has, after more than a century of use, suddenly become a wonder drug for the prevention of heart attacks, what can we make of the equally enthusiastic use of fish oil?

The foundation for the belief that fish oil might prevent heart disease was laid by two Danish physician-scientists, Jorn Dyerberg and Hans Olaf Bang. They were aware that for several thousand years, the Inuit peoples of Northern Canada and Greenland ate a diet rich in the fat of fish and marine mammals such as whales and seals and virtually devoid of fruits and vegetables. By the lights of modern nutrition, a very unhealthy diet indeed. Yet, like users of aspirin, the Inuit, when cut, tended to bleed longer than others.[14] Something in the Inuit diet diminishes clot formation and that something is now known to be yet another prostaglandin discovered by Salvador Moncada, John Vane, and their coworkers. It is called prostacyclin and its formation is promoted by the *omega*-3 fatty acids found abundantly in the Inuit diet.[15]

In its wonderful complexity, our bodies create from the essential fatty acids one member of the prostaglandin family which increases the clotting of the blood, thromboxane, and another, prostacyclin, which opposes this effect. For most of us most of the time, these opposing forces are kept in a delicate balance and our blood flows on. Now to the tough question: should we be fooling with that balance by taking aspirin every day along with a fish oil supplement? The answer is important because if we subdue our clotting mechanisms too much, we increase the risk of a stroke due to bleeding in the brain. In addition, the well-known ability of aspirin to irritate the stomach can lead to fatal bleeding in that organ. Nonetheless, as has already been noted, 81 mg of aspirin has been recommended for most of us and I, for one, have taken that advice. Can the same thing be said for fish oil?

Throughout this book, you will detect my bias against dietary supplements. This bias is based in my belief that most of us most of the time throughout our lives are provided all necessary nutrients by eating a variety of foods as close to their natural state as is compatible with pleasurable eating. In addition, many supplements provide a vitamin or mineral or other nutrient in a quantity greater than what is normally provided by the diet or is much in excess of any known deficiency. At that point, supplements should be regarded as drugs and, as drugs, we should have knowledge both of efficacy, the power to do good, and adverse effects, the power to do harm. For example, as I will describe more fully later, many a person has failed to realize that vitamin A, a deficiency of which in the developing world leads to blindness in countless children, is, in excess, a poison. Finally, my anti-supplement bias is further strengthened by the virtual absence of regulation by the Food and Drug Administration due to the Dietary Supplement Health and Education Act discussed in chapter 2.

Despite my general aversion to supplements, might fish oil be an exception? I have already mentioned the Inuits and their tendency to bleed a bit longer than others, a sign of a somewhat reduced tendency to form blood clots. But this alone cannot explain the current enthusiasm for fish oils and what some have called "the Eskimo diet." No, we must couple this with a statement by Drs. Bang and Dyerberg in their initial report in 1971 which referred to "the very low incidence of heart disease...in Greenlandic Eskimos."[16] Despite the fact that the statement has been quoted in the medical literature countless times since, it is almost certainly based on faulty data.[17] As early as 1940, an experienced Danish physician who had long practiced in Greenland noted a high incidence of heart disease among the Inuit.[18] Subsequent epidemiological studies have confirmed that observation.[19] Simply put, "the Eskimo diet" does not appear to be good for Eskimos.

With respect to the use of fish oil supplements, there are two populations we want to consider: those with pre-existing heart disease or diabetes and those, the majority of us, who appear to be healthy. For the first group, the American Heart Association and the American College of Cardiology Foundation in 2011, no doubt influenced by Bang and Dyerberg, provided this guideline: "it may be reasonable to recommend *omega*-3 fatty acid from fish or fish oil capsules (1 gram per day) for cardiovascular disease risk reduction for all patients with established heart disease or seriously elevated triglycerides."[20] However, the Heart Association also noted that the evidence for this recommendation is "less well-established." Indeed, following issuance of the guideline, the results of two investigations published in 2012 failed to find any benefit from supplementation with 1 gram per day of fish oil in persons with heart disease or diabetes.[21, 22] In a tribute to the power of advertising, this absence of evidence of benefit has not slowed the use of fish oil supplements. It has been estimated that 10% of the American adult population took one in 2014 at a cost of several billion dollars.

If any benefits of fish oil for those with preexisting heart disease or diabetes have yet to be proven, the situation for healthy people is murkier yet. However, there presently is underway in the United States the Vitamin D and Omega-3 Trial (VITAL) under the leadership of JoAnn E. Manson, chief of the Division of Preventive Medicine at Brigham and Women's Hospital Boston and Professor of Women's Health at Harvard Medical School.[23] Dr. Manson's study will include 20,000 men over the age of 50 and women over the age of 55 without evidence of heart disease or cancer who will randomly be assigned to one of four treatment arms: (1) 1 gram of fish oil plus placebo pill, (2) 2,000 IU of vitamin D plus one placebo, (3) fish oil plus vitamin D, and (4) two placebos. We may hope that VITAL will, in a few years, definitively answer the question of whether healthy people reduce their risk of cancer or heart disease by taking fish oil or vitamin D either alone or in combination. Preliminary results of the trial are not expected until 2017.

So far I have hardly mentioned linoleic acid, the prototypic essential *omega*-6 fatty acid. Linoleic acid is found in abundance in a variety of vegetable oils such as corn, sunflower, safflower, flaxseed, and soybean oils. Each of these oils is for sale on line and in health food stores as supplements accompanied by lavish claims for a variety of health benefits. First let it be said that the biological systems mediated by the products of *omega*-3 and *omega*-6 fatty acids fatty acids are so devilishly complex that virtually unlimited speculation is possible. One such speculation is that since linoleic acid is the precursor for arachidonic acid which can be converted into inflammatory prostaglandins, any increased intake of *omega*-6 fatty acids is harmful. Many of those who provide nutritional advice to the general public have taken this speculation to be truth and urge decreased intake of *omega*-6 fatty acids with an increase in *omega*-3. In contrast, in 2009 the American Heart Association urged *higher* intake of *omega*-6 fatty acids as a way to decrease the risk of heart disease.[24]

Some argue that what is important is the ratio of *omega*-6 fatty acids to *omega*-3 fatty acids in the diet. What about increasing *omega*-3 to alter that ratio? On this issue, countless conflicting findings could be cited. One report that caught my eye was published in 2013 in the *Journal of the National Cancer Institute*. It was found that men with the highest levels of *omega*-3 fatty acids in the blood had an elevated risk of prostate cancer.[25] In this sea of uncertainty, the most prudent course is to avoid supplements of either *omega*-3 or *omega*-6 fatty acids and place our faith in a balanced diet rich in both of these essentials.

Anyone who lives in New York City knows of yet another category of fat, the evil trans fats. Low levels of trans fats occur in nature, primarily in animal products, but most are introduced by man. Years ago in response to concerns about saturated fats in butter and their effects on cholesterol levels, a number of polyunsaturated vegetable oils were converted into semi-solid margarines by a process called hydrogenation. In doing so, trans fats are produced. In addition to making oils into solids and thus suitable as substitutes for butter, partial hydrogenation has the very great advantage of extending the shelf-life of a variety of snack foods and permitting longer use of oils for deep-frying; think French fries. One such margarine advertised itself as "Heart Smart." Only much later was it recognized that these margarines, because of their high content of trans-fats, were in fact, as Nigel Hawkes put it, "Heart Stupid." The evidence for that came from 85,000 participants in the Nurses' Health Study. They completed dietary questionnaires in 1980 and were followed for eight years. When the data were analyzed by Walter Willett and his colleagues at the Harvard School of Public Health it was found that products made with partially hydrogenated vegetable oils were significantly associated with a higher risk of heart disease. Indeed, trans fats appear to be even worse than saturated fats in this respect.[26] In addition, more recent studies suggest a sinister role for trans fats in diabetes and inflammation. Thus began the war on trans-fats.

As might be expected, the international food industry has opposed the removal of trans-fats from processed foods. They cite increased costs and more rapid rancidity thus shortening the shelf life of their many products. As the tobacco industry before it, these interests have in many places blocked regulation; the United Nations' panel on non-communicable diseases for example has taken no position despite urging to do so by the World Health Organization. On the other hand, by 2009, Denmark, Austria, and Switzerland had enacted a complete ban. In this country, the Food and Drug Administration in 2003 required packaged foods to be labeled with their content of trans fat. (It should be noted that "0 grams trans fat" really means less than 0.5 gram.) Three years later, New York City's Board of Health took more direct action. It announced a phasing out in restaurants of the city of trans fats in frying, baking, or cooking or in spreads with complete elimination in 2008. Some called this a win for the Food Nazis, those who would restrict the freedom of the American people to eat as they wish, an example of government as the enemy. However, others pointed out that trans fats have no redeeming nutritional virtues and that their reduction or elimination saves lives. Happening as it did in New York City, the ban on trans fats generated increased awareness of the problem throughout the country and, more important, contributed to the preemptive actions of companies such as Burger King, McDonalds, Taco Bell, Long John Silver's, and Wendy's to reduce or eliminate trans fats in their products on a national basis and proudly to advertise that fact. In November 2013, the Food and Drug Administration announced their plan to remove the designation of "Generally Recognized As Safe" (GRAS) from trans fats and to eliminate the labeling of less than 0.5 gram trans fat as "0 trans fat." The Grocery Manufacturer's Association expressed strong opposition and, as of this writing, no final decision by the FDA has been issued.

"Julia Child, goddess of fat, is beaming somewhere." Those were the words of Mark Bittman in his article, "Butter is Back", in the *New York Times* on March 25, 2014. It came just a week after the publication of a study in the *Annals of Internal Medicine* that found no association between the consumption of saturated fat (think meat, cheese, and other animal products) and the risk of heart disease. The authors were Rajiv Chowdhury and his colleagues of the University of Cambridge and other leading institutions in England, the United States, and the Netherlands.[27] They had reviewed the results of studies involving more than 600,000 people and, with their conclusions, brought joy to the hearts of chefs for whom sugar, salt, and fat are the cornerstones of fine cooking. Unlike the chefs, the sellers of fish and krill oil supplements could not have been pleased. The study could detect no virtue in these supplements rich in *omega*-3 fatty acids. Indeed, the only clear-cut finding was that trans-fats are bad for us. Dr. Chowdury and his colleagues close by suggesting that current cardiovascular guidelines "may require reappraisal."

I hope that it is clear by now that nutritional science is not exact science and that official guidelines on the most appropriate amount and kinds of fat we eat are ever subject to change as new data are gathered. Nonetheless, despite current uncertainties, a prudent course can be plotted. Multiple lines of evidence indicate that partial replacement of saturated fat from animal products with plant-derived mono- and poly-unsaturated fats is a good idea.[28] The DASH and Mediterranean diets described in chapter 8 admirably accomplish that end. As to fish oil, until Dr. Manson's *omega-3* trial is completed in a few years, avoid supplements and go straight to the source. Eat fish as often as your budget allows.

Salmon is perhaps the best of the fatty fish but tuna, mackerel, herring, lake trout, catfish, pollack, cod, flounder, and sardines are rich in *omega-3* fatty acids as well. My favourite crustacean sources are shrimp and crab. Though we tend to associate *omega-3* fatty acids with fish, they are found in plants as well. For example, ounce for ounce, walnuts contain nearly 5 times that of salmon. Tofu, or bean curd, dear to the heart of vegetarians but abhorred by many, is comparable to tuna as a source. So long as vitamin B_{12} intake is adequate, vegans, who eat no fish whatsoever, tend to have very favourable risk profiles for heart disease.[29, 30]

CHAPTER 6

NUTRITION

6.3 Protein
Too much of a good thing?

Of the three macronutrients, only protein has an unblemished reputation among the general public. After all, protein is the substance of muscle and many of us yearn for more shapely or more massive muscle. Protein supplements are advertised in every body-building and weight-lifting magazine. Countless commercial messages from milk producers, cattlemen, and other commercial interests tell us that we need protein.

Popular notions about protein are as likely to be erroneous as are those of just about any other aspect of nutrition. This is not a new phenomenon. Around 1850, Baron Justus von Liebig, an influential German chemist, stated that protein is the sole source of energy for the contraction of muscle. Despite a series of experiments in the second half of the 19th century that disproved the idea, many continue to think of protein as "energy food." Though it is true that the body can use protein for energy if fat and carbohydrate are lacking, protein is essential in the diet only as a source of amino acids. If no protein were ever used for energy, we would be none the worse for it.

Physically, all proteins are structured like strands of pearls in which each pearl corresponds to an amino acid and the string that connects one to another is a chemical link called a peptide bond. When we eat meat, the muscle of an animal, we cannot make direct use of the proteins contained therein. Instead, our digestive enzymes, themselves proteins, break the chemical bonds and release the amino acids. It is the individual amino acids, not the protein as a whole, which are absorbed from the gut.

The structure of proteins and the facts of digestive physiology make nonsense of the often-heard claim that eating larger quantities of a particular protein will cause more of that protein to appear in the body. Consider superoxide dismutase. It is an enzyme, a protein which facilitates essential biochemical reactions in our bodies. The function of superoxide dismutase is to protect cells against the damaging effects of oxygen. Disorders of that function have been implicated in numerous diseases. For example, some persons suffering from Lou Gehrig's Disease (amyotrophic lateral sclerosis) carry a genetic mutation which limits the production of super oxide dismutase. No means to correct that loss has yet been discovered. Undeterred, advertisements for superoxide dismutase supplements say that they will extend your life and you are told to swallow one to three capsules per day. What you are not told is that your gut doesn't read advertisements. Superoxide dismutase will be digested like any other protein. To be sure, my body will manufacture the enzyme, as our species has done throughout its history, but the quantity is quite independent of the commercial product I have eaten. A similar fantasy is that eating large amounts of a single amino acid will promote synthesis of proteins containing that amino acid. Shelves in places like Walmart and GNC are filled with "protein supplements" with vague and not so vague promises that this is the way to build muscle. What is not said is that it is exercise that stimulates muscle growth (chapters 4 and 5) and that protein in excess is simply added calories to be converted to fat.

Once it was recognized that all proteins are made up of amino acids, scientists could begin to ask questions about the relative importance of each amino acid. It is now known that of the 21 amino acids that make up all of the various proteins of the body, only nine are essential for man, i.e., like vitamins and essential fatty acids, they cannot be produced by the body and must be provided by our food. An ideal dietary protein would contain all of the essential amino acids in the exact proportions required by the body. The degree to which an actual protein conforms to this ideal is referred to as the protein's "quality."

"High quality protein" has a nice sound to it and, given a choice, we would certainly be inclined to choose high quality over low. But this is not always a good idea. The reason is that most measures of protein quality have been based on the ability of a protein to produce a high rate of growth in young rats or farm animals. In planning a diet for a human being with a life expectancy of perhaps ninety years, several factors other than growth rate have to be considered.

Beef is a high quality protein, i.e., it provides the essential amino acids in proportions that are close to what our bodies need. However, beef is not necessarily a good choice as a primary source of protein for humans. It is not the beef protein that is at fault but the saturated fat that comes with it. As we have already seen in our discussion of fats, it is thought that saturated fat may contribute to elevated levels of LDL-cholesterol, a risk factor for heart disease and stroke. In addition, in chapter 13, we will consider the epidemiological evidence for a link between red meat and several forms of cancer. Vegetables, on the other hand, provide protein of relatively low quality but it is not accompanied by much in the way of saturated fat. In addition, vegetables bring along with the protein a number of other desirable nutrients and thus can be said to be a better choice from a nutritional standpoint. Others would add that the extensive use of animal protein raises issues with respect to the environmental costs of raising animals as well the humane treatment of those animals.

In choosing a source of protein, we also may want to consider the number of calories that it provides. A quart of whole milk gives us more than half of our daily protein requirement. It also will contribute about 650 calories. On the other hand, a quart of skim milk containing exactly the same amount of protein has only 320 calories. If we are interested in feeding starving people, providing whole milk is a much better idea because they have need of a source of energy as well as of protein. But, if we are typical Americans fighting a never ending battle against our waistlines, the difference between a quart of skim and a quart of whole milk works out to be about a half pound of fat a week.

Millions of people throughout the world are protein deficient. The disease that they suffer has been given the Ghanian name, kwashiorkor. Victims may retain substantial amounts of body fat, yet they are severely malnourished and will soon die if untreated. The appearance of children is especially deceptive. The puffy faces, thickened limbs, and potbellies they exhibit are not signs of overfeeding, as many who see photographs of these truly starving bodies so readily assume, but instead signify the abnormal accumulation of fluid in their bodies. Because the human immune system is dependent upon protein synthesis, bacterial and viral infections of all kinds are a constant threat to the lives of those with kwashiorkor.

In the United States, protein malnutrition is seen most often in children and the elderly. In the latter group, the deficiency may lead to progressive confusion, a symptom that has sometimes been interpreted as a sign of Alzheimer's disease, a condition to be discussed in chapter 12. Although it is sometimes directly caused by poverty, protein deficiency in America is more often simply the result of a poor choice in foods. Laurence Finberg has called this the triumph of ignorance over affluence. The money paid for an order of French fries at a fast-food counter would provide enough protein for a day if it were used instead to buy milk.

How much protein do we need? One hundred and fifty years ago, Edward Smith, a British physician and physiologist, estimated the human requirement to be 80-90 grams per day (2.8-3.2 oz). The figure has moved steadily downward since then. The World Health Organization and the Institute of Medicine, an arm of the National Academy of Sciences in this country, are in agreement that men and women of all ages should get about 0.8 grams of protein per kilogram of body weight per day.[1] For me at 180 pounds (81.8 kg) that works out to be 65 grams (2.3 oz.) To see just how easy that is to obtain, consider this menu: 2 ounces (1/4 cup) of tuna fish, 8 ounces of skim milk, 2 slices of whole wheat bread, 1 egg, 6 ounces of yogurt, 2 tbsp. of peanut butter, 1 cup of raisin bran, ½ cup kidney or baked beans, 2 ounces of tofu, and 2 tablespoons of almonds. In one day, these modest amounts of a variety of foods provide a total of 65 grams of protein and all of the essential amino acids. For those of a carnivorous inclination, a 6 ounce beef steak alone provides 42 grams of high quality protein.

During pregnancy or for those regularly engaged in vigorous physical activity, a modest increase in protein intake is a good idea.[1] But, as can be seen from the example I have provided, even a 100% increase requires no heroic measures, i.e., none of the protein powders, bars, shakes, or drinks which surround us at most commercial fitness centers and in every super-market. Recently the American Armed Forces weighed in on this mat-ter. A meeting was held in November 2012 at the U.S. Army Research Institute of Environmental Medicine. The resulting consensus statement recommended that soldiers in the field, warfighters was the term they used, consume 1.5 to 2.0 grams of protein per kilogram body weight, roughly twice our value of 0.8 grams per kilogram. However, noting that nearly 20% of all active duty personnel regularly use protein supplements, the statement went on to urge that all protein come from whole foods rather than from commercial supplements, with their risk of contamination.[2]

Vegans, those who eat no foods of animal origin, need not risk pro-tein deficiency if a proper variety of plant foods is consumed. Although an individual vegetable protein may be poor in one or more of the essen-tial amino acids, simply eating combinations of vegetables will provide all of the essentials. For example, Scott Jurek is a vegan; he eats no animal products. He also holds the American record for distance run in a twenty-four hour period, 165.7 miles, and three times has won the Spartathlon, a 152 mile ultra-marathon held in Greece.[3]

A dramatic example of the use of vegetable protein to prevent kwashiorkor was provided by Nevin Scrimshaw. Already the possessor of a Ph.D. degree in physiology from Harvard, Scrimshaw received his medical training during World War II at the University of Rochester where his mentors advised against a career in nutrition. Fortunately, he did not heed them. In the 1950's he led a group that invented a protein-rich food made from cottonseed meal and gave it the name Incaparina.[4] Later his group used peanut flower and wheat to make a similar product to fight protein-deficiency in India.

The fact that a purely vegetarian diet can deliver adequate protein should not lead us to believe that all such diets are without risk. As with a variety of other nutritional insults, the young and the frail old are most likely to be harmed. Years ago, Drs. Eric Shinwell and Rafael Gorodischer treated some of the children born into a strictly vegetarian religious cult in Israel.[5] Of 25 infants brought to their hospital, three were dead on arrival and five others died within hours of admission. Seven of the babies displayed the classic signs of protein deficiency. After weaning at about three months of age, no milk had been provided. Instead, the major constituent of the infants' diet had been a dilute "milk" made from soybean flour. Despite persistent efforts over a three-year period, the physicians were unable to induce the leader of the group to modify their dietary practices. At the other end of the age spectrum are the frail elderly who may benefit from a modest increase in protein intake coupled with strength training. I would note however that an increase in protein intake in the absence of strength training will do nothing for the frail, whether elderly or not.

An oft-repeated fallacy regarding protein, often directed against those who eat no animal products, is that each meal must contain all of the essential amino acids in just the right proportions. This idea seems to have originated in the early 1940's with the realization that protein synthesis in the body's cells requires the simultaneous presence of all of the essential amino acids. Thus, it is reasoned that we must eat a completely balanced array of all the essential amino acids each time we consume protein. But there is another source of protein to be considered. The fact is that all of us, vegetarians included, are auto-cannibals. Each day, in addition to the protein of my food, I digest about 70 grams of the high quality protein of my body.[6] It comes from spent digestive enzymes, cells sloughed from the stomach and intestines, and a variety of other proteinaceous debris. What reaches my liver is a mix of amino acids derived both from my diet and from the recycling of my very self. Thus, in the short run, the liver is able to pump an optimal mixture of essential amino acids into the bloodstream even when there are large fluctuations in the protein content of individual meals.

Need we be concerned about protein in excess? Probably not up to about twice the recommended amount of 0.8 g/kg/day. As I noted above that works out for me to be just 2.3 ounces. But we should be concerned about the source of the protein. In 1910, about half of dietary protein came from vegetables but today more than two-thirds is of animal origin, with beef, poultry, and pork the major contributors. The epidemiological evidence in support of the benefits of the DASH and Mediterranean diets (chapter 8), both of which include only modest amounts of animal products, suggests that a return to the animal/vegetable ratio of a century ago would be of value.

In chapter 7, I will tell you that obesity and diabetes are major risk factors for kidney disease. For people with diabetes or early-stage kidney disease, the American Diabetes Association recommends limiting protein intake to 0.8 to 1.0 gram of protein per kilogram of body weight (roughly 10 percent of energy intake).[7] The late Conrad Elvehjem, one of America's greatest nutritional scientists, once said that as far as protein is concerned, minimal and adequate and optimal are all the same thing. Unfortunately this message has been lost on many, especially the young. A study by Dr. Maria Eisenberg and her colleagues found that, among nearly three thousand boys and girls in the Minneapolis/St. Paul area with an average age of 14 years, 35% had used protein powders, shakes, or bars in 2011.[8]

Looking back at what I have written, I fear that you may suspect that I am a closet vegetarian at best or a vegan at worst. I am not. I grew up on a meat and potatoes diet before anyone cared much about saturated fat, cholesterol, and such. Also, I confess elsewhere in this book to a love for an occasional filet mignon with baked potato and butter. Having said that, I believe, as a scientist, that the evidence coming at us from many directions strongly urges a reduction in our intake of animal protein in the form of red meat, processed meat, and the burgers offered us by fast food franchises. For those like me who cringe at the thought of life without steaks, chops, and roasts, let meat be the crowning glory of your major meals rather than the mainstay of each and every breakfast, lunch, and dinner.

NUTRITION

6.4 Carbohydrates
Sugar is not a poison.

Earlier I mentioned that for decades saturated fat has been regarded as the major villain in American nutrition. Now auditioning for that role are the carbohydrates, more specifically, sugars, the simplest of the carbohydrates. How can it be that a carbohydrate, a member of the macronutrient family long considered the bedrock of the healthiest diets, is now assailed in books with titles such as *Pure, White, and Deadly* and *Suicide by Sugar*? We are told by a few evangelical nutritionists and writers that sugar is as addictive and as harmful to the body as is alcohol and that cupcakes may enslave us as surely as does cocaine. Fructose, the simple sugar found in fruits and vegetables, is singled out for special scorn and called by one author *Sweet and Vicious*. To address these claims and others like them, I will begin with a bit of the basic science of carbohydrates and then go on to establish how carbohydrates, including fructose and other sugars, fit into a healthy diet for the long run.

Using the table below as a guide, let us begin with a few definitions and a brief consideration of how carbohydrates are handled by our digestive systems.

Carbohydrate	Other name	Complexity	Simplest unit(s)
glucose	dextrose	monosaccharide	glucose
fructose	fruit sugar	monosaccharide	fructose
sucrose	table sugar	disaccharide	glucose, fructose
lactose	milk sugar	disaccharide	glucose, galactose
maltose	malt sugar	disaccharide	glucose, glucose
starch	plant starch	polysaccharide	glucose
glycogen	animal starch	polysaccharide	glucose
cellulose	fiber	polysaccharide	glucose

Carbohydrates take their name from the fact that they are made up of carbon and water (hydros). They may be called "simple" or "complex" depending upon how many individual units are strung together. Glucose and fructose are simple carbohydrates; were they any simpler, they would lose their outstanding sensual characteristic, a sweet taste. When glucose and fructose are joined together, a new carbohydrate, sucrose, is formed. Although sucrose is commonly called "sugar", confusion will be avoided if we remember that all of the many simple carbohydrates with a sweet taste are sugars. The Latin word for sugar is *saccharum* so we sometimes refer to sugars as saccharides; glucose and fructose are thus monosaccharides, sucrose a disaccharide, and so forth. When many glucose units are strung together, we speak of a polysaccharide or complex carbohydrate.

We previously have seen how dietary fat and protein are broken down in the gut, absorbed, and then reassembled in the body as human protein or fat. The same thing happens with digestible carbohydrates. We can use the potato as an example. When eaten, the plant starch contained in the potato is rapidly broken down into glucose, absorbed from the gut, passes through the liver, and then enters the blood to be distributed throughout the body. Several things then can happen to the potato-derived glucose. Much of it is taken up by muscle where it can be converted into ATP, the direct fuel of muscle contraction, as discussed in chapter 4. The glucose that goes to the brain will serve as that organ's sole source of energy. Any glucose left over can simply be stored for future use in the form of glycogen. In this process we convert the plant starch of the potato to our own animal starch; both are complex carbohydrates; both serve as a source of glucose. However, these glycogen storage sites are relatively small and, when full, the excess glucose will be converted into fat. Alas, as most of us are aware, our capacity for fat storage is virtually unlimited.

If it was table sugar that I had eaten, the sucrose is broken down into glucose and fructose and the glucose handled in a fashion identical to that described for potato-derived glucose. Fructose, whether from sucrose or more directly from a fruit or vegetable, is treated somewhat differently. It too is absorbed from the gut but on reaching the liver it is converted by a series of steps largely into glucose where it may be stored as glycogen or converted into fat. This peculiarity of fructose metabolism is the basis for many of the claims for the toxicity of sugar cited above. More about those in a moment.

If my account of the fate of table sugar or of a potato sounds simple, I assure you that it is not. Indeed, hundreds of different biochemical mechanisms are involved. A primary orchestrator of these events is insulin, a hormone secreted by the pancreas. Total absence of insulin as occurs in type 1 diabetes is incompatible with life. The reason is that without insulin, our cells are starved of the glucose they need to survive. Far more common than type 1 diabetes is the situation in which insulin is present but its functions are disrupted. This is called type 2 diabetes and, for reasons not yet fully understood, it is closely connected with obesity. Indeed, there is good reason to believe that obesity is the primary risk factor for type 2 diabetes and, when uncontrolled, all that it entails including heart disease, blindness, and amputations of the extremities. This issue will be discussed more fully in chapter 7.

When glucose enters the bloodstream from whatever dietary source, cells of the pancreas referred to as *beta* sense its presence and, in response, secrete insulin. Circulating throughout the body, insulin produces a myriad of effects. Principal among these is to cause changes in muscle and other cells which allow them to take up glucose. If insulin is absent or deficient, too little glucose enters the cells and the excess remains in the blood. One consequence of this excess is that some of the free glucose will be excreted in the urine where it signals the presence of diabetes mellitus, literally, honey-sweet diabetes. But more sinister than sugar in the urine is the fact that chronic exposure to excess glucose causes irreversible changes in blood vessels.

The cause of type 1 diabetes is straightforward, the *beta* cells of the pancreas are destroyed and insulin therefore is absent. Before the discovery of insulin by Frederick Banting and Charles Best of Toronto in 1922, type 1 diabetes meant an early death.[1] Type 2 diabetes is in a sense more complex and less well understood. The secretion of insulin in response to dietary glucose, the passage of that glucose into cells for production of energy, and the subsequent drop in insulin levels appears simple enough. However, this mechanism can be overwhelmed by excess glucose in a phenomenon called insulin resistance. The cells for which glucose is to provide energy no longer fully respond, blood glucose levels rise, and, to compensate, more insulin is released. Thus, in the early stages of type 2 diabetes, glucose levels may be normal but only in the presence of abnormal amounts of insulin. This cannot go on forever; soon the *beta* cells become unable to respond to the demands placed on them for insulin and we enter into the mature form of type 2 diabetes with an elevated level of blood glucose and the pathological changes that follow. The mechanism by which insulin resistance develops is unknown but its consequences are clear. Most important for you and me is the fact that obesity is the clearest risk factor for insulin resistance and resultant type 2 diabetes.

If it is obesity that causes type 2 diabetes and we can become obese by excess energy intake in the form of fat or protein or carbohydrate, how have we arrived at the point where today some tell us that sugar is the root of nearly all evil?

The current vilification of sugar can be traced to a young physician named Thomas Cleave, the ship's doctor aboard HMS *King George V* during World War II. One of the most common medical problems he encountered among the sailors was constipation. Just as had the ancient Greeks before him, Cleave treated the condition with pure bran, a form of fiber that is almost entirely composed of cellulous hence indigestible unless you happen to be a cow. From this humble beginning, Cleave developed the idea that many human diseases are the consequence of improper diet. More specifically, he proposed that when carbohydrate crops---whether grains or fruits or vegetables or sugar cane---are consumed in large quantities, they produce disease. His list included varicose veins, deep venous thrombosis, hemorrhoids, dental decay, obesity, diabetes, coronary heart disease, stomach ulcers, gout, hypertension, appendicitis, diverticulitis, hiatal hernia, and acne rosacea; there is something there for nearly everyone.

A second English physician, John Yudkin, had similar but more focused views, hypothesizing that sugar is the cause of heart disease.[2] Following World War II, Yudkin would become Professor of Nutrition and Dietetics at the University of London. With respect to fat, Yudkin and Cleave believed that vegetable oils were bad while fat derived from animals, being both natural and unrefined, could do no harm. Cleave argued that undigested material in the large intestine leads to disease, a notion at the heart of the still flourishing but largely irrational business of cleansing colons. Despite his earlier prescription of bran to sailors, the virtues of soluble and insoluble fiber as discussed below eluded him. Both men wrote provocatively titled books for the general public. Yudkin's in 1972 was called *Pure, White, and Deadly*[3] followed in 1974 by Cleave's *The Saccharine Disease*[4].

The books by Drs. Cleave and Yudkin were pretty much ignored by the medical establishment as well as by the general public and sugar remained under the radar for most Americans. That all changed with the publication in 1975 of a book by William Dufty called *Sugar Blues*[4]; it remains in print today and nearly two million copies have been sold in the United States alone. Dufty began his career as an organizer and speech writer for the United Auto Workers, became a columnist for the *New York Post*, and, in 1956, collaborated with Billie Holliday in writing her biography *Lady Sings the Blues*. That same year, in his role as newspaper columnist, Dufty met Gloria Swanson who advised him that "sugar is poison." Twenty years later, he became Swanson's sixth husband and the couple began a nationwide tour promoting *Sugar Blues*.

A few quotations from the paperback cover of *Sugar Blues* will give you the flavor of the book. "Like opium, morphine and heroin, sugar is an addictive destructive drug...If you are overweight or suffer from migraine, hypoglycemia, or acne, the plague of the sugar blues has hit you...Exposing sugar, the killer in your diet..."

In my view, *Sugar Blues* is a sometimes entertaining mixture of science, pseudoscience, hyperbole, name dropping, flimflam, and just plain ignorance. Nonetheless, sales of the book were brisk and remain so today. In addition, *Sugar Blues* has inspired numerous clones with colorful titles; among them are *Suicide by Sugar, Overcoming Sugar Addiction, The Hidden Truth Behind America's Deadliest Habit,* and *Sugar Shock: How Sweets and Simple Carbs Can Derail Your Life.*

The contemporary wrinkle put on the *sugar is poison* story told by Drs. Cleave and Yudkin and others and expanded upon by Dufty is to condemn not only sucrose but to elevate fructose to the pinnacle of toxicity. You will recall from earlier in this chapter that fructose or fruit sugar is a monosaccharide that comprises one half of the sucrose molecule. Free fructose is also found in a wide variety of fruits and vegetables. While fructose in relatively small quantities has been a part of the human diet for thousands of years and sucrose has been a major instrument of international trade since the seventeenth century, it is only relatively recently that what is called high fructose corn syrup (HFCS) was introduced into the American diet. To make it, corn starch is digested to release free glucose which is then converted to fructose. HFCS is then created by adding back glucose to produce a roughly 50-50 mixture of fructose and glucose or about the same proportion as found in table sugar derived from sugar cane or sugar beets. Thus, the "high fructose" of HFCS is a bit misleading; aside from the fact the glucose and fructose are present as free monosaccharides in HFCS, it contains about the same proportions of glucose and fructose as in sucrose. For the food industry, the primary merit of HFCS is its lower cost.

In the 21st century, the two people who have done the most to advance the notion that we should fear sugar in general and fructose in particular are a California pediatrician named Robert Lustig and Gary Taubes, a science writer. On May 26, 2009, Dr. Lustig presented a public lecture entitled *Sugar: The Bitter Truth*. His talk later appeared on YouTube where it has been viewed by millions. The Lustig lecture is one and a half hours long with roughly the middle portion devoted to the well-established biochemical details of glucose and fructose metabolism. The front and rear ends of his engaging talk are filled with provocative statements.

Dr. Lustig opens with an expression of hope that by the end of the story "I will have debunked the last thirty years of nutrition information in America." With respect to obesity, we are told that "obesity has nothing to do with calories" and that "eating less and exercising more does not prevent or reverse obesity because a calorie is not a calorie." In Dr. Lustig's pantry there are good foods and bad foods. Fructose in his view is not only bad; it is "a poison." Indeed, its toxic effects on the liver are judged to be the same as those of alcohol or, putting it more directly, "Coca Cola and Budweiser are the same." "Fructose is alcohol without the buzz." Whether in sucrose or HFCS, he tells us that fructose causes all features of the metabolic syndrome including high blood pressure, heart disease, and type 2 diabetes: "eat all foods raw and you will cure type 2 diabetes in a week." We are told that a "high fructose diet is a high fat diet", "we are being poisoned in every processed food" and, directly threatening our lemonade, the pronouncement that "there is no such thing as a good sugar beverage." In closing, Dr. Lustig says that "I stand here today to recruit you in the war against bad food."

Gary Taubes brought the Lustig message to the readers of the *New York Times Magazine* on April 17, 2011 in a cover story called *Sweet and Vicious, The case against sugar*. In it, Taubes recites the claims of Lustig but, should you not be sufficiently fearful, he goes on to add that "If it's sugar that causes insulin resistance,…then the conclusion is hard to avoid that sugar causes cancer." (He supports neither the premise nor the conclusion with evidence.) A subsequent article directed at the scientific community by Lustig, Laura Schmidt, and Claire Brandis was entitled *The Toxic Truth About Sugar*. The piece appeared in *Nature*, a well-respected British scientific publication, on February 7, 2012.[6]

What do others think of the Lustig/Taubes crusade against fructose? YouTube viewers seem convinced; likes outnumber dislikes by nearly 50 to 1. The scientific community, in responding to the *Nature* article, was less enthralled. Some pointed out that obesity is on the rise in many countries in which fructose consumption has changed not at all. Others regarded the equating of fructose with alcohol as nonsense. Many strongly disagreed with Lustig's pronouncement that "eat less and exercise doesn't work" with respect to obesity. David Katz, founding director of Yale University's Prevention Research Center, was blunt: "The notion that sugar is evil…is, in a word, humbug."[7]

There will always be individuals, varying greatly in their credibility, on both sides of an issue. Let's consider someone called by Mr. Taubes "the world's foremost authority" on the subject of fructose. He was referring to Luc Tappy, a medical scientist at the School of Medicine of the University of Lausanne in Switzerland. Dr. Tappy in 2012 said this: "There is no evidence that fructose is the sole, or even the main factor in the development of these (metabolic) diseases…public health measures should broadly focus on the promotion of healthy lifestyles generally with restriction of both sugar and saturated fat intakes, and consumption of whole grains, fresh fruits and vegetables rather than focusing exclusively on reduction of sugar intake."[8]

My personal view is that Dr. Lustig and Mr. Taubes have taken some interesting but highly speculative hypotheses and elevated them to the level of a dogma little different from that of Cleave and Yudkin and Dufty before them. It is most certainly not my intention to overly defend sugar as a component of the diet. In isolation, sucrose and high fructose corn syrup provide energy without anything else, so-called empty calories. No vitamins or minerals or fiber accompany the eating of refined sugar. In the form of soft drinks and the ubiquitous energy drinks, too many calories are consumed too readily. Indeed, in a perfect world, we would not consume sugars other than those found in unprocessed fruits and vegetables and those required for delightful eating. The hypothesis most attractive to me and for which an extensive scientific literature provides support is that obesity drives the metabolic diseases which are ascribed to fructose by Dr. Lustig. Two things are certain: the first is that caloric excess from any source is the cause of obesity and the second is that if I am obese and physically unfit, fructose is the least of my worries.

Mark Twain liked to talk about "things we know that ain't so." Is any harm done if the public is told that sugar "primes the brain for addiction" or that "fructose is a poison" and it turns out it ain't so? If claims such as these frighten people into reducing sugar intake might we gain ground on obesity? I am reminded of a girl who, when told that marijuana makes you crazy, replied "I don't see what's wrong with pot. All my friends smoke it and none of them are crazy." If the same girl, when told that Coca Cola, a drink she and her friends consume regularly with no apparent harm, contains poison, might she be inclined to reject all of the valid information she is provided about healthy eating and the dangers of obesity? If fructose, the natural sweetener of fruits and vegetables, is poison, does it not follow that these wonderful components of a healthy diet are to be avoided? A very bad idea indeed.

An apocryphal story has it that Herman Boerhaave, a celebrated Dutch physician of the 18th century, left behind a book that contained all of the secrets of his medicine. Every page was blank but one. On it was written: "Keep the head cool, the feet warm, and the bowels open." The last third of that prescription brings us back to fiber, that complex carbohydrate about which we so far have said little. Indeed, you might immediately wonder why we should care at all about indigestible things.

Concurrent with Dr. Cleave's development of his hypothesis of a "saccharine disease", a group of his fellow British-trained physicians was gathering evidence that would lead to quite different conclusions. More important, their ideas would be solidly rooted in observation, unencumbered by any general philosophy of life or of medicine.

During World War II, Dr. Alexander Walker of the South African Institute for Medical Research in Johannesburg began to observe the effects of high fiber diets on stool bulk and frequency of defecation in the Bantu of South Africa. In addition, Walker observed that despite a number of dietary deficiencies, the Bantu rarely suffered a large number of diseases that caused much sickness and death among Europeans. [8] For example, heart disease was much less common. In 1958, Walker was visited by Dr. Hugh Trowell, who for many years had been a medical missionary in Uganda. In his talks with Walker, Trowell became convinced that fiber influences diseases of the colon. In 1960, he published a book extending his list to seven other colonic disorders and 32 "non-infectious diseases of unknown origin rarely reported in rural blacks but common in Western populations."[10] Trowell, Walker, and others began to use the collective term "diseases of civilization."

Denis Burkitt assured himself a knighthood and a place in medical history when in 1957 he described a peculiar malignant disease of the lymphatic system in Ugandan children that is now known as Burkitt's lymphoma.[11] But it is his contribution to our present understanding of the nutritional role of dietary fiber that interests us here.

In 1967, Richard Doll, Professor Medicine at Oxford, introduced Dr. Burkitt to Dr. Cleave and his notion of a saccharine disease. Suddenly, the indecipherable complexity of the African epidemiology of colonic and venous disorders was simple for Burkitt. Fiber was the answer. The "diseases of Western civilization" weren't caused by a mysterious poisonous action of sugar. They were diseases of deficiency---a deficiency of fiber.

It was Burkitt's insight and advocacy that in large measure moved "the fiber hypothesis" from obscurity to the forefront of scientific and popular nutrition. For American medicine, the turning point was the appearance of a paper by Burkitt, Walker, and their colleague Neil Painter in the *Journal of the American Medical Association* for August 19, 1974.[12] It was titled simply "Dietary Fiber and Disease." In the decade following its publication, a consensus developed regarding fiber. Simply stated, the American population would benefit from an increased intake of fiber. That consensus often has been misinterpreted by popular writers and by those in the "health food" industry. To this day, many still equate fiber with cereal bran when in fact that is but one form of fiber.

As already noted, fiber is not a uniform material. It is composed of many components, the specific effects of which are largely unknown. It is useful to divide plant fiber into two categories based upon water solubility. The prototypical insoluble fibers are wheat bran, a carbohydrate, and lignin, a non-carbohydrate. The water-soluble carbohydrate fibers include pectin and a variety of plant materials called gums. Though it is true that citrus fruits are rich in pectin and that oat bran is an abundant source of gums, we should not forget that all fruits and vegetables present a complex mixture of fibers. For example, the much maligned potato is a good source of both lignin and pectin.

Division of fibers into soluble and insoluble categories is of considerable practical significance. This is illustrated by an investigation conducted Drs. K. L. Wrick, Daphne Roe, and their colleagues at Cornell University's Division of Nutritional Sciences.[13] They studied the effects of cabbage fiber (a rich source of pectin), purified cellulose, and wheat bran, either course or fine, in healthy men over a period of 80 days. The four sources of fiber had quite different effects on mouth-to-anus transit time, stool bulk, and ease of defecation. Fine-ground bran and cellulose were associated with hard, dry, difficult-to-pass stools. In contrast, course bran and cabbage fiber made for ease of defecation despite the fact that they had quite different effects on stool bulk. To understand these results, we need briefly to consider the mechanics of stool formation and some of the strange forms of life that inhabit our bodies.

Upon first feeding by breast or bottle, humans begin to develop a population of bacteria that soon exceeds in number the cells of the body itself. From mouth to anus alone there reside some 100 trillion bacteria, referred to collectively as the microbiome. The quantity and kinds of these bacteria rise and fall with what we eat, the state of our health, and the kinds of drugs we are taking. The specific contributions of these alien life forms remain largely unknown but suggestive links, both positive and negative, have been presented for obesity, heart disease, and a variety of immune disorders. One thing is certain, these microbes are largely anaerobic; they derive their energy for growth and multiplication by fermentation, the same process that causes bread to rise and beer to brew and corn mash to become whisky.

Now let us return to course bran and cabbage fiber. These represent the two general methods for prevention of constipation. Course bran is left largely undigested and unfermented, absorbs water, and results in a bulky soft stool. Cabbage fiber produces a soft stool but with considerably less bulk. The reason for this difference is that cabbage fiber is extensively fermented by bacteria of the gut. The bacteria multiply enormously and the stool that is passed is in large measure made up of the soft bodies of these bacteria with her high water content.

If course bran and cabbage fiber are so different in the way they are handled by the gut, a question that naturally comes to mind is "which form of fiber is preferable?" Should we add generous amounts of crude fiber to our usual diet or should we obtain our fiber from a variety of cereals, fruits, and vegetables? If defecation were the only issue, it wouldn't much matter. It is not the only issue. There are abundant epidemiological correlations between habitual consumption of diets rich in a variety of fibers, the DASH and Mediterranean diets of chapter 8 come to mind, and a decreased risk of colon cancer, heart disease, obesity, and diabetes. I said "epidemiological correlations"; causal links are more elusive. Nonetheless, all signs point to significant benefits from natural fiber. I emphasize *natural* because no study has ever shown an association between isolated fiber supplements and decreased disease risk. The association has always been with *foods* rich in fiber: whole grains, bran cereals, fruits, vegetables, dried peas and beans.

Carbohydrates should be the primary source of calories in the foods we eat. But if energy were the only thing we were looking for in a carbohydrate, a simple sugar such as sucrose would do as well as the complex carbohydrates found in cereals, fruits, and vegetables. There are at least three reasons why complex is better than simple. First of all, sucrose is a pure source of energy and brings with it no other nutrients. Second is the concept of dietary fiber. Insoluble fiber passes through the body undigested but epidemiological studies have linked a high content in the diet with a diminished incidence of diseases of the digestive tract including colon cancer. Currently of even greater interest is soluble fiber, the type that is fermented in the gut by the trillions of bacteria which normally reside there. Third, there is abundant epidemiological evidence that persons who eat diets rich in fruits and vegetables live longer and healthier lives. Although much remains to be learned about these matters, it is difficult to argue against a shift in dietary content away from excess protein and fat to a variety of carbohydrates both simple and complex. As for Coke, Pepsi, sports drinks, and all other beverages sweetened with sucrose or high fructose corn syrup, substitute water and save your sugar calories for a slice of pie or cake or whatever other sweet delicacy you may crave.

I will close this chapter with some advice from an editorial in the *Journal of the American Medical Association*: "…in reasonable amounts sugar is both wholesome and nutritious…(it) should be eaten in moderate quantities."[14] Those words appeared on August 16, 1913. Still good advice after more than a century.

NUTRITION

6.5 Vitamin A and *beta-carotene*
Of polar bears and flamingos

An infant is brought to the visiting American physician. She has seen children like this before and is not surprised when the interpreter tells her that the baby is sick and doesn't open his eyes. A quick examination confirms her fears: the child is blind. Behind the closed lids the corneas have dissolved into a shapeless jelly. The scene is repeated every day in Southeast Asia, Africa, India, Brazil, Central America, wherever children are starving. The specific cause is a lack of vitamin A. A half million of the world's children are rendered permanently blind each year by this readily correctable deficiency disease.

Our knowledge of vitamin A did not begin with blind children but with a more benign condition, the inability to see at night. Most have had the experience of entering a darkened movie theater and stumbling over those already seated. We have no problem upon leaving; those around us are clearly visible then. We have "gotten used to the dark." The process by which our eyes shift from seeing things in bright light to night vision requires the presence in the retina a substance called visual purple or rhodopsin. Vitamin A (retinol) is an essential component of visual purple.

Night blindness, the failure to adapt to dim light, and its cure, juice squeezed from liver, were described 3,500 years ago by an anonymous Egyptian physician. Many years later, but still before the birth of Christ, Hippocrates prescribed raw ox liver dipped in honey.

Fisherman in various parts of the world discovered the efficacy of seagull or codfish liver. Despite this practical knowledge, it remained for Georg Wald and his colleagues to demonstrate that vitamin A is directly involved in the synthesis of visual purple. Wald's investigations began in the early 1930's at the Kaiser Wilhelm Institute in Berlin and were completed in the Biological Laboratories of Harvard University. For his discoveries, Dr. Wald was awarded the Nobel Prize for Physiology or Medicine in 1967.[1]

To explain the sightless child whom we met at the beginning of this chapter, we must consider night blindness as but the first in a series of ocular changes that occur when too little vitamin A is available. The second step is called xerophthalmia. Xero, as in Xerox, comes from the Greek word for dryness. Xerophthalmia begins as simple dryness of the eyes but quickly progresses to softening of the cornea and total blindness. Accompanying these structural changes in the eye is a diminished resistance to infection; measles is a common cause of death among blinded children. Even a modest degree of deficiency may adversely affect immune function.

If, in the 21st century, hundreds of thousands of children are blinded each year by vitamin A deficiency, we might imagine that xerophthalmia and its tragic consequences are new to medical science. This is hardly the case. On October 3, 1923, Dr. C. E. Block, Professor of Medicine at the University of Copenhagen, read a paper before the World's Dairy Congress in Washington, D.C.[2] He reviewed what was known about xerophthalmia prior to 1910: epidemics in Brazil, Russia, and Japan; always among poor children and always in conjunction with a near-starvation diet. He told his listeners of xerophthalmia in animals. Finally, he summarized his experiences with poor children in Denmark.

A child taken from its mother's breast and fed little or no milk, butter, cream, fruits, or colored vegetables soon becomes listless and apathetic. Growth stops and weight loss begins. Infections of all kinds but especially of the skin and urinary tract are likely. Night blindness progresses to xerophthalmia and eventual blindness if death from infection does not intervene. Yet, Dr. Block concluded, all of these effects are readily prevented by providing fresh milk, butter, or cod liver oil.

Dr. Block's remarkable presentation rested in large measure upon the work of Elmer Verner McCollum. Born in 1879 on a farm in Kansas, McCollum would become the most influential nutritionist of his time. After training at the University of Kansas and at Yale University, he joined the faculty of the College of Agriculture of the University of Wisconsin in 1907. With a dozen rats purchased with his own money McCollum began to answer the question of why animals and humans cannot live on diets containing only protein, fat, carbohydrates, and minerals. Just six years after his arrival in Wisconsin, McCollum together with Marguerite Davis reported a growth-promoting factor in egg and in butter; they called it "fat-soluble A."[3]

Shortly after the appearance of the report by McCollum and Davis, supporting evidence was published by Lafayette Mendel, McCollum's teacher at Yale. But Mendel and his colleague, Thomas Osborne, went further. They showed that blindness in animals fed lard as the only source of fat could be prevented by butter.[4] The idea that blindness associated with human starvation might have a similar cure was subsequently refined and focused by McCollum. He wrote in the 1918 edition of his book, *The Newer Knowledge of Nutrition*, that xerophthalmia occurs in humans as a result of a specific lack of fat-soluble A.[5] Nearly a century later, none question that conclusion yet, on the day that you read this sentence, several thousand children will be blinded for want of this substance.

For his part, McCollum was happy to call the anti-xerophthalmic factor "fat-soluble A." It neatly differentiated it from "water-soluble B", the anti-beriberi factor we will talk about in the next section of this chapter. By this time many influential figures in nutrition had begun to accept the unifying notion of Casimir Funk that there existed a whole class of vital nutritional factors. The three for which substantial evidence then existed would thus be called vitamine A, vitamine B, and vitamine C, the anti-scurvy factor. The "e" was later dropped from "vitamine."

Elmer McCollum was persuaded to use the term in the 1922 edition of his book and universal usage soon followed.

By 1920 all agreed that vitamin A is a fat-like material found in things such as butter and egg yolk. Because of the color of these foods and because of the inactivity of fats such as lard and almond oil, Harry Steenbock, a colleague of McCollum's at Wisconsin, proposed that vitamin A is carotene, the yellow pigment of butter and egg yolk.[6] Others rejected the notion because some colorless fats had high vitamin A activity. The solution to this puzzle came with the discovery that carotene is a "provitamin", a precursor substance that is converted into vitamin A in the body. Conclusive proof was provided in 1929 by Thomas Moore in England. He showed that rats with no preformed vitamin A in their diets were able to maintain adequate levels of the vitamin when fed carotene.[7]

We now know that there are more than 400 different carotenoids. They give us the yellow of egg yolk and butter and the orange of carrots but also lobster-red, flamingo-pink, and salmon. Just as their hues are varied so too is the pro-vitamin A activity of the carotenoids. The most active is called "all-*trans*-*beta*-carotene" or simply *beta*-carotene and all others are measured against it.

Beta-carotene is the predominant carotenoid in green leaves and carrots, making each an excellent way to avoid vitamin A deficiency. Upon eating your daily salad, a very good idea, *beta*-carotene passes to the intestine where some is absorbed unchanged and some is converted to a form of vitamin A. (As a part of their singular nature, cats are unable to cleave *beta*-carotene. In 1971, Donald McLaren and Beatrice Zekian of the American University of Beirut described a 10-year-old Lebanese Arab girl who was cat-like with respect to *beta*-carotene and who, like a cat, required preformed vitamin A in her diet.[8] This is surely a rare condition in humans.)

Few attempts have been made to determine the exact human need for vitamin A. An important reason for this is illustrated by a World War II study done in Sheffield, England. Sixteen volunteers were fed a vitamin A and carotene-deficient diet and observed closely for possible effects. After eight months, blood retinol levels were lower in half of the subjects. After 11 months, three developed night blindness. Others showed no signs of deficiency even after staying on the diet for more than two years.[9]

A fact of life for all clinical investigators is that no two human beings are exactly alike in their response to a particular diet or drug or treatment. But the Sheffield results showed a degree of variation between subjects that is truly remarkable. The probable explanation lies in the fact that in times of plenty our bodies set aside a large amount of vitamin A for future use. One estimate is that the typical American has enough to last for two years; some of us may be carrying around a ten-year supply. A happy situation for those about to be cut off from their usual supply of vitamin A but a real problem for scientists who wish to study deficiency in normal volunteers in the laboratory.

The British work was far from a complete loss. Based upon the response of those few who developed night blindness and upon changes in blood levels when vitamin A was returned to the diet, it was estimated that the minimal protective amount was 390 micrograms (1,287 International Units) and a probably adequate intake would be 750 micrograms (2,475 IU). These estimates provided a point of reference for all subsequent work and are not far from the present recommendations to be discussed below.

Preformed vitamin A is found almost exclusively in animal tissues. Liver is by far the richest source but eggs and whole milk provide the vitamin as well. However, each of these food items carries with it a penalty. In addition to vitamin A, each contributes to our daily intake of saturated fat and, in the case of eggs, a significant amount of cholesterol. We will consider cholesterol and saturated fat in the context of heart disease in chapter 14. For now we will assume that we don't want to increase our intake of either in our quest for vitamin A.

When all of the saturated fat is removed from whole milk, all of the vitamin A is removed as well. But read the label on a container of skim milk; each cup has nearly twice the amount of vitamin A found in whole milk as it comes from the cow. This feat has been accomplished by adding back a larger amount of vitamin A than was originally present. As unnatural as it sounds, this is food processing and food additives at their best. An undesired element of the diet, saturated fat, has been removed and a desired one has been provided in a palatable and widely consumed form.

As little as a single egg a day and a pint of skim milk will provide about all of the preformed vitamin A anyone needs. The rest of the requirement should come in the form of carotene. Indeed, vegans, those who consume no animal products at all, get along perfectly well with virtually no pre-formed vitamin A in their diets. The best guide to the carotene content of fruits and vegetables is their color. A white potato contains none whereas a sweet potato has a two-day supply. Green, yellow, orange, and red fruits and vegetables are sure to provide the pro-vitamin but in quite variable amounts. Those that give us our daily need or more in a single serving are broccoli, cabbage, chard, collards, kale, cantaloupe, pumpkin, mango, and spinach. There is even some preformed vitamin A in spinach. My personal choice is the carrot; eat even a small one each day and you needn't trouble yourself further about carotene. On cooked versus raw, there's little to suggest that cooking is a problem but, as always, time, water, and temperature, should be kept to a minimum. In view of the abundance of carotene and vitamin A in foods around us, it is remarkable that many Americans are deficient. Of greatest concern are children and the elderly whose diets too often contain too little milk and too few vegetables.

Later I will say a bit about *beta*-carotene and vitamin A supplements but first we will consider the fact that when it comes to vitamin A, more is definitely not better. Polar bears and humans have shared the Arctic for a very long time. The flesh of the bear has occasionally sustained humans and, on occasion, vice versa. From this extended association has come the sure knowledge among Eskimos and others of the region that the liver of the polar bear is poisonous and should not be eaten. European explorers have been rediscovering that fact on a regular basis for the last 400 years. Despite these many years of experience, it was not until 1943, 30 years after McCollum and Davis, that the toxic element of bear liver was identified as vitamin A.[10]

There are many tales of human intoxication with vitamin A that could be told but we will consider just one. It happened a long time ago but is still relevant today. Sarah, a woman of 21 years, was admitted to a hospital in New York City on July 24, 1945. Her chief complaints were double vision, headache, and nausea. During her stay of a month and a half, no effective treatment was provided but she was given a diagnosis: brain tumor. Six days after her discharge from the first hospital Sarah entered a second. There she revealed that for the past two years she had been taking vitamin A for her dry and scaly skin. She had begun with 7,500 micrograms a day but soon increased the dose to 150,000 micrograms with an occasional day at twice that amount.

Among Sarah's examining physicians was a neurosurgeon. He thought her problems were caused by increased pressure of fluid surrounding her brain. To relieve that pressure he removed a piece of her skull and drained off some of the fluid. After recovery from her surgery she left the hospital but soon returned because chest pain and numbness in her pelvic area had been added to her previous problems. This time Sarah spent two months in the hospital. She was treated with thiamine and radiation therapy but remained unimproved and undiagnosed. A neurologist favored the idea that a brain tumor was spreading.

Sarah entered her third hospital on February 10, 1947. There a neurosurgeon covered the previously made hole in her skull with a metal plate. Treatment then included "fever therapy"—intentional infection with typhoid fever in an attempt to correct what had now been diagnosed as encephalitis, an inflammation of the brain. She was discharged on April 7th only to be admitted to still another hospital a month later.

Two symptoms were noted at hospital number 4: First, Sarah's pain was less severe if she remained motionless. To capitalize on that fact she was placed in a cast that ran from the nipple line to mid-thigh. Second, she was still taking 500,000 IU of vitamin A each day for her skin condition. Her physicians saw no reason to discontinue it. A neurologist suggested a possible viral infection of the nervous system.

Sarah entered her fifth hospital just five months after leaving the fourth. Pain in her joints had become so severe that she was able to walk only with great difficulty. A diagnosis of generalized infectious arthritis was soon made and she was discharged to the outpatient department for continued physiotherapy. For the next five years she was treated by chiropractic and osteopathic methods, continued to take her vitamin A, and lived in constant pain.

On February 5th, 1953 Sarah came under the care of Alexander Gerber at the Jewish Hospital of Brooklyn.[11] For the first time, the possibility of vitamin A poisoning was considered. All supplemental vitamin A was stopped. From that day her health began to improve. Within two months her skin texture was nearly normal and she had regained an appetite for food. For the first time in more than eight years she was free of pain.

Many years have passed since Sarah began her adventure with vitamin A but the lessons to be learned from her odyssey are no less fresh today.

(1) vitamin A in excess is a poison.

(2) Intoxication with vitamin A can produce myriad effects: nausea, dry and peeling skin, pain in bones and joints are but a few. Increased pressure on the brain may cause signs and symptoms that, as in Sarah's case, are easily interpreted as the effects of brain tumor or infection.

(3) A general principle for both physicians and patients is that whenever a person becomes ill in mind or body for no apparent reason, every drug and dietary supplement must be evaluated as a possible cause.

It may appear reasonable to some readers for the Federal government to step in and protect the public from this essential but nonetheless toxic substance. The Food and Drug administration in 1973 attempted to do just that. It was proposed that all vitamin and mineral supplements containing more than 150% of the recommended daily allowance be classified as drugs and hence subject to regulation. The courts would not permit the FDA to act. The FDA next focused on vitamin A. A regulation was published requiring a physician's prescription for any daily dose in excess of 3,300 micrograms. In what their chief counsel called "a humiliating defeat", the FDA lost again in court.[12] We retained our right to poison ourselves with vitamin A.

"Teratology" is an uncommon word; the Greek *teras* means monster. Teratology is the science of monsters. In 1953, S. Q. Cohlan reported that rats given large amounts of vitamin A gave birth to malformed pups.[13] Since then, the teratogenic effects of vitamin A have been proven in several species and multiple case reports have linked excess vitamin A intake to human malformations. It is for this reason that the Teratology Society, a group devoted to the study of the origins of malformations, recommends that *beta*-carotene be the primary source of vitamin A for women in their reproductive years.[14] The human body is well able to regulate the conversion of *beta*-carotene to vitamin A and there is no known instance of birth defects following excess intake of *beta*-carotene.

Although deficiency of vitamin A is a leading cause of blindness in less affluent nations, it is an excess of the vitamin that poses the greater hazard to Americans. While it is true that few of us are likely to be poisoned by too much polar bear liver, toxic amounts can be found in every vitamin store and catalog. Current recommendations are that men and women over the age of 50 take in about 3,000 International Units of vitamin A per day with no more than half coming preformed in things such as skim milk and eggs. As was noted earlier, vegans ingest virtually no preformed vitamin A yet maintain adequate levels via the carotenes in fruits and vegetables.

The fact that some segments of the population have marginal intake of carotenes and vitamin A and the seemingly ineradicable notion that more is better have led many to seek dietary supplements. The makers of such supplements have been only too willing to oblige. The current recommendations are 900 and 700 micrograms per day for men and women over the age of 50, respectively.[15] A typical vitamin A supplement for sale on-line or in a vitamin store provides 3,000 micrograms and products containing 7,500 micrograms (25,000 IU) per capsule are not uncommon. Thus, it is very easy to exceed the currently specified upper limit for safety of 3,000 micrograms. Indeed, a recent study of postmenopausal women found that long-term intake of preformed vitamin A in excess of about 2,100 micrograms increases the risk of osteoporosis and hip fracture.[16] As I noted earlier, we retain the right to poison ourselves with vitamin A. Anyone determined to use a supplement should choose *beta*-carotene. You may take on an orange hue but vitamin A levels will nicely be controlled by the wisdom of your body. Indeed, until recently, it was believed that *beta*-carotene could do no harm. Today we are not so sure.

More than thirty years ago, a rhetorical question was asked: Can dietary *beta*-carotene materially reduce human cancer rates? After all, correlational studies had suggested that persons who consume more fruits and vegetables have a lower risk of cancer. Among those raising the issue were Sir Richard Peto and Sir Richard Doll, the two men most responsible for sounding the alarm about smoking and lung cancer.[17] A few years later, two studies were undertaken, one in Finland and the other in the United States. Both investigations used cigarette smokers as subjects and both examined the effects of *beta*-carotene supplements. In the U.S., the study was stopped 21 months earlier than planned when it became evident that the risk of lung cancer and death was *increased* by *beta*-carotene.[18] In Finland, cancer of the lung, prostate, and stomach *increased* with the use of *beta*-carotene.[19] Might similar effects be seen in non-smokers? That question has not yet been answered.

NUTRITION

6.6 Thiamine (vitamin B$_1$)
Beriberi and polished rice

Beriberi is a disease that takes its name from the Singhalese word for weakness. Percy Netterville Gerrard, district surgeon of the Federated Malay States civil service, gave us in 1904 the following description.[1] "Picture yourself a skeleton, with a parchment-like wrinkled skin…drawn over it, weary dilapidated individual, apparently a picture of misery, with a staff to assist his tottering footsteps if the power of locomotion still remains to him." Later workers would also note a variety of behavioral disturbances: decreased attention span, personality changes, depression, lack of initiative, and poor memory. (Colonials readily interpreted the more subtle effects of beriberi as a reflection of inborn characteristics of the natives.)

Under various names, beriberi has been known in the Orient for thousands of years. In Japan it was called kake, a rare condition found almost exclusively among the wealthy. That exclusiveness began to erode in the 17th century with epidemics occurring in Tokyo and other cities. By 1870, beriberi was a nationwide problem whose incidence would increase for the next 50 years. It was an officer of the Japanese Naval Medical Service who had provided clear evidence in the 1880's of a nutritional cure for beriberi.

The Japanese warship *Riujo* sailed from Japan in 1882 with a crew of 276. After stops in New Zealand and Chile, she arrived in Honolulu. During the voyage of 272 days, 60% of the men suffered from beriberi and 25 died of the disease.

Dr. Kanehiro Takaki was in 1882 a junior medical officer recently returned from five years of study at St. Thomas's Hospital Medical School in London. He had observed that beriberi was rare in the Royal Navy despite voyages of equal length and generally comparable living conditions. In seeking differences between British and Japanese sailors, Takaki focused on their respective diets. The British consumed large amounts of animal protein whereas the principal component of the Japanese diet was polished rice. When separated from the leaves and stalks of the plant, a grain of rice remains encased in its indigestible hull. Hand grinding will remove the hull but the pericarp or "bran coat" is left behind. The resulting "brown rice" is edible but becomes rancid in storage. When steam-driven milling machines became available, large quantities of rice could be stripped of their bran coats and buffed to produce gleaming white "polished rice" that could be stored indefinitely.

Dr. Takaki hypothesized that beriberi was caused by a deficiency of nitrogen in the diet. Protein is the only significant source of nitrogen. This hypothesis was tested in 1884 when the warship *Tsukubu* retraced the path of the ill-fated *Riujo*. At Takaki's insistence, *Tsukubo* carried with her ample supplies of meat and dried milk. By voyage's end, none of the crew had died of beriberi and signs of the disease had been seen in only 14. Meat and dried milk became a part of the diet of the Japanese sailor and beriberi was virtually eliminated from the Emperor's fleets.[2, 3] Non-oceangoing Japanese were less fortunate. (In recognition of his achievement, Dr. Tanaki was later named Director-General of the Medical Department of the Imperial Japanese Navy and elevated to the peerage as Baron Takaki.)

Despite Takaki's success in preventing beriberi by dietary means, others must be credited with recognizing the true nature of the disease and for providing a specific remedy. For several hundred years, the Netherlands controlled a vast area of the Pacific, the Dutch East Indies. As a result, Dutch medical officers had ample opportunity to study beriberi in the prisons and insane asylums of Kuala Lumpur, Djakarta, and elsewhere. By the 1880's, their interest centered on the influence of rice. It was known that prisoners fed polished rice were 250 times more likely to develop beriberi as were those fed brown rice. Christiaan Eijkman, a Dutch physician on the island of Java, showed in 1887 that a beriberi-like condition occurred in chickens fed polished rice but the chickens were cured by feeding them a water extract of brown rice.[4] Eijkman thought that a toxin in rice was being unmasked in the conversion of brown rice to polished rice. For his work, Eijkman shared the Nobel Prize for Physiology or Medicine for 1929 with Sir Frederick Gowland Hopkins, a British pioneer in the study of vitamins.[5]

It remained for Eijkman's successor on Java, Gerritt Grijns, to suggest the true cause of beriberi. He proposed in 1909 that an essential substance was being removed from rice during the milling process and that it was a deficiency of this substance that caused beriberi.[6] Furthermore, the essential substance was not confined to rice. Beriberi was also prevented by water extracts of green peas, beans, and meat.

The Japanese experience could now be explained. Beriberi remained a scourge of the rich so long as only they could afford the lovely whiteness of polished rice. Technology in the form of steam-driven milling machines brought polished rice, and beriberi to the common man. Takaki's achievement in ridding the Japanese navy of beriberi did not result from the introduction of more animal protein into the diet but to the water-soluble substance that happened to come along with the protein.

The protective substance found in rice and other foods had come to be called the "antineuritic factor", a reference to the neuritis of beriberi in which both sensory and motor functions are impaired hence accounting for the "tottering footsteps" noted by Gerrard. To distinguish it from the previously discovered "fat-soluble A", some referred to it as "water-soluble B." A more euphonious name was needed and Casimir Funk, a Polish biochemist, provided it. Funk realized in 1911 that water-soluble B belonged, together with fat-soluble A and water-soluble C , to a new class of food factors. He named this class "vitamine", a contraction of vital amine. As noted earlier, the "e" was soon dropped. Water-soluble

B this became vitamin B and, when other water-soluble vitamins were found, vitamin B_1. With the identification of its chemical structure in 1926, the official name, thiamine, was given.[7] Vitamin B_1 and thiamine refer to the same chemical substance.

We still occasionally find someone referring to thiamine as antineuritic factor. Confusion may result. While a student at the Culinary Institute of America, my elder daughter showed me one of her textbooks, the English translation of Prosper Montagne's *Nouveau Larousse Gastronomique*, subtitled The World's Standard Encyclopedia of Food, Wine, and Cookery. The book describes vitamin B_1 as an "antineurotic factor" and goes on to say that "absence of vitamin B_1 from the diet gives rise to neurotic complaints." Though the words neuritic and neurotic differ by but a single letter, their meanings and implications are far different. I can't help wondering how many gourmets, professional chefs, and other readers of *Larousse* have been led to treat their anxiety with thiamine. (I have never seen the French edition of the book, so I don't know if the error was by the author or by the translator.)

The Recommended Dietary Allowance for thiamine for adults is 1.1 to 1.2 mg per day with an increase to 1.4 mg during pregnancy and lactation.[8] Although a number of studies have found thiamine deficiencies in the institutionalized elderly, this is most likely a reflection of overall poor nutrition. For this reason, there is no increase in the RDA as we age. No toxicity has been associated with thiamine in excess and no upper limit has been recommended.

Because the signs of beriberi include the loss of appetite, constipation, and fatigue, many constipated, tired, people with poor appetite have been led to believe they need more thiamine. This is rarely the case. Though it has often been suggested that marginal thiamine deficiency is common in the United States, a number of surveys have failed to support that idea. The probable reason for our relatively good thiamine status is the nearly universal practice of fortifying flour with thiamine. Check the label of Wonder Bread, one of those pure white homogeneous products so abhorred by advocates of natural foods, and you will find that it provides as much thiamine as any whole-grained bread. This is a case in which a food additive is not a bad thing. However, this is not meant as an endorsement of the practice of refining and fortifying. Much more is lost in the refining of cereal grains than thiamine.

The classic descriptions of beriberi provided us by the Dutch and British physicians of the Malay Archipelago were surely contaminated by the effects of multiple vitamin and macronutrient deficiencies. However, there is no reason to doubt that the major signs of beriberi are caused by lack of thiamine. In a Japanese investigation, otherwise well-fed subjects were limited to 0.3 mg of thiamine per day. Clear-cut signs of beriberi appeared after about three months. If thiamine intake is reduced to near zero, effects may be seen much more rapidly. Another Japanese study detected changes in heart function after only one week. This is consistent with the fact that thiamine, like other water-soluble vitamins, is stored in the body in only limited amounts.

Four forms of thiamine deficiency disease are generally recognized. The first type, infantile beriberi, occurs in babies nursed by thiamine-deficient mothers.[9] It is a frequent cause of death in areas of the world where gross malnutrition is common. The person described in the opening paragraph ("...dilapidated...picture of misery...with...tottering footsteps") suffered from the second variety of the disease which was then and is still called "dry beriberi." When thiamine deficiency is somewhat more profound, the third manifestation of the disease, "wet beriberi", results. It takes its name from the accumulation of fluid in the body; Gerrard asks us to "imagine a patient swollen beyond recognition."

The fourth and final form of thiamine deficiency is seen almost exclusively in alcoholics: the Wernicke-Korsikoff syndrome.[10] Alcoholics often carry the double burden of an inadequate diet and alcohol-induced impairment of thiamine absorption. Although some aspects of Wernicke-Korsikoff syndrome respond favorably to treatment with thiamine, others appear to reflect permanent damage to the brain. Fortification of alcoholic beverages with thiamine to prevent the syndrome has often been proposed but never implemented.

The major natural sources of thiamine are the bran coats of cereal grains, fresh vegetables, especially green beans and peas, pork, beef, and organ meats. In addition, many processed foods have had thiamine added to them. I've already mentioned the fortification of flour and, if you read the labels on typical breakfast cereals, you will find lots of thiamine there as well.

Those who can't shake the idea that more is better and are tempted to buy one of those supplements advertising 500 mg of thiamine should be aware that at least 98% of that thiamine goes right down the toilet. Even with depletion to the point of beriberi, our bodies are able to absorb only about 10 mg of thiamine per day.

Despite the ease of meeting the RDA for thiamine, we should keep in mind that the vitamin can be lost from foods during cooking. Though we might imagine that thiamine would be destroyed by heat, the major culprit seems to be water. Thiamine-enriched flours are little affected by baking or toasting but significant losses can occur when pasta is cooked in water. The vitamin simply dissolves in the water and is drained off. The general rules to be followed are to use a minimum of water, to cook no longer than necessary, and to make use of as much of the cooking water as possible.

Some foods contain substances that either inactivate thiamine or block its actions. This interesting bit of information is sometimes brought to public attention by those with vitamins for sale. In fact, we have little reason to be worried. In some fish there is an enzyme that destroys thiamine but cooking inactivates the enzyme. There is no question that tea and coffee contain small amounts of anti-thiamine chemicals but they are doubtful importance for human nutrition. Some years ago a study was conducted in Thailand among natives who chew tea leaves all day and drink large amounts of tea as well. It was found that thiamine levels were only slightly lower than normal and no signs of deficiency were seen. I would note however that there is a weight loss potion that contains horsetail (*Equisetum arvense*), an herbal product which has significant anti-thiamine activity.

For those who may succumb to advertisements for 500 mg thiamine tablets, it is fortunate that no harm is likely to be done. The only reports of thiamine toxicity followed injection of the vitamin in alcoholics and in those cases it is difficult to determine the source of the problem.

I began this chapter with the statement that "Colonials readily interpreted the more subtle effects of beriberi as a reflection of inborn characteristics of the natives."Today, such thoughts would be labeled racist. Instead, an advertisement will ask "Are you tired, depressed, and have a poor memory? Then you need our 500 mg thiamine supplement." Both statements are equally lacking in merit.

NUTRITION

6.7 Niacin (vitamin B$_3$)
Pellagra and madness

When Christopher Columbus reached the West Indies, corn had been a part of the diet of Native Americans for at least 5,000 years. Columbus could not have imagined that by introducing corn into Europe he would lay the groundwork for pellagra, a disease that would spread across the Continent and would, in the first third of the 20th century, kill tens of thousands of poor whites and blacks in the United States.

The characteristics of pellagra are usually remembered as the three D's: dermatitis, diarrhea, and dementia. A fourth should be added: death. Early signs such as weakness and lack of energy are easily confused with laziness and deficiency of character, a not uncommon interpretation when they appeared in mill workers and tenant farmers. Writing in 1940 J. P. Frostig and T. D. Spies said "men previously strong, courageous, and enduring became shaky, weary, and apprehensive even before the generally recognized signs of pellagra develop…(it) breaks down the morale…" Insomnia, depression, and impaired memory often progressed to delusions, hallucinations, and dementia. Twenty-five percent of the patients admitted in 1910 to an insane asylum in South Carolina were found to have pellagra.

Unlike beriberi, pellagra is not an ancient disease. It was first observed in 1735 by Gaspar Casal, physician to Philip V of Spain.[1] It takes its name from the Italian *pelle ruvida*: rough skin. That is too mild a term. The skin lesions of pellagra are terrible to behold. I particularly recall the photograph of a girl, perhaps seven years of age, with a ribbon in her neatly combed hair, whose hands and face were swollen and cracked by pellagra. Typical changes in the skin of the neck and upper chest are still referred to as "Casal's necklace." As the disease progresses, the effects upon the nervous system become more obvious, with irreversible insanity the ultimate phase.

The cause of pellagra eluded scientists for hundreds of years but its association with corn was evident to all. Although Casal suspected that pellagra was caused by faulty nutrition, most theories of the 18th and 19th centuries suggested a toxin or germ in spoiled corn. The public health officials of France took a pragmatic approach: they discouraged the eating of corn and the disease virtually disappeared in their country.

In formulating his concept of vitamins in 1911, Casimir Funk had proposed that scurvy, beriberi, rickets, and pellagra were deficiency diseases. We have seen in the preceding section how water-soluble B had been shown to have anti-beriberi properties and, for a time, many believed that the matter of vitamin B to be settled. However, in the constant ferment that is science, evidence began to accumulate that vitamin B was not a single substance but a group of substances, the B complex. Thus began what Leslie Harris has called "this long history of disentanglement." It would eventually yield thiamine, niacin, riboflavin, pyridoxine, pantothenic acid, and biotin.

Although pellagra was probably present in the United States in the early 1800's and surely occurred in Civil War prisoners, it was not generally known to the medical profession until 1907 when George Searcy described 88 cases in an Alabama insane asylum.[2] So long as only those living in institutions, mainly the orphans and the insane, were affected by pellagra, not much note would be taken of it. However, within two years of Searcy's report, pellagra had been identified among workers in more than twenty states. By 1914, pellagra was epidemic in the American south particularly among sharecroppers and in the textile mills. Political pressure to do something about it became irresistible.

In March of 1914, Joseph Goldberger was a 40-year-old physician in the United States Public Health Service. When he was assigned to study pellagra, he was already a 15-year veteran of investigations into measles, parasitic worms, diphtheria, malaria, typhus, typhoid, dengue and yellow fever. Although the cause of pellagra was obscure, most American authorities believed it to be an infectious disease. Given Goldberger's past experience with insect carriers of disease and the prevailing belief in a microorganism as the cause of pellagra, his natural inclination may have been along those lines. His genius is revealed by the fact that three months after beginning his investigations, he published a paper in which he concluded that pellagra is not infectious, the cause is dietary, and it can be prevented by an increase in the consumption of fresh meat, eggs, and milk.[3]

Goldberger's hypothesis met considerable resistance. The Pellagra Commission of the State of Illinois had concluded just three years earlier that pellagra was caused by infection with a microorganism and, in 1912, the Thompson-McFadden Pellagra Commission in South Carolina had reached the same conclusion.[4] Goldberger knew that his hypothesis had to be tested. He did so in three ways.:

(1) The children of an orphanage in Jackson, Mississippi received additional meat, eggs, milk, beans, and peas for a period of two years. Pellagra, which had been rampant, disappeared. When the money ran out and the children's diets returned to "normal", the disease came back.[5, 6]

(2) He put a group of prisoner's at the Rankin farm of the Mississippi State Penitentiary on a diet like that of the pellagrans; signs of the disease appeared after three months.[7, 8]

(3) He tested the infectious nature of pellagra in himself, his wife, and fourteen of his colleagues. They injected themselves with the blood of pellagrans and swallowed capsules containing nasal secretions, bits of dead skin, urine, and feces of pellagrans. They did not catch pellagra.[9]

By the end of 1915, Goldberger had demonstrated, in his words, the complete prevention of pellagra by diet alone. We might imagine that pellagra ceased from that time to be a public health hazard. It did not. In 1916, pellagra was the second leading cause of death in South Carolina. During the years 1924 through 1939, no fewer than 2,000 and as many as 8,000 Americans died of the disease. W. Henry Sebrell, one of Goldberger's early associates, estimated that there were 250,000 cases in 1928.[10]

Why did pellagra continue to kill Americans long after Goldberger demonstrated its dietary basis? Some would argue that the application of all advances in science requires the passage of time to win over those who hold other beliefs. Leslie Harris, former director of the Dunn Nutritional Laboratory of the University of Cambridge, thought otherwise: "The explanation is economic, not scientific...It is a sad commentary that while these people were dying from a dietary deficiency, at the same time in other parts of the country food was being burned or thrown into the sea because of overproduction." It is a still sadder commentary that we in the United States still find ourselves uncertain as to the extent of hunger in America. In the midst of enormous stockpiles of food, we are still confronted with malnutrition in significant numbers of children, pregnant women, and old people.

There are many in our society who today question the value of animal research in solving the puzzles of human disease. Goldberger had no such doubts. He recognized that blacktongue, a disease in dogs, was analogous to human pellagra and could be produced by the pellagran diet. After eight years of experimentation with the dog model, Goldberger and his associates concluded that "...there is a heretofore unrecognized or appreciated dietary factor which we designate as factor P-P...", the pellagra-preventative factor. It soon became clear that factor P-P was in fact a previously unrecognized vitamin. The British called it vitamin B_2 to distinguish it from the anti-beriberi factor, vitamin B_1. In 1929, the year of Goldberger's death, the American Society of Biological Chemists honored him by naming the pellagra-preventative factor vitamin G.

Nicotinic acid had been known to chemists since 1897. It takes its name from the fact that it shares a part of the nicotine molecule, the addictive substance in tobacco cigarettes. Funk had isolated nicotinic acid from rice polishings but, because it was inactive against beriberi, little note was taken of it. It was not until 1936 that nicotinic acid was shown to be important to the function of several enzymes and to be required for the growth of a number of microorganisms. Only then did interest arise in the possibility of a nutritional role for nicotinic acid. In 1937, it was shown that nico-tinic acid cured blacktongue in dogs[11] and that same year the cure of pel-lagra in humans was reported at the Central Society for Clinical Research in Chicago.[12] Goldberger's pellagra-preventative factor was nicotinic acid.

The need for another name for nicotinic acid soon became evident. When the proposal was made in 1939 to fortify bread with nicotinic acid, a headline read "Tobacco in Your Bread." Confusion of nicotinic acid with nicotine, the alkaloid of tobacco, was inevitable. To remedy the situation, the Food and Nutrition Board declared that nicotinic acid should henceforth be called niacin.

Despite the success of niacin in curing pellagra, there were still a number of puzzling aspects. How, if the pellagra-preventative factor is niacin, are niacin-poor foods able to prevent pellagra? This is the way that Conrad Elvehjem put the question to Willard Krehl, one of his grad-uate students: "Why is it that milk, which contains very little niacin, cures and prevents pellagra in man and blacktongue in dogs while corn, which is very much richer in niacin, is a major factor in the production of pellagra?." As would any good scientist, Krehl answered the question with an experiment. He fed tryptophan, an essential amino acid, to dogs maintained on a pellagrous diet. They grew normally and remained healthy.[13] Later it was learned our bodies convert tryptophan into niacin. Indeed, no preformed niacin is required in the diet if adequate trypto-phan is present.[14] This is exactly what Dr. Goldberger had accomplished by feeding meat, eggs, milk, and legumes to his Mississippi orphans. Even today, one sometimes sees the niacin requirement expressed as nia-cin equivalents where 60 mg of tryptophan equals 1 mg of niacin.

A second puzzle: why did pellagra not appear in the native peoples of the Americas? In Mexico, for example, all of the conditions for pellagra

117

seemed present: poverty, lack of animal protein, and a corn-based diet. The answer lies in a discovery made more than three thousand years ago by an unknown genius in what is now Guatemala. When corn is soaked and cooked in an alkaline solution, structural changes occur such that the resulting cornmeal forms dough suitable for cooking when water is added. The process is called nixtamalization, a term derived from the Aztec word for ashes, *nextli*, the source of the alkaline solution, and *tamalli*. Unknowable at the time was the fact that the process also converts niacin in the corn to a form that is readily absorbed by the human body. Had the sharecroppers of South Carolina adhered to this ancient method of preparation, they would have been spared the curse of pellagra.

The many sources of niacin and tryptophan in the typical diet and fortification with niacin of most flour together with the fact that niacin is quite resistant to destruction by cooking or in storage, makes it easy to insure an adequate intake of the vitamin. Recall that Goldberger had no trouble eliminating the disease in his orphans simply by adding meat and milk to their fare. Despite these facts, our friendly health food store or online site is pleased to offer us still more of the vitamin in the form of supplements containing as much as 1,000 mg per tablet; that's about 50 times the currently recommended daily value for niacin in a single tablet.[15] The rationale for using such huge amounts comes not from prevention of pellagra but from a curious connection between niacin and cholesterol.

The title of this chapter connects pellagra and madness. It is thus appropriate that the discovery of niacin's anti-cholesterol effects had its roots in a department of psychiatry. In 1939, Rudolf Altschul was a Jewish physician driven from Czechoslovakia by the German invasion. As fate would have it, Dr. Altschul found himself in far-off Saskatoon, Canada, where a new medical school had been created. There he encountered Abram Hoffer, a psychiatrist interested in treating schizophrenia with niacin. Hoffer reasoned that if a deficiency of niacin results in the madness of pellagra then niacin might ameliorate the madness of schizophrenia.

Though trained as a neuropsychiatrist,, Altshul's interests had moved toward heart disease in general and the idea that lowering cholesterol might be of benefit. Over the next decade and a half, first in rabbits, then in a group of medical students, and finally in patients, Altshul found that large amounts of niacin caused a modest decrease in serum cholesterol. In his medical students, a dose of 4,000 mg per day was used.[16] In 1958, the Council on Drugs of the American Medical Association recommended the use of niacin as a treatment for elevated cholesterol.

It took about fifteen years for Hoffer's treatment of schizophrenia with niacin to be thoroughly discredited by the psychiatric community though there are still those who subscribe to the notion of megavitamin therapy for mental illness. In contrast, the use of niacin to lower LDL cholesterol, "bad cholesterol", and to elevate HDL cholesterol, "good cholesterol", became an established part of medical practice. The use of niacin for this purpose was further boosted by the publication in 1987 of an enormously popular book, *The 8-Week Cholesterol Cure,* by a journalist named Robert Kowalski. The subtitle of his book was *How to lower blood-cholesterol by up to 40 percent without drugs.* Without drugs? When used in doses several hundred times greater than the amount needed to prevent pellagra, niacin is a drug with a full spectrum of effects. Many discontinue its use because of the intense flushing that it can elicit. Indeed, its cholesterol-lowering properties are independent of its activity as a vitamin. The real virtue of niacin for do-it-yourselfers is that it can be bought in unlimited quantities without a prescription. I am all for self-reliance in matters of health, but do-it-yourself cardiology has all the appeal for me as does do-it-yourself brain surgery. (Mr. Kowlaski died in 2007 at the age of 65 of heart disease.)

The use of niacin to reduce serum cholesterol has been overshadowed by the discovery of a class of drugs called the statins. They will be discussed more fully in chapter 14. Nonetheless, Forbes magazine estimated that more than $1 billion was spent in 2012 on just a single niacin formulation, Abbott Laboratories' Niaspan, an extended-release version of the vitamin.

It will be interesting to see how sales of niacin progress, whether on line, in drug stores, or as prescribed by a physician, in the next few years. It turns out that Niaspan in combination with a statin is no better than a statin alone and is associated with a number of adverse effects.[17] A second study, published in 2014, was even more damning. The investigation had the imposing title Heart Protection Study 2-Treatment of HDL to Reduce the Incidence of Vascular Events (HPS2-THRIVE).[18] More than 25,000 men, age 50-80 years, who already had heart disease were treated with a placebo or with Tredaptive, Merck's extended release form of niacin, together with a drug to reduce flushing of the skin. As expected, LDL cholesterol levels fell and HDL cholesterol levels rose. However, there was no significant improvement in the cardiovascular health of the participants who received niacin. What was significant was an increase in adverse effects including a 9% increase in the risk of death. In an accompanying editorial, Donald M. Lloyd-Jones of the Northwestern University School of Medicine wrote that "niacin must be considered to have an unacceptable toxicity profile for the majority of patients...it should not be used routinely."[19] In light of this evidence, any continued use of the vitamin in large quantities, whether by prescription or over the counter, will be a tribute to marketing not medicine.

CHAPTER 6

NUTRITION

6.8 Riboflavin (vitamin B₂)
A vitamin for depression?

Riboflavin takes its name from *flavus,* the Latin word for yellow, and *ribose,* a simple sugar. Although a wide variety of water-soluble yellow dyes was studied by biochemists more than a century ago and, in retrospect, signs of riboflavin deficiency had been seen for many years, it was not until the late 1930's that agreement was reached on riboflavin's status as a vitamin. Several reasons for this long delay can be suggested. Riboflavin deficiency does not produce a dramatic and life-threatening disease such as beriberi or pellagra. Diets that are deficient in riboflavin are likely to lack other essential nutrients as well, so that a mixed deficiency disease is seen. Finally, the chemistry of the vitamin B complex turned out to be far more difficult than could be imagined by those who first described "water-soluble B."

The history of riboflavin is inextricably linked with thiamine, the anti-beriberi vitamin, and niacin, the pellagra-preventative. Indeed, signs now recognized as resulting from riboflavin deficiency were long regarded as a part of the syndrome of pellagra. When riboflavin was isolated in 1933, its role in human nutrition was not clear.[1] Only after niacin was shown to be the pellagra preventative factor could the crucial experiments be undertaken.

When volunteers were fed the Goldberger pellagra diet plus supplements of thiamine, niacin, and vitamin C, full blown pellagra did not appear. Instead, the lips became red and sore and cracks appeared at the angles of the mouth. These signs, formerly associated with pellagra, disappeared completely when riboflavin was added to the diet. Riboflavin was finally ready to join thiamine and niacin in the growing family of B vitamins.

The present view of riboflavin deficiency suggests the following sequence. First there is sore throat and then the lips, mouth, and tongue feel as if on fire. The angles of the mouth become dry and cracked. The skin of the face, especially the nose, is inflamed. Finally, the deprived individual may become anemic.

A particularly interesting and persistent idea is that riboflavin deficiency is related to depressed mood. This notion seems to have arisen in the early 1970's during nutritional studies by the United States Army at Fitzsimons General Hospital in Denver.[2] Six male conscientious objectors were put on a liquid diet for 8 weeks. Riboflavin intake was estimated to be less than 0.1 mg per day or about 5% of the current recommendation. Because of the short duration of the study, no classical signs of deficiency were expected and none were seen. However, a widely used measure of emotional status, the Minnesota Multiphasic Personality Inventory (MMPI), revealed a number of changes consistent with depression. In the many years since that observation was made, numerous investigations have sought a link between riboflavin status and depression particularly in the elderly and in women who have recently given birth.

Might it be that normal people neglect their diet, become riboflavin deficient, and, as a result, become depressed? Or might it be that those who are depressed lose interest in eating and become vitamin deficient? Put another way, are we depressed because we don't eat well or do we not eat well because we are depressed? Presently there are no certain answers to these questions but it is plausible that the brain is susceptible to the effects of deranged nutrition as is any other organ of the body. A dramatic example of course is provided by pellagra. However, no such convincing evidence exists for riboflavin. With respect to the prevention of postnatal depression, a thorough analysis in 2013 of all previous studies found no evidence to recommend supplementation with riboflavin as a preventative measure.[3]

When the Recommended Dietary Allowances were first issued in 1943, the value for riboflavin was 0.7 mg per 1,000 calories or about 1.9 mg. The intervening years have seen that number move up and down over a fairly narrow range. Most recently, distinctions have been made on the basis of age, sex, pregnancy, and lactation but again within a narrow range 0f 1.2-2.0 mg per day with the highest intake for women who are pregnant or nursing.[4] With respect to 100 mg supplements, little harm is likely to be done but it should be noted that the best recommendation is that all of your riboflavin, like virtually all of your vitamins, should come from dietary sources. Pure riboflavin deficiency is quite rare due to its wide distribution in eggs, dairy products, nuts, mushrooms, and green vegetables of all kinds.

NUTRITION

6.9 Pyridoxine (Vitamin B$_6$)
Not just for morning sickness

By 1930 there remained no doubt that "water soluble B" was a complex mixture of several essential nutrients. Thiamine, the anti-beriberi vitamin, was easily distinguished from the rest of the B complex by its rapid inactivation by heat. Teasing out the rest of the B vitamins would prove much more difficult. Workers around the world used a variety of diets to induce deficiencies in mice, rats, dogs, and various other species. They then attempted to cure their animals with factors that had been isolated by diverse chemical techniques. In contrast with the sanitized, straight-line version of science often taught to students, real-life science takes time. More than a decade was spent sorting out just six of the B vitamins. As each factor was isolated in chemically pure form, it could be tested in the animal models.

Rats fed diets in which the only B vitamin is thiamine soon develop skin problems. Among others, Paul Gyorgy of the University of Cambridge used this dermatitis in rats as a model for pellagra. On February 4, 1933, Gyorgy proposed the existence of a "rat pellagra preventative factor" that he designated vitamin B$_6$. It cured rat dermatitis. But animal models are just that, models of human disease. Their validity must be assessed in man. After Goldberger's pellagra-preventative factor was shown to be niacin, the vitamin was found not to cure rat dermatitis. The rat dermatitis model of pellagra was invalid.[1]

Paul Gyorgy is not remembered as the discoverer of a cure for human pellagra. But fame, if not fortune, came to Paul Gyorgy nonetheless. His vitamin B_6 turned out to be a chemical, first synthesized in 1939, called pyridoxine.[2] Soon after, it was found that vitamin B_6 is a collective term for three different chemicals: pyridoxine, pyridoxal, and pyridoxamine. They are present in differing amounts in a variety of foods but the human body converts them all into the same product. The usual form found in vitamin supplements is pyridoxine. As with the other B vitamins, the biochemical functions of vitamin B_6 are quite diverse and complex. Certainly a primary role has to do with the metabolism of amino acids.

The first indication that vitamin B_6 might be essential in human nutrition came, oddly enough, in patients with pellagra. Dr. Tom Spies and his colleagues in 1939 at the University of Cincinnati College of Medicine observed that some disorders in pellagrans didn't respond to niacin, thiamine, or riboflavin but were cured by vitamin B_6.[3] However, there remained no direct evidence of the essentiality of the vitamin. Following World War II, an attempt was made to correct this situation. W. W. Hawkins, a biochemist at the University of Saskatchewan put himself on a diet that contained "all necessary vitamins with the exception of vitamin B_6."[4] After 55 days, Dr. Hawkins had lost nine pounds, an effect he attributed to the "unpalatability" of the diet. Toward the end of the 55 days, he did note "an unusual degree of depression and mental confusion", effects he thought worthy of further investigation.

The next attempt to produce vitamin B_6 deficiency in humans was made by Selma Snyderman and her colleagues at the Department of Pediatrics of the New York University School of Medicine during the winter of 1948-1949. Their subjects were two "mentally defective infants" aged 2 and 8 months. After being on a diet devoid of pyridoxine for 76 days, the younger of the infants suffered convulsions. When pyridoxine was given, the convulsions stopped. Early in the experiment, the older baby showed signs of anemia. Both babies had been tiny at the start of the experiment. After 130 days, neither had gained appreciable weight. The conclusions of Snyderman and her colleagues were that pyridoxine is needed for normal growth, for red blood cell formation, and for the appropriate electrical activity of the brain.

In passing it should be noted that the experiments described in these two infants could not ethically be repeated today. Indeed, even at the time the work was done, the investigators appeared ambivalent. In their initial report in 1950, it was stated that the deficient diet was "given for therapeutic reasons" though these reasons were never spelled out. Three years later in a lengthier publication, it was said that "this study was designed to determine if pyridoxine was indeed required in the human and what the signs and symptoms of such a dietary restriction would be in the growing infant."[5] They felt justified in using the two infants because they were "severely mentally defective." Furthermore, the babies would be receiving "very specialized nursing and medical care." Such arguments would be unlikely to sway a human subjects review committee of today.

In 1951, the American Medical Association reviewed all of the existing evidence on vitamin B_6. They noted the experiments in animals that suggested that the vitamin was essential for mice, rats, dogs, chickens, pigs, and calves. Regarding the need in humans, not much was said. The AMA cited the apparent value of the vitamin in pellagrans who didn't respond fully to the other B vitamins, Hawkin's attempt at self-deprivation, and Snyderman's infants. Their conclusion was that there was indeed a human requirement for pyridoxine. No attempt was made to provide a quantitative estimate of that need.

Without a Recommended Dietary Allowance, mere statement of the belief that vitamin B_6 is essential for humans would have little effect on physicians, nutritionists, or the American public. Few multivitamin tablets of the day even included pyridoxine. More dramatic testimony was needed.

Beginning in the early 1950's, a peculiar convulsive disorder arose among infants in various parts of the United States. Peculiar in the sense that the children seemed not to suffer the ancient disease of epilepsy and no other cause could be found. They were healthy at birth and remained so for several months. The convulsions then began. The babies were treated with the standard anticonvulsant drugs of the day, apparently with good effect.

The solution to the puzzle of the convulsing babies was provided in back-to-back articles in the January 30, 1954 issue of the *Journal of the American Medical Association.*[6, 7] Drs. Clement J. Maloney and A. H. Parmalee of Los Angeles and David B. Coursin, a physician in Lancaster, PA, described 60 babies who had two things in common. All suffered unexplained convulsions and all had been fed a liquid formula called SMA. In 1951, Wyeth Laboratories of Philadelphia, the maker of SMA, instituted more rigorous sterilization of their product. In their desire to kill bacteria, they had unwittingly destroyed virtually all of the natural vitamin B_6 that had been present. The SMA-fed infants thus provided the first convincing demonstration that pyridoxine is a dietary essential for humans.

Despite the clear evidence that vitamin B_6 is required by babies, progress toward a Recommended Dietary Allowance was slow. It was not until 1963 that the Food and Nutrition Board suggested a tentative value of 1.5-2.0 mg per day. A half century later, that value is virtually unchanged with a 2.4 mg recommendation for all adult men and women and a slight increase during pregnancy and lactation.[8] There remains little doubt that overt deficiency of vitamin B_6 is a rare event that is usually associated with general malnutrition. It can be produced in pure form only under extreme conditions such as prevailed in the babies fed exclusively a pyridoxine-free formula. For nearly all of us, our need is easily met by a varied diet. Rich sources include cereal grains, legumes, nuts, carrots, spinach, peas, potatoes, milk, cheese, eggs, fish, and meat. An average banana alone provides about one-third of our daily need for pyridoxine plus other good things as well.

But if adequate vitamin B_6 is so easily obtained in the diet and the RDA of about 2 mg per day readily achieved, why are tablets containing as much as 500 mg sold on line and in every vitamin store? The answer is that pyridoxine has, over the years, been used as a drug to treat a wide variety of ailments with varying levels of success. As a dietary supplement, it is of course not subject to stringent control by the Food and Drug Administration. Speculation is allowed to run free.

On the positive side, it has long been known that isoniazid, an anti-tuberculosis drug, inactivates pyridoxine and that supplementation with the vitamin is a good idea in TB patients receiving that drug. Also, the vitamin B_6 status of infants who experience convulsions is routinely tested and supplements provided when needed. Indeed, a rare, genetically based form of epilepsy is pyridoxine-dependent.[9] Clearly these are situations in which excellent general medical care is required. In contrast, there are a large number of conditions amenable to self-treatment with pyridoxine and many have been tempted to do so. We may recall that when W. W. Hawkins deprived himself of pyridoxine for 55 days, he noted "an unusual degree of depression and mental confusion." Unfortunately, pharmacological doses of pyridoxine have proven ineffective either in relieving depression or improving acuity.[10] Similarly disappointing results have been observed in schizophrenia, diabetic neuropathy, Lou Gehrig's Disease (amyotrophic lateral sclerosis), anxiety, autism, fatigue, and Parkinson's disease. Modest, if not totally convincing, success has been reported for premenstrual syndrome[11] and carpal tunnel syndrome.[12]

Should you be tempted to take massive doses of pyridoxine, you should be aware of a study published in the *New England Journal of Medicine* entitled "Sensory neuropathy from pyridoxine abuse. A new megavitamin syndrome."[13] It appeared on August 25, 1983. Prior to that time it was widely assumed that no dose of pyridoxine was toxic. The senior author was Herbert Schaumburg of Albert Einstein School of Medicine in New York City.

Dr. Schaumburg and his colleagues described seven adults who had been taking 2,000-6,000 mg of pyridoxine per day. All had developed difficulty in walking and had begun to lose feeling in their hands and feet. One, a 26-year-old woman, had been told that the vitamin was a "natural" way to rid herself of excess water during a part of her menstrual cycle. Over the course of a year she had increased her daily dose from 500 to 5,000 mg per day. By the time she sought medical attention, she could walk only with the help of a cane, had trouble handling small objects, and had severe sensory impairments. Stopping the vitamin, she slowly improved but even after seven months she was not completely recovered. There is nothing natural about taking hundreds or thousands of times the RDA of any vitamin. Presently, as a refinement of the RDA's, an upper tolerable limit of 100 mg per day of pyridoxine is specified.[14]

Although this book is dedicated to optimal aging, the use of pyridoxine in pregnant women is worthy of a few lines to illustrate the sometimes complex interactions between medicine, human frailty, and the law. A nearly universal experience during the first trimester of pregnancy is some degree of nausea. For those women in whom vomiting is so severe as to threaten the health of mother and embryo, many remedies have been tried over the years. In 1956, a combination of two drugs plus pyridoxine was introduced under the trade name Bendectin. Later, the formula was simplified to include just pyridoxine and doxylamine, an antihistamine, and, by 1980, a quarter of all pregnant women were taking Bendectin.

William McBride, an Australian gynecologist, was one of the first to suggest, in late 1961, that thalidomide might damage a developing embryo. For this observation he received many awards, both honorary and monetary. In 1962 he was named Australian of the Year. Two decades later, Dr. McBride again gained worldwide attention with a paper describing birth defects caused by Bendectin (In Australia, the trade name was Debendox.)

It is an unfortunate fact that human reproduction is regularly accompanied by birth defects. With millions of women around the world using Bendectin it was inevitable that the use of the drug would coincide with the birth of some fraction of less-than-perfect babies. Following McBride's announcement, lawyers descended on Merrell Dow Pharmaceuticals with claims of causation and demands for damages. Dr. McBride was a frequent expert witness for the claimants.

Under the weight of these suits, Bendectin sales were stopped in 1983. A decade later, Dr. McBride underwent what Robert Milliken called "one of the most spectacular falls from grace the medical world had seen." The Medical Tribunal of New South Wales ruled that he had exhibited "reprehensible conduct" in falsifying data to support his claims about the dangers of Bendectin.[15] Subsequently, his license to practice medicine was suspended for five years. To this day, no epidemiological evidence has appeared suggesting that pyridoxine is teratogenic. In April 2013, the Food and Drug Administration approved the sale of a combination of 10 mg of doxylamine and 10 mg of pyridoxine, the same formulation as was used in Bendectin, for the treatment of morning sickness. The new trade name is Diclegis.[16]

Despite the widespread distribution of vitamin B_6, the content of any one food item is usually small and there probably are significant losses during commercial food preparation. As with all other water-soluble vitamins, prolonged cooking with lots of water can remove much of the pyridoxine content. It would be easy to suggest that all of us take a daily supplement. But I won't. A mixed diet rich in whole grains, fruits, and vegetables that includes modest amounts of meat, fish, and poultry will provide more than adequate amounts of all the B vitamins. Achievement of such a diet is well worth the effort. With the exception of women suffering from morning sickness, to focus upon pyridoxine for supplementation is a foolish distraction.

NUTRITION

6.10 Pantothenic acid
Burning feet and gray hair

The origin of the notion that pantothenic acid can prevent or reverse gray hair was a paper presented at the annual meeting of the American Chemical Society by a pair of Norwegian scientists named Gilbrand Lunde and Hans Kringstad. The year was 1939 and their provocative title was "The anti-gray hair vitamin, a new factor in the vitamin B complex."[1] They proposed the name vitamin B_x. Their subjects were rats. In fact, their vitamin B_x was pantothenic acid, a substance shown six years earlier by Roger Williams, an American biochemist, to be essential for the growth of yeast. The name given the vitamin comes from the Greek *pantothen*, "from all sides", an indication of its widespread distribution in living things.

By the early 1940's, pantothenic acid had an accepted role in animal nutrition but nothing was known of human needs. The curtain then rose on World War II. Though it would not be fully appreciated for several years after the war's end, the period 1941-1945 provided the first clear evidence that pantothenic acid is required by humans, a need shared by lower forms of life.

When Hong Kong fell to the Japanese on Christmas Day 1941, there began a massive study of human malnutrition. The unwilling subjects were troops of the British garrison. They soon would be joined by American, Dutch, Canadian, and Australian soldiers in places like Singapore, Java, and the Philippines—wherever the first wave of Japanese victory washed. Fed a generally inadequate diet based on polished rice, it is not surprising that signs of beriberi, pellagra, and riboflavin deficiency began to appear by the spring of 1942. In addition, a peculiar syndrome called "burning feet" began to be seen throughout the prisoner of war camps of the Far East. Nearly 40% of the Americans at Cabanatuan POW camp on Luzon were known to be affected by December of 1942.

John Simpson, a captured medical officer of the British Royal Air Force, described burning feet in the camps of Java. "Through the day the men were comparatively free of pain. Nights, however, were spent massaging the feet or incessantly walking in the compound. Other men sat with their feet in a bucket of water; they were a pathetic sight during their long nocturnal vigils."[2]

Prisoners transported to the Japanese home islands sought relief on the cold brick floors of their barracks. In the bitter winters of Honshu this contributed to frostbite, gangrene, and eventual amputation. With understatement worthy of a British officer, Dr. Douglas Denny-Brown wrote that "... confinement in prison camps, on extremely limited diets for extended periods of time, has unwittingly provided data on the effect of dietary insufficiencies, on a scale that experimental medicine can hardly hope to emulate."[3]

A few of the captive physicians were aware that burning feet had been reported in various groups of soldiers, laborers, and prisoners as early as 1828 and that a dietary cause had been suggested a hundred years before World War II. In the Japanese prison camps, it soon became evident that the condition was not an aspect of beriberi or pellagra since neither thiamine nor niacin was curative, nor was riboflavin of any use. It remained for Corish Gopalan, a research assistant in the Stanley Hospital of Coonoor, South India, to provide the answer. Working among the very poor and obviously malnourished people of the area, Dr. Gopalan demonstrated that pantothenic acid is a specific cure for burning of the feet caused by a nutritional deficiency. His results appeared in the January, 1946 issue of the *Indian Medical Gazette*.[4]

A diet such as that found in the Japanese prison camps leads to multiple deficiencies and very complex effects. For this reason, scientists much prefer to study subjects in which only one essential nutrient is missing. Beginning in 1951, William Bean and Robert Hodges of the University Hospitals of the State University of Iowa fed convicts from the Anamosa (Iowa) State Reformatory a variety of diets lacking pantothenic acid.[5] They were unable demonstrate an unequivocal deficiency syndrome. Only after the diets were combined with a drug that blocks the actions of pantothenic acid did the prisoners become ill. They tired easily, were irritable, and suffered vague stomach upsets. More significantly, several complained of burning sensations in their feet. (Current ethical standards no longer permit most experimentation on prisoners.)

In the absence of a clearly defined and reproducible deficiency disease, it remains difficult to say just how much pantothenic acid humans really need. In 1942, Roger Williams, its discoverer, concluded that we can get along nicely with 11 mg per day. He based this on the pantothenic acid content of what everyone agreed, in 1942, was a good diet: fruits, vegetables, whole grains, and somewhat more meat and dairy products than are now fashionable. As I write this in 2014, the Food and Nutrition Board of the National Academy of Sciences does not specify a Recommended Dietary Allowance nor has an upper limit been determined. An adequate intake is 5 mg for all adult men and women with a slight increase during pregnancy (6 mg) and lactation (7mg).[6]

A century ago, Thomas Clifford Allbutt, a distinguished British physician, said that "a man of thirty, if he be of liberal education, can read the very newspapers themselves without much harm."[7] Thus reassured, though Sir Thomas could not have foreseen the internet, I will now mention a few of the claims made by present day purveyors of vitamin supplements. We are told that pantothenic acid will add ten years to your life and that it relieves stress, listlessness, and fatigue. Furthermore, the vitamin will relieve hay fever, arthritis, and headaches. But, as the advertisements say, "wait, there's more." Pantothenic acid will cure acne, regulate cholesterol levels, improve athletic performance, strengthen the immune system, promote weight loss, and (you knew this was coming) ease burning feet. What about gray hair? It is unquestionably good for the gray hair of pantothenic acid-deficient rats but will do nothing for the human variety. Anyway, to meet these needs, Puritan Pride offers 500 mg tablets, a mere 5,000 percent of the amount regarded as adequate. Fortunately, such doses are unlikely to do harm. Equally unlikely is the possibility of any benefit being derived.

Even nutritional hypochondriacs (and I include myself in that number) must put pantothenic acid deficiency far down on their list of worries. There is virtually nothing we eat that doesn't contain at least a trace of the vitamin. Whole grain cereals and legumes such as beans and peanuts are especially rich sources but substantial amounts are also found in fruits, vegetables, milk, and meats of all kinds.

NUTRITION

6.11 Biotin
Did Rocky know about avidin?

In the predawn Philadelphia darkness, Sylvester Stallone's Rocky Balboa staggers to his refrigerator. He cracks five eggs into a glass and drinks the mess down. The viewer's gag reflex is activated. Rocky starts off on his morning run secure in the belief that he is fortified with raw animal energy at its best. Rocky has never heard of "egg white injury."

In 1922, Margaret Averil Boas was a research fellow at the Lister Institute in London. Her main interests were the role of calcium and phosphorus in the diet of rats. To minimize those minerals, she fed her rats dried egg white as their sole source of protein. Within three weeks the animals began to lose their hair, their skin became rough and inflamed, and eventually they died. Following up this observation, which others had made before her, Boas conducted a brilliant series of experiments. She found that some foods contain a substance able to protect against injury from egg white; she called it "protective factor X."[1] The material was water-soluble and in many respects resembled McCollum's previously described vitamin B. However, closer examination revealed that her factor X differed from both the anti-beriberi and pellagra-preventative factors.

Following the publication of Boas' work in 1927 many others took up the search for the identity of factor X. Among them was Paul Gyorgy, whom we met earlier during his work with pyridoxine. By 1931, Gyorgy had purified factor X to the point that he was confident that it was in fact a previously unknown vitamin. He proposed to call it vitamin H. (H was simply the next available letter because, two years earlier, the Americans had honored Goldberger by calling his pellagra-preventative factor, vitamin G. Neither letter designation is used to any great extent at present.) Animals could be fed raw eggs without any harm so long as there was sufficient vitamin H in the diet.

Gyorgy, who by this time had moved from England to the Babies and Childrens Hospital of Cleveland, could get no satisfaction until he knew the chemical identity of vitamin H. He was aware of the isolation in Germany in 1936 of a factor essential for the growth of yeast; it had been given the name biotin from *biotos*, the Greek word for life. Gyorgy and his collaborators, Vincent du Vigneaud and Donald Melville of Cornell University College of Medicine, were struck by the similarity of distribution and chemical properties of vitamin H and biotin and by mid-1940 concluded that they were in fact identical.[2] Two years later, du Vigneaud determined the chemical structure of biotin.[3] (Dr. du Vigneaud received the 1955 Nobel Prize in Chemistry for his synthesis of oxytocin, a substance popular today in pop psychology as the "love hormone.")

The missing piece to the puzzle, the nature of the toxic material in eggs, was provided by a group at the University of Texas. Roger Williams, the discoverer of pantothenic acid, together with Robert Eakin and William McKinley, found that chicks fed raw egg white had much less biotin in their tissues despite adequate amounts in the diet. They concluded that there is something in egg white that makes biotin of the diet unavailable for use. Later they showed the material to be a protein for which they suggested the name avidin.[4] As predicted, avidin is inactivated by heating; cooked eggs do not lead to biotin deficiency.

On October 8, 1941 a retired Italian-American laborer was admitted to Boston City Hospital. He was identified only by his initials RM. (I would like to think that his first name was Rocco.) He had a number of things wrong with him but the most obvious was the fiery red color of his face and half the rest of his body. RM was attended to by Robert Williams, a junior physician at the hospital. Dr. Williams would later describe RM in the *New England Journal of Medicine*.[5] I quote from that account: "Since adolescence the patient had been extremely fond of raw eggs, putting one or two into each glass of wine that he took...During the six years preceding admission he had drunk from one to four quarts of wine daily. In order to have a sufficient number of eggs for his drinks, he deserted his family and moved to the country so that he could maintain his own chicken farm. During this period he ate from two to six dozen raw eggs per week...Sometimes he ate nothing but wine and eggs for one or two days..."

Although Dr. Williams provided a vivid account of suspected biotin deficiency in man, credit for the unequivocal demonstration of the syndrome goes to V.P. Sydenstricker. Even before RM was admitted to Boston City Hospital, Dr. Sydenstricker and his colleagues at the University of Georgia School of Medicine had begun experiments in human volunteers.[6]

Three white men and a black woman were put on a diet low in biotin. Other B vitamins, iron, calcium, and vitamins A and C were given as supplements. To reduce biotin still further, avidin in the form of 200 grams (about 7 ounces) of dried egg white were added to the diet. Over the course of 11 weeks, a variety of signs and symptoms appeared. All of the subjects developed dry and flaky skin. More remarkable were the mental changes: mild depression at five weeks was followed by sleepiness, lack of energy, and, in two of the subjects, anxiety. The experiment was terminated when all of the subjects lost interest in eating. Rapid recovery followed the addition of 150 micrograms of biotin to the diet.

For anyone able to take food by mouth, biotin deficiency is not an easy state to attain. Since 1942, there have been fewer than a dozen instances reported in the worldwide medical literature. All have involved the eating of large numbers of raw eggs. Indeed we might be inclined to doubt the reality of a biotin deficiency syndrome were it not for the fact that rash and hair loss has been seen in patients maintained for long periods on intravenous fluids containing no biotin. In addition, there is a rare inborn error of metabolism in which biotin is not absorbed. Babies born with this condition develop a scaly rash and lose their hair when only a few months of age.[7] In the United States, babies are now routinely screened for the presence of this disorder.

It seems a bit odd that biotin deficiency does not develop on even the most bizarre diets as long as they don't include raw eggs. A possible explanation comes from a curious observation made years ago: humans excrete more biotin than they take in. The likely explanation is that some of the trillions of bacteria residing in our digestive tracts are able to synthesize biotin and a portion of it is absorbed by our bodies.[8]

The biotin-deficiency syndrome induced by the eating of raw egg whites is quickly reversed by biotin. But recall that the syndrome may include skin rash, loss of hair, anxiety, depression, fatigue, and insomnia. Millions of us with adequate intake of biotin suffer from one or more of these conditions. Might it be that a biotin supplement would be helpful? For those who would sell us such supplements, the answer would certainly be an unequivocal yes. For example, Puritan's Pride, a purveyor of vitamins, offers tablets containing 7,500 micrograms of biotin. That is 25,000 percent of the adequate intake value of 30 micrograms suggested by the Food and Nutrition Board of the National Academy of Sciences.[9] Fortunately, no direct harm is likely to be done. Biotin appears to be non-toxic and excessive amounts will be excreted in the urine.

I said that no direct harm will result. But what if I have been seduced by a print or on-line claim that biotin is an effective treatment for type 2 diabetes or hair loss or fatigue or acne or any of the other common conditions for which it has been touted as a cure? A recent web site tells us that biotin is "a natural source for helping combat pain and depression." The danger lies not in taking unnatural amounts of biotin but in the potential for ignoring other, truly effective, approaches to these ailments.

NUTRITION

6.12 Vitamin B$_{12}$
Dr. Castle's predigested hamburger

Anemia is a condition in which the blood is unable to carry sufficient oxygen from the air we breathe to the tissues of the body. The three nutritional factors most commonly associated with anemia are vitamin B$_{12}$, folic acid, and iron. We will first consider B$_{12}$.

During the 19th century a number of British physicians described a form of anemia that so often ended in death that it was given the name "pernicious." The most famous person interested in the disease was Thomas Addison of London and we still find reference to Addisonian pernicious anemia.[1] In 1824, the Scotsman J. S. Combe suggested that pernicious anemia is caused by "some disorder of the digestive organs."[2] Combe's idea would give birth to a cure for pernicious anemia; gestation took 100 years.

From the time of its first description there were those who treated pernicious anemia by dietary means. In general, these efforts met with little long-term success and, in the absence of any unifying hypothesis regarding the origin of the disease, there was little incentive to pursue them. Instead, investigators tended to focus on possible defects in bone marrow, the tissue that produces red blood cells, or upon bacterial infection of the gut. Only after scientists became comfortable with the idea of vitamins and the possibility that deficiencies might cause disease was there sustained interest in dietary factors.

The August 14, 1926 issue of *The Journal of the American Medical Association* carried an article entitled "Treatment of Pernicious Anemia by a Special Diet."[3] The authors were George R. Minot, 40-year-old chief of the medical service at Boston's Huntington Memorial Hospital, and William P. Murphy, only 34, a physician in private practice.

Minot's interest in pernicious anemia began in 1912 when, as a resident physician at the Massachusetts General Hospital, he entertained the thought that the disease might be caused by an inadequate diet. Others before him had regarded diet in rather general terms: the patient with pernicious anemia perhaps needed an especially nutritious foods or easily digested ones. The spark of genius that Minot brought to the question was that food might have some "direct effect on blood." He was encouraged in this line of thinking by experiments done in the early 1920s at the University of Rochester by George Hoyte Whipple and Frieda Robsheit-Robbins. They made dogs anemic by periodic bleeding and showed that specific foods, especially liver, were able to stimulate the formation of hemoglobin, the essential iron-containing protein of red blood cells.[4]

Drs. Minot and Murphy begin: "This paper concerns the treatment of 45 cases of pernicious anemia in which the patients were given a special form of diet." The most striking feature of the diet was the inclusion of 4 to as much as 12 ounces of calf, beef, or lamb liver. By today's standards, this would not be considered very healthy. Not healthy? All 45 of Minot and Murphy's patients quickly improved in appearance and function. After a month, their red blood cell counts had more than doubled; in the most profoundly anemic, the increase was nearly fourfold.

We have become accustomed to the calling of press conferences to announce medical "breakthroughs." Today's media-oriented physicians and scientists should blush at the words of Minot and Murphy: "...time may show that the specific diet used, or liver or similar food, is no more advantageous in the treatment of pernicious anemia than an ordinary nutritious diet. Let this be as it may, at the present time it seems to us...that it is wise to urge pernicious anemia patients to take a diet of the sort described."

Their modest words were met with enthusiasm around the world. Though doubts would persist for several decades about the implications of their experiments, most soon accepted as fact that, indeed, a cure for pernicious anemia had been found. In 1934, the Nobel Prize for Physiology or Medicine was awarded to Minot, Murphy, and Whipple, the first Americans to be so honored.[5]

If pernicious anemia is a disease curable by diet, why don't we all need to eat a half pound or so of liver to avoid anemia? William Castle, an assistant resident physician at the Thorndike Memorial Laboratory of the Boston City Hospital, thought he had an answer to that question. Even before the Minot and Murphy diet, Castle was convinced that there was a causal relationship between pernicious anemia and an abnormality in the secretions of the stomach. The way he proved his hypothesis is vividly described in the title of his December 1929 paper: "The effect of the administration to patients with pernicious anemia of the contents of the normal stomach removed after the ingestion of beef muscle."[6] The "beef muscle" was hamburger; Dr. Castle provided "the normal stomach."

The experiment began with Castle eating 10 ounces of lean beef. An hour later he emptied his stomach. The recovered material was incubated to a clear liquid state and then fed by tube to a patient with pernicious anemia. When repeated on a daily basis, this procedure had remarkable effects. The patient looked and felt better and there was an increase in red blood cells and hemoglobin. Neither normal human gastric juice nor beef digested in the absence of human gastric juice had a beneficial effect. Dr. Castle concluded that "some unknown but essential" interaction must occur between beef, extrinsic factor, and gastric juice, the intrinsic factor.

If Castle was correct, all that remained was to learn the chemical identity of the extrinsic and intrinsic factors. It proved more difficult in the doing than in the saying. By 1937 extrinsic factor had been identified in milk and eggs in addition to beef muscle and liver but progress toward purification was slow indeed. The major problem was that no one knows how to test for activity of extrinsic factor except in patients with pernicious anemia. They were in short supply and not always willing to be experimented upon. After all, Minot and Murphy had already provided a cure for their disease. As we have come to expect in science, help came from an unlikely place.

Mary Shorb was professor of poultry husbandry at the University of Maryland when she discovered that the growth of a bacterium called *Lactobacillus lactis Dorn* depended on a factor found in liver.[7] The bacterium could fill in for hard-to-find pernicious anemia patients.

With Dr. Shorb's microbiological assay to guide them, a group of chemists at the Research Laboratories of Merck and Co. made rapid progress toward isolation of extrinsic factor. In the April 16, 1948 issue of the journal *Science*, they described small red needles of a pure chemical to which they gave the name vitamin B_{12}.[8] In the same volume, Randolph West of Columbia University College of Physicians and Surgeons reported three pernicious anemia patients who responded well to the injection of as little as 3 micrograms of vitamin B_{12}.[9] The vitamin behaved in all respects like the anti-pernicious anemia factor of liver. Vitamin B_{12} was the extrinsic factor.

Clinically the problem of pernicious anemia was solved. Vitamin B_{12} could be injected thus avoiding all problems of absorption from the gut. The fascinating physiological question of the nature of the intrinsic factor was answered only slowly but it turned out that Castle's hunch was correct. We now understand the intrinsic factor to be a protein secreted by specific cells in the stomach. Vitamin B_{12} entering the stomach combines with the protein and the complex is carried to the far end of the small intestine where it is absorbed via specific receptors. Victims of pernicious anemia suffer not from a lack of vitamin B_{12} in the diet but from an inability to secrete the intrinsic factor essential for its absorption.[10]

Before leaving these medical classics, something more needs be said about Minot and Murphy. I've already mentioned that doubts persisted for years about just what it was that their Nobel Prize-winning diet had done. First of all, Whipple showed in 1936 that his anemic dogs benefited from liver because of the iron it contains. Pernicious anemia patients lack vitamin B_{12}, not iron. It was humanity's good fortune that the liver diet is also rich in vitamin B_{12}. But liver does not contain intrinsic factor, the B_{12} should not have been absorbed and so, for a second reason, the Minot-Murphy diet should not have worked.

Forty years after the liver diet was introduced, Ragnar Berlin and his colleagues at the Linkoping University Medical School in Sweden solved the puzzle. They found that about 1% of vitamin B_{12} given by mouth is absorbed even in the absence of intrinsic factor.[11] Minot and Murphy had cured pernicious anemia because their diet provided B_{12} far in excess of that needed by normal people but just the right amount for those unable to secrete intrinsic factor.

All of the vitamin B_{12} required by humans is produced by bacteria whose humble abodes are soil, sewage, and the far end of our guts. Though it is true that some members of the animal kingdom eat their own feces (the fancy word for it is coprophagy), there are many good reasons why we humans avoid soil, sewage, and the contents of our large intestines. Instead we allow animals to eat bacteria-laden food, the bacterial B_{12} is incorporated into the tissues of the animal, and we then consume the animal or its renewable parts such as milk or eggs. This is a neat system for all but those who don't want to eat animal parts; more about them in a moment.

Just exactly how much vitamin B_{12} most of us need in our diets has been a matter of controversy for many years. The first attempt to set a value was in1989 when the World Health Organization suggested 2 micrograms per day. Little has changed since then. Presently, the Food and Nutrition Board in the United States lists 2.4 micrograms per day for all adults with the exception of pregnant and nursing women for whom the values are increased to 2.6 and 2.8 micrograms, respectively.[12] For purposes of food labeling, a Daily Value of 6 micrograms is used. Thus, for example, if the side panel of your morning cereal box says that a single serving provides 25% of the DV, that translates to1.5 micrograms.

Surveys of the American diet indicate that the typical meat-eater has an average daily intake of 5-15 micrograms of vitamin B_{12}. For those who regularly eat organ meats such as liver, the value may be as high as 100 micrograms. Although the recommended values for vitamin B_{12} are on a per day basis, daily intake of the vitamin is not required. Substantial amounts are held in reserve and, when intake is reduced, our bodies become quite parsimonious; a greater percentage is absorbed and less is excreted. Even with a total lack of the vitamin in the diet, a person with maximal stores to begin with has enough B_{12} to last 2 to 10 years.

In multiple places in this book, I make it clear that I am generally opposed to the use of dietary supplements of any kind. It is, I believe, far better to devote our energy to insuring that our regularly eaten foods provide all of the essential nutrients. However, for all of us over the age of 50, vitamin B_{12} is an exception. It has long been recognized that, as we age, there is a tendency for our stomachs to become less acidic. For perhaps 20% of us, this change in acidity is sufficient to decrease the efficiency with which we absorb vitamin B_{12}. Recognition of this fact prompted the Food and Nutrition Board to recommend in 1998 that persons over 50 regularly consume foods fortified with the vitamin or take a B_{12} supplement. This suggestion, which was repeated in 2010, took on added importance with the recognition that some drugs commonly used in the elderly represent an added hindrance to our vitamin B_{12} status.

I mentioned that there is a natural decline in stomach acidity with age. For those who suffer from gastroesophageal reflux disease (GERD), this normal process is intentionally augmented by the use of a family of drugs called proton pump inhibitors. Well-known representatives of the family are Previced, Prilosec, and Nexium. While useful in treating GERD, an undesired effect is interference with the absorption of B_{12}.[13] A second offender is metformin, an oral anti-diabetic drug that has been a mainstay in the treatment of type 2 diabetes for many years.[14] The issue of whether a drug-induced deficiency of B_{12} contributes to diabetic neuropathy is unsettled but an authoritative review published in 2013 in the *New England Journal of Medicine* recommends the use of a vitamin B_{12} supplement of 500-1,000 micrograms every day for all those taking metformin or a proton pump inhibitor.[15]

Now a few words about vitamin B_{12} and vegans, those among us who eat no animal products. Let me begin with the story of a 6 ½-pound baby boy born to a 26-year-old woman living in Southern California. He was a happy and healthy infant for the first four months of his life. Then he sickened. He became progressively less active and soon lost the ability to move his head. Feeding at his mother's breast held little interest for him. His weight dropped to 13 pounds. He was irritable but cried little. At 6 months of age he fell into a comatose state, unresponsive even to painful stimuli.

The boy was near death when first seen by Dr. Marilyn Higginbottom and her colleagues at the University of California Medical Center in San Diego.[16] Laboratory tests revealed a profound anemia together with other evidence of deficiency of vitamin B_{12}. A transfusion of red blood cells provided some relief and injections of B_{12} were then begun. Within four days the boy was alert and smiling. He began to gain weight and his reflexes slowly returned to normal.

The cause of the boy's near-fatal encounter with vitamin B_{12} deficiency was not hard to find. Beginning at age 18, his mother had eaten no animal products---no meat, no eggs, no fish, no milk---and she took no vitamin supplements. Despite this she was not anemic and her B_{12} blood level was in the low normal range, testament to the body's ability to conserve the vitamin. Nonetheless, her breast milk, the only source of the vitamin for her baby, simply did not contain enough B_{12} for his needs.

Vegetarianism can be an emotional subject. The avoidance of animal products is for many a matter of religious or moral principle. This does not mean that vegan mothers or their exclusively breast-fed babies need risk vitamin B_{12} deficiency. Animals are but carriers of the vitamin. Bacteria are the actual source. The "synthetic" form of B_{12} found in nearly all vitamin supplements is derived from bacterial ferments. The

Vegetarian Society of the United Kingdom says this: "Vitamin B_{12} is essential to the development and growth of your baby...It is especially important for vegans to include a reliable source of B_{12} in the diet during pregnancy...If you feel that your intake of vitamin B_{12} is inadequate, then a supplement is highly recommended."[17] As to non-animal dietary sources, a seaweed called purple laver or nori in Japan is reputed to be a rich source.

To this point I have acted as if anemia were the only consequence of deficiency of vitamin B_{12}. In fact the brain and spinal cord are directly affected as well. This often results in numbness, tingling, and pain in the hands and feet, together with poor coordination. The condition may progress to the point that unaided walking becomes impossible. More difficult to describe and less constant in their appearance are a variety of behavioral effects including changes in mood, poor memory, confusion, and hallucinations. In the past, these consequences were sometimes interpreted as mental illness. Numberless poor souls have been sent to mental institutions for lack of a proper diagnosis of pernicious anemia.

Before leaving this fascinating vitamin, I want to mention an unusual but interesting source of deficiency. In chapter 11, we will visit the history of nitrous oxide as a pain-relieving and anesthetic agent. It remains today a useful drug widely used in dentistry. But, like so many psychoactive drugs, it has a darker side. To illustrate this, I will use a story I tell regularly to third year dental students at the university at which I work. It involves a dentist who, at age 29, began to self-administer nitrous oxide for its pleasurable and stress-relieving effects. He regularly indulged for an hour a day, seven days a week. Two years after beginning his use of nitrous oxide he noted twitching of his toes, a stiff neck, and a zinging sensation down his spine. After four years, he experienced a loss of balance, weakness and numbness of his legs, and impotence. Ultimately, he was unable to walk unassisted. Nitrous oxide had induced all the neurological signs and symptoms of pernicious anemia. It did so, not by interfering with absorption of B_{12}, but by directly inactivating the vitamin. Recreational users of laughing gas, beware.[18]

CHAPTER 6

NUTRITION

6.13 Folic acid
Lucy Wills in the slums of Bombay

Lucy Wills graduated in 1920 from the London School of Medicine for Women, the first school in England to train those of her sex to be physicians. Dr. Wills gained her place in medical history not in London but in a less elegant part of the Empire, the slums of Bombay. She went out to India, she said, to meet the Viceroy, to see the Himalayas, and to identify what was killing women in pregnancy.[1]

Among the poor pregnant women in Bombay, a severe and often fatal form of anemia was not uncommon. The picture of the disease in the blood and bone marrow of its victims was that of Addisonian pernicious anemia. With the discoveries of Minot and Murphy and Castle, the matter appeared closed. The anemia was cured by the liver extract.

Wills was not satisfied. She wanted to know the exact nature of the missing factor. She fed a diet like that of the poor of Bombay to rhesus monkeys and they became anemic. When crude liver extracts were added to the diet, the monkeys, like their human counterparts, were cured. But then a curious thing occurred. As Dr. Wills and her colleague Dr. Barbara Evans made the extracts purer, they began to lose their anti-anemic properties. More curious yet, the same thing happened in her patients; the purest liver extracts were inactive. Most curious of all, the purest liver extracts could still cure Addisonian pernicious anemia.[2]

Dr. Wills' conclusions now have the appearance of inevitability but at the time they were bold indeed.

(1) Bombay's anemia of pregnancy is different from that which medicine called pernicious anemia.

(2) Crude liver extracts contain something else than the extrinsic factor of Castle. Others would call this something else by the name "Wills factor."

In the last chapter we saw how the key to the chemical identification of vitamin B_{12} was Mary Shorb's discovery that *Lactobacillus lactis Dorn* depended upon it for growth. In a similar fashion another bacterium would lead us to the identity of Wills factor.

While Lucy Wills worked in India, scientists in the West were learning more and more of the nutritional needs of other life forms. Bacteriologists laid claim to the discovery of such odd entities as vitamins B_{10} and B_{11}, norite eluate factor, *Lactobacillus casei* factor, and factor SLR. From studies in animals came vitamins M and B_c, and factors 1, U, R, and S. All of these, together with Wills factor would eventually be shown to be one form or another of a chemical isolated in 1941 by Herschel Mitchell and his colleagues at the University of Texas. Beginning with four tons of spinach and *Streptococcus lactis* as their guide, they obtained a substance they named folic acid, from the Latin word for leaf, *folium*.[3] After its chemical structure was determined, a more proper, if less euphonious name was given: pteroylglutamic acid. "Folacin" properly refers to all of the various active forms of folic acid of which there are more than 100.

The strikingly similar changes in the blood that occur when we are deficient in either folic acid or vitamin B_{12} suggest a common cause. Today most accept the explanation called the folate trap hypothesis. When too little B_{12} is present, folic acid is trapped in an inactive form and folate deficiency arises. The anemia seen when we are B_{12} deficient is thus identical to that when too little folic acid is present in the diet.

By 1945, the anti-anemia properties of folic acid were well established. Some went so far as to suggest that folic acid was a safe and effective substitute for liver extract in pernicious anemia. This was a serious error. The problem is illustrated by a patient, identified only by the initials "OK", treated by Drs. Robert Heinle and Arnold Welch in

Cleveland in 1946.[4] A conclusive diagnosis of pernicious anemia had been made and, in keeping with the latest in therapeutic advances, he was treated with 10 mg per day of folic acid.

New treatments have always had an attraction for both physician and patient. This is especially true today when every minuscule advance is heralded in a press conference as a "breakthrough." Cynics say that one should always rush to use a new therapy because someone soon will show that it doesn't work. Anyway, OK was put on folic acid and within a week all signs of his disease were improved. He had more red blood cells and he both looked and felt better. But Mother Nature was playing a not very funny joke on OK and his doctors. Three months after starting the folic acid treatment, numbness began to spread from OK's elbow downward. He could neither tie his tie nor button his shirt. When his legs began to lose their feeling, it was obvious to even the most optimistic that a change in therapy was needed. They went back to old fashioned liver extracts and improvement began almost at once.

It is now recognized that large amounts of folic acid can correct the anemia caused by vitamin B_{12} deficiency while neurological damage goes on. We shall see in a moment how this fact complicates the question of what constitutes an appropriate folic acid supplement.

Despite the fact that folic acid is widely available in our foods, there are a few situations in which deficiency is likely to occur. The first was illustrated in 1961 by Victor Herbert, then a physician at Boston City Hospital. At that time no one knew what a pure deficiency of folic acid looked like; in a natural setting it is nearly always confounded by multiple deficiencies. Dr. Herbert put himself on a diet in which all foods had been boiled three times. By discarding the water after each boiling, most of the water-soluble vitamins were lost. He then added back all but folic acid.[5]

Although he had an estimated intake of only 5 micrograms per day and a steady decline in the level of folate in his blood nothing very dramatic happened to Dr. Herbert for three months. He then started to have trouble sleeping. He became forgetful and progressively more irritable.

Finally, after nearly four and one-half months, the expected anemia appeared. By then taking pure folic acid as a supplement, Herbert concluded that his need for the vitamin was about 50 micrograms per day.

Cultures in which foods are habitually boiled or heated for long periods are in fact replicating the experiment of Dr. Herbert. But even among people who destroy most of their folic acid in cooking, a second factor is usually present before overt deficiency appears. That factor is a greater than normal need for the vitamin.

Pregnancy is far and away the most common situation in which humans experience an increased need for folic acid. Magalie, a 24-year-old woman seen by Drs. Mortimer Greenburg and Shirley Driscoll at the Lemuel Shattuck Hospital in Boston illustrates the point.[6] She had never liked fruits and vegetables and, living in a free country, she ate none, apparently without ill effects. Then came pregnancy. Several months after conception, Magalie became severely anemic. Laboratory tests revealed a deficiency of folic acid.

One of the essential functions of folic acid is to participate in the synthesis of new genetic material.For this reason, rapidly dividing cells are most in need of it. A baby growing in its mother's womb is a lovely example of a mass of rapidly dividing cells. As a result, lack of enough folic acid is the most common form of malnutrition among pregnant women, especially among poor pregnant women. Magalie's marginal diet was good enough for her alone but her baby's need pushed both of them into severe anemia. Worse, even when anemia is not present, folic acid deficiency is associated with miscarriage, excessive bleeding, fetal malformations, and generally poorer health of both mother and child. (Other classes of rapidly dividing cells are seen in cancer. It occurred to Sidney Farber in the mid-1940's that if cancer cells could be starved of folate they would die. From that idea was developed aminopterin, an anti-folate drug he used in treating childhood leukemia.[7] Dr. Farber is regarded as the father of cancer chemotherapy. The center he founded in Boston carries his name, the Dana-Farber Cancer Institute, as does Farber Hall, the building in which I have worked for a half century.)

Given the history of folic acid we have just considered, it is mildly surprising that a recommended intake was not suggested until 1968. The value given then was 400 micrograms with modest adjustments upward during pregnancy and while nursing. In the years that followed, a major point of contention was how to balance the obvious benefits of the vitamin with its risks. The observation that large amounts of folate could mask the neurological effects of vitamin B_{12} deficiency made a deep impression upon leading American physicians. In the 1960's, the Food and Drug Administration ruled that multivitamins containing more than 100 micrograms of folic acid could be obtained only by prescription. As a result, most makers of multivitamins removed folic acid entirely from their products. Magalie, our pregnant lady in Boston, had taken a multivitamin popular at the time. Unfortunately, it contained no folic acid.

Every mother-to-be prays that her baby will be perfect in every way. A cruel fact of life is that not all prayers are answered. For example, about 3,000 babies are born each year in the United States with what are called neural tube defects. The cells in the developing embryo that are destined to become the brain and spinal cord begin as a flat sheet which then folds to form the neural tube 28 days after conception. When the closing of the tube is incomplete, portions of the brain and spinal cord are exposed at birth. Consequences evident at birth may include blindness, paralysis, and death.

The suggestion that folate deficiency might be a factor leading to neural tube defects was first made in 1975 and, a few years later, studies were undertaken to test the hypothesis. Initial interventions were done in women who had already given birth to an infant with a neural tube defect in the hope that risk in subsequent pregnancies could be reduced by a folic acid supplement. Reporting in 1980, R. W. Smithells and his colleagues in Ireland and England found that supplementation with folate before and during pregnancy reduced the incidence by more than 85%.[8] A dozen years later, the same protective effect was demonstrated in women who had not previously given birth to a child with a neural tube defect. It was time for a change in attitude toward folic acid supplements.

In response to the data linking folic acid deficiency with neural tube defects, two things happened. First, the Food and Drug Administration eliminated the need for a physician's prescription for folic acid in excess of 100 micrograms. Second, in 1996, fortification of foods with folate was begun. Prior to fortification of grains, it was estimated that 26% of the population had inadequate folate intake. This fell to less than 1% after fortification. Check your box of Cheerios and you will find that 1 cup now provides 50% of the Daily Value for folate.

Combine fortification with abundant natural sources such as green vegetables, beans, peas, orange juice, and berries and the RDA of 400 micrograms per day is easily met.[9] Nonetheless, any woman for whom pregnancy is even a remote possibility is advised to take a modest folic acid supplement, something on the order of 200-400 micrograms. Recall that neural tube defects may arise prior to a woman being aware that she is pregnant. In addition to the well-established link between folate and neural tube defects, studies conducted in the early years of the 21st century are highly suggestive of an association between maternal folate deficiency and an increased risk of autism and developmental delays.[10]

NUTRITION

6.14 Vitamin C
Scurvy, Dr. Pauling, cancer, and colds

There are two quite distinct stories that must be told regarding vitamin C. The first is concerned with a deficiency disease, scurvy, its practical eradication, and the identification of the responsible vitamin. The principal characters are a British sea captain, two Norwegian scientists, and a group of guinea pigs. The second vitamin C story has Linus Pauling, twice winner of the Nobel Prize, in the leading role.

Scurvy is a disease in which small pools of blood appear beneath the skin, the mouth and eyes and skin become dry, the hair falls out, the gums bleed, and there is eventual loss of teeth. An individual with scurvy is weak and lethargic, everything aches, and there are periods of anxiety and depression. Death may come slowly from infection or suddenly when a weakened blood vessel bursts in the brain.

It is thought that scurvy was present in ancient Egypt, in Rome, and in Greece, during the Crusades, and in many other times and places. But it was with the great voyages of exploration that scurvy presented itself in full detail. Vasco da Gama, the first European to reach India by sea, returned to Portugal with only one-third of his original crew; most of the rest had succumbed to scurvy. There was hardly an expedition lasting more than a few months that was not affected.

Over the years, many remedies for scurvy were suggested. In the early 1500's Jacques Cartier was advised by the Indians of Canada to use a brew made from spruce needles or sassafras or arbor vitae. Admittedly, many of the proposals for treating scurvy, particularly those that involved prolonged heating or fermentation, were almost certainly without value. Nonetheless, it is evident that by the seventeenth century many men of the sea knew how to cure scurvy. In 1600, Captain James Lancaster of the East India Company suggested lemon juice and, in books intended for use by ship's surgeons, the value of fresh fruits and vegetables for treating scurvy was acknowledged. In 1617, John Woodall referred to the juice of the lemon as a precious medicine. Sir Richard Hawkins, in his account published in 1622 of voyages in the Pacific, spoke of "the plague of the sea" and recommended "sower oranges and lemmons."

Given this state of knowledge, why then did sailors continue to suffer and die from scurvy in all navies of the world? Admiral George Anson of England's Royal Navy set out around the world in 1740 with six ships and a combined crew of 1,955. Four years later he returned with his flagship and 900 men. Scurvy had gotten most of the rest. The answer to our question is that the minds of naval officers and landlubbers alike were unprepared for the idea that intimate details of the diet could be of consequence in health and disease. We must remind ourselves that the word vitamin did not enter our language until the early years of the 20th century.

In the year 1780, the Royal Naval Hospital at Portsmouth cared for 1,457 sailors suffering from scurvy; in 1806 there were but 2. A single change in the diets of all men of the Royal Navy was responsible for this remarkable decline. Beginning in 1795, all men at sea for longer than six weeks were to receive one ounce of lemon juice per day. The story of how this change took place illustrates two things. First, it is a lovely example of well-designed scientific research and, second, it illustrates the importance of advocacy.

On the 20th of May, 1747, HMS *Salisbury* was at sea with twelve of her crew sick with scurvy. The ship's surgeon was a 31-year-old Scotsman named James Lind. On that day, Dr. Lind began what Duncan Thomas called "the first deliberately planned therapeutic trial ever undertaken." He assigned two of the sick men to each of six treatments. These were

(1) sea water, (2) vinegar, (3) cider, (4) nutmeg, (5) citrus fruits, and (6) an elixir containing sulfuric acid.

By the end of six days, none but the two receiving the fruit had improved. One of the latter was returned to duty and the other assigned as a nurse to the remaining ten. Unfortunately, Lind's demonstration of the efficacy of citrus fruit was to be of little value to men of the sea for many years. He did not publish his findings until six years later.[1] More important, the Royal Navy officially ignored his cure for scurvy for nearly a half century.

As valuable as was the work of Dr. Lind, credit for the virtual eradication of scurvy from the British Navy must go to James Cook, a man Allan Villiers called "that extraordinary sea genius." Whereas Lind was an obscure surgeon who left the naval service shortly after his tour on *Salisbury*, Cook was an officer of the line who had commanded vessels in voyages around the world and was the first European to reach Australia and the Hawaiian Islands. More important, he managed to bring back nearly all those under his command. It is doubtful that Captain Cook thought in terms of any single factor, what we now call a vitamin, keeping his men safe from scurvy but he surely believed that some aspect of the diet or of general hygiene was of importance.[2] He fed fruits and vegetables to all members of his crew. At every opportunity he obtained fresh water and food. He insisted on the highest standards of personal and shipboard cleanliness.

Whatever it was that Cook was doing, it worked; scurvy was eliminated on all ships that followed his customs. In 1786 he was elected a fellow of the Royal Society and awarded the Copley medal for his conquest of scurvy.

But, then as now, bureaucracies often had a glacial quality. Not until nine years later did Sir Gilbert Blane, First Lord of the Admiralty, order the use of lemon juice in all ships of the Royal Navy. Another forty years would elapse before passage of the Merchant Seaman's Act which required lemon juice in the rations of merchant sailors. Isabella Leitch called it the first formal action to institute a dietary recommendation as public policy. British seaman, as well as Englishmen at large, became known as limeys because of a misidentification of the Navy's lemon juice as that of the lime. Unfortunately, limes provide only about one-third as much of the anti-scorbutic factor. The unhappy consequence was that scurvy broke out on several British ships in 1845 after an enterprising governor of Bermuda talked an admiral into substituting Bermudian limes for lemons.

Despite British success in preventing scurvy, nutritional deficiencies continued to diminish the effectiveness of the navies of the world. In the early 1900's, Axel Holst and Theodore Frolich began their studies of a deficiency disease in the Norwegian fishing fleet called "ship- beriberi."[3] It was their great good fortune to eventually choose the guinea pig for study. When they fed polished rice to their animals with the expectation of inducing beriberi, they observed instead a disease "identical in all essentials with human scurvy."

Following the observation that guinea pigs, like humans, are susceptible to scurvy, very rapid progress was made in characterizing the anti-scorbutic factor. In some foods, the factor was destroyed by heating. This provided an explanation for what had been a puzzling observation. Infantile scurvy occurred more often in babies fed according to the highest nutritional standards of the day: foods well-cooked and milk carefully sterilized.

The existence of an anti-scorbutic factor was not immediately accepted by all. Part of the delay arose from the failure to recognize that humans, monkeys, guinea pigs, and a few birds are unique in their dependence on an external source of the factor; rats simply won't do as a model for man. Nonetheless, by 1919, a prominent British authority felt justified in listing three "accessory food factors": fat-soluble A, water-soluble B, and water-soluble C. The case for the existence of vitamin C was essentially closed that same year when an extract assayed for efficacy in the guinea pig was found to cure scurvy in children. The finishing touches were added between 1928 and 1932 when it was shown that a reducing agent isolated from adrenal glands and cabbage was identical with lemon anti-scorbutic factor. When its chemical structure was established, the factor was given the name ascorbic acid, a term now used interchangeably with vitamin C.[4]

What is the human requirement for vitamin C? The first systematic attempt to establish that value was conducted in England toward the end of World War II under the direction of Hans Krebs, a Jew forced from Germany with the rise of Hitler. Nineteen men and one woman lived on a diet that provided less than 1 mg of vitamin C per day. After 17 weeks, signs of scurvy began to appear and became progressively worse. The minimum supplement needed to abolish all signs of scurvy was 10 mg per day and subjects remained healthy at that dose for an additional 14 months. Lesser amounts did not cure the scurvy; larger amounts appeared to add nothing. To be safe, the Krebs group suggested that a daily intake of 30 mg would be appropriate.

In the United States, there has been continuing controversy. Set at a value of 75 mg in 1943, it moved downward to 45 mg in 1974. Today, more detailed suggestions are made such that the recommended intake for adult males is 90 mg, for adult females 75 mg with an increase to 85 mg and 120 mg during pregnancy and lactation, respectively.[5] For food labeling purposes, the Daily Value is set at 60 mg.

Many years ago, John Crandon, a young surgeon at Boston City Hospital with an interest in scurvy, put himself on a diet of cheese, crackers, bread, eggs, beer, and chocolate plus vitamin supplements with the exception of vitamin C.[6] After four months, signs of scurvy appeared. I tell you this because, if your diet is like Dr. Crandon's, you may wish to consider a supplement. Otherwise, it is a simple matter to obtain more than enough vitamin C from a diet rich in fruits and vegetables.

Just 4 ounces of orange juice provide 60 mg. Despite the fact that many of us are remarkably unwise in our choice of foods, signs of scurvy are rarely seen in the United States except in alcoholics and grossly malnourished infants and old people. These facts have not deterred those who would sell us vitamin C in supplement form and one easily finds tablets providing 1,000 mg of the vitamin. Fortunately, even at that level, harm is unlikely to be done because any excess will be excreted in the urine. Whether any good will result is less certain. Most claims for benefit are based not on the use of supplements but are derived from studies of populations in which consumption of fruits and vegetables is high. With few exceptions, I much recommend the latter course.

And now we arrive at the second story of vitamin C: Linus Pauling, Irwin Stone, the common cold, and cancer. About 1935, reports began to appear concerning vitamin C and immune function. It was used to treat infections such as pneumonia, whooping cough, and rheumatic fever. However, a review of the subject that appeared in the *Journal of the American Medical Association* in 1938 could find no value for vitamin C in these diseases.[7]

In 1966 Irwin Stone was an obscure 59-year-old chemist from Staten Island, New York. (He is not to be confused with Irving Stone, author of biographies of van Gogh, Darwin, Michelangelo, and others.) Stone proposed that we all suffer from "hypoascorbemia", a fancy way of saying too little vitamin C in our blood. In Stone's words, hypoascorbemia is "a very important factor in the incidence and mortality of diseases, of the aging process, and in the extent of the human life span." In a book published in 1972 called *The Healing Factor*, Stone suggested that vitamin C might be useful in treating colds, polio, hepatitis, herpes, bacterial infections, cancer, heart disease, vascular disorders, arthritis, rheumatism, aging, allergies, glaucoma, cataracts, ulcers, kidney and bladder disease, diabetes and hypoglycemia, the effects of poisons, toxins, smoking, stress, wounds, bone fractures, shock, difficulties of pregnancy, and mental disorders.[8] Later he proposed treating narcotic addicts with vitamin C and, in 1983, suggested it as a cure for AIDS.

The world does not pay much attention to the likes of Irwin Stone. His ideas might have gained currency in the netherworld of pop nutrition but little more. Linus Pauling, on the other hand, is a man to be reckoned with. Twice winner of the Nobel Prize, for chemistry in 1954 and for Peace in 1962, Pauling was both a distinguished scientist and a world-shaking activist. In a book published in 1970 called *Vitamin C and the Common Cold,* Pauling advocated the use of several grams (several thousand milligrams) per day in order to attain "the best health."[9] The public response was overwhelming and, for a time, drug and vitamin stores had only bare shelves where the vitamin C supplements previously rested. There was obvious appeal to an idea endorsed by a Nobel laureate that a harmless natural substance obtained without a physician's prescription could banish the common cold. But, as is said in so many television advertisements, "Wait, there's more." As a bonus, Professor Pauling suggested that the vitamin might also be good for back problems and heart disease and would produce a general sense of well-being.

The medical establishment was not enthusiastic about *Vitamin C and the Common Cold.* The opinion of reviewers ranged from "near quackery" to "a brilliant but speculative venture." Nearly all reviews by medical scientists raised the question of why a scientist of Pauling's stature had gone to the public with ideas that had no convincing support but would, nonetheless, be accepted uncritically by millions of people. Critics would suggest that the answer lay in Pauling's ego and the attention the book would gain him. My personal opinion is that Pauling wished to force the establishment to test adequately his hypothesis that vitamin C prevents or cures colds. If that was his goal, he succeeded. Over a period of three years beginning in January 1972, a series of large-scale clinical trials was conducted by Terence Anderson and his colleagues at the University of Toronto.[10] Several thousand persons were enrolled and doses as high as 5,000 milligrams per day were given. When all the data were gathered and analyzed, the authors, in an admirably conservative assessment, concluded that colds had not been prevented but that a small beneficial effect in terms of severity of illness had been demonstrated.

Earlier, I mentioned a review that could find no value for vitamin C in treating a number of different infectious diseases including the common cold; that was 1938. Seventy-five years later (2013), a review of all available evidence by the much respected Cochrane Group in England was kinder. While saying that there is no evidence that vitamin C supplementation reduces the incidence of colds, "it may be useful for people

exposed to brief periods of severe physical exercise."[11] The latter statement was based on studies in marathon runners, skiers, and soldiers on
subarctic exercises. Kinder still, after acknowledging conflicting evidence
regarding the effect of vitamin C on the duration and severity of colds,
the review group concluded that, considering the low cost and safety of
the vitamin, "it may be worthwhile for common cold patients to test on
an individual basis whether therapeutic vitamin C is beneficial for them."
Not all agree but there you are. We are about as close to the truth as we
are likely ever to get.

The common cold is not a trivial matter but it pales in comparison
with cancer. Thus, the idea that vitamin C cures cancer is worth comment because of the fearful nature of the disease and the all too common
futility of its treatment. In 1971, Ewan Cameron, a physician at the Vale
of Leven Hospital in Loch Lomanside, Scotland, began to treat cancer
patients with vitamin C. He reasoned that the vitamin would strengthen
"the intercellular ground substance" of normal tissue and thus permit it
"to resist infiltration of malignant tumors."[12] Daily doses ranged from
10,000 to 50,000 milligrams per day. Some benefit was claimed for all
forms of cancer. Not surprisingly, Cameron's claims came to the attention of Linus Pauling.

F. Hoffmann-LaRoche, Ltd. is a venerable Swiss pharmaceutical
house with a global presence. Among other holdings, it is the owner of
Roche USA and of Genentech, a major force in medical biotechnology.
As the first industrial producer of vitamin C, the company has an interest in promoting its use. For a time, this took the form of a small newspaper called *The Good Drugs Do*. It was, in the words of the company,
"specifically prepared for the waiting rooms of American physicians to
provide patients with accurate information about drugs, vitamins, and
foods their physicians may prescribe." An issue which appeared in June
1975 was devoted entirely to vitamin C. In it, Linus Pauling stated that
"when a Scottish physician gave 10,000 milligrams per day to terminal
cancer patients, they felt better and lived longer. In a controlled study of
100 cancer patients by the same physician, long term survival increased

fifty fold." Pauling was of course referring to Ewan Cameron. Over the next few years, Pauling and Cameron joined forces to publish three articles in the prestigious *Proceedings of the National Academy of Sciences of the United States of America*. According to the authors "There is little doubt...that treatment with ascorbate is of real value in extending the life of patients with advanced cancer...addition of ascorbate to treatment regimens at an earlier stage might well have a much greater effect, increasing the average survival time by several years." [13, 14, 15]

The initiation of government-funded medical research in the United States is often as much a matter of politics as it is of scientific judgment. Under ordinary circumstances Cameron's work in Scotland would have been ignored by the American medical establishment in general and the National Cancer Institute in particular. His studies were too poorly designed and carried out to be taken seriously. However, Pauling's well-publicized advocacy led to intense political pressure on the National Institutes of Health to conduct an adequate trial. As a result, a contract was entered into by the NIH with the Division of Medical Oncology of the Mayo Clinic in Rochester, MN.

The results of the Mayo Clinic trial were published in the September 29, 1979 issue of the *New England Journal of Medicine*.[16] The title chosen by Drs. Edward T. Creagan, Charles G. Moertel and their colleagues tells the story: "Failure of High-Dose Vitamin C to Benefit Patients with Advanced Cancer." Some 150 patients were randomly assigned to either placebo or 10,000 milligrams of vitamin C per day. In what is called a double-blind trial, neither the patients nor their doctors were aware of who received what. When the code was broken, no differences in adverse events, improvement of symptoms, or survival were found.

How can we explain the difference between the results of Cameron on the one hand and the Mayo investigators on the other? One interesting possibility is suggested by the outcome of a group of 27 patients at the Mayo who initially elected to enter the study but later changed their minds and received neither placebo nor vitamin C. As a whole, this group survived for only half as long as those who took part. The explanation of this is uncertain. The point is that if this group has been compared with those who had received vitamin C, the vitamin would have appeared to double survival time when in fact it did nothing at all.

Linus Pauling's explanation for the failure of the Mayo investigators to confirm Cameron's findings was that the patient population was different. In a letter to Drs. Creagan and Moertel, Dr. Pauling stated that of the 100 patients treated in Scotland, only four had received prior drug treatment and only 20 had received radiation. Pauling expressed his belief that prior drug treatment "may have negated the benefits of vitamin C" for the Mayo Clinic patients. Creagan and Moertel, as good scientists, could only reply that, based on Pauling's statement, their study groups were indeed different.

Dr. Pauling, his faith in vitamin C intact, did just what he had done with the common cold: he went public. In 1979, the Linus Pauling Institute of Science and Medicine published a book by Cameron and Pauling called *Cancer and Vitamin C*; two years later it was republished as a paperback.[17] The authors once again expressed their belief that high-dose vitamin C has value "for essentially every cancer patient." I believe it fair to say that scientific and medical authorities in this country and elsewhere were united in their skepticism about vitamin C as a cancer treatment. But the general public is notoriously suspicious of "the medical establishment." Furthermore, only a tiny fraction of those who read the book by Cameron and Pauling were aware of the details of the Mayo Clinic study; the *New England Journal of Medicine* is not to be found at the supermarket checkout. Pressure on elected officials and upon physicians responsible for the treatment of cancer patients was intense. Once again, the National Cancer Institute turned to the Mayo Clinic.

Results of the second attempt by the physicians at the Mayo Clinic to verify the claims of Cameron and Pauling were presented on January 17, 1985 in the *New England Journal of Medicine*.[18] One hundred patients with advanced colorectal cancer received either 10,000 milligrams per day of vitamin C or placebo; once again, a double-blind experimental design was used. In accordance with Dr. Pauling's criticism of the earlier investigation, none of the 100 patients had received any prior treatment with anticancer drugs. The results were unequivocal: "No patient had measureable tumor shrinkage, the malignant disease in patients taking vitamin C progressed just as rapidly as in those taking placebo, and patients lived just as long on sugar pills as on high-dose vitamin C."

One might think that the two stakes driven into the heart of the Cameron/Pauling hypothesis by the Mayo Clinic studies would have settled the matter of vitamin C as a treatment for cancer. They did not. There are two reasons for this. First of all, in the absence of curative treatments for numerous forms of cancer, many will seek unproven alternative approaches. They will be encouraged in their search by the continued presence of books encouraging such treatments. These include not only the original *Cancer and Vitamin C* by Cameron and Pauling, both of whom are now dead, but also by the regular appearance of the same arguments restated by others.

The second reason we will continue to see the issue of vitamin C and cancer in the media is the relatively recent observation that the intravenous administration of the vitamin can achieve much higher blood levels than is possible with even the enormous oral doses advocated by Pauling.[19] Indeed, Cameron in 1991 published "A protocol for the use of vitamin C in the treatment of cancer" in which he suggested that all cancer patients be treated initially by the intravenous route. Unfortunately, as of this writing there is no evidence that the intravenous administration of vitamin C has any beneficial effect on cancer.

NUTRITION

6.15 Vitamin D
Hormone or vitamin?

Steven Spielberg, *Jaws*, and numerous aquaria have made most Americans aware of the sinuous grace of a shark moving through the water. Much of that ease of movement comes from the shark's lack of bones. Their skeletons are made of cartilage, a soft and flexible material, a material so admirably suited to life in the oceans that sharks have changed little in millions of years.

A cartilaginous skeleton would never do for us. Humans live in air, not water; we feel the force of gravity much more keenly than does the shark. Dense, strong, rigid bones are needed to support the weight of our bodies. Although our bones begin as cartilage or soft membranes, calcium and other minerals are soon laid down to form our skeletons. So long as we have adequate calcium in the diet and are exposed to modest amounts of sunlight, the formation of bone will proceed in a perfectly normal fashion. The need for calcium seems obvious; the role of sunlight we soon shall consider.

The disease state that results when bones are improperly calcified has various names. In children it is called rickets, in adults, osteomalacia. The consequences of rickets in growing children are dramatic. The spine and leg bones bend under the body's weight. In its most severe form, breathing and movement are impaired.

Although rickets was described by Hippocrates, mankind's struggle with the disease really began less than 400 years ago and then only in a very limited area of the world. The first detailed description appeared in the mid-seventeenth century. On the Continent, it was called the "English Disease" because of its prevalence in that country. By 1850, rickets had become a major source of disability and early death among the children of the great cities of Western Europe and Great Britain. Those who survived it were marked for life by bowed legs and misshapen teeth. Poverty was an inconstant factor. The children of factory workers and the unemployed were often afflicted yet rickets never occurred in even the poorest of farm children. It was indeed a disease of the city.

Armand Trousseau was in 1860 Physician-in-Chief of the Hotel Dieu, Paris' best and most famous hospital. Although he was known around the world for his descriptions and analyses of many diseases, he had a particular interest in rickets. His ideas about the disease were based partly in an observation made 30 years earlier by his countryman, Jules Guerin, that puppies raised in darkness soon became rachitic. The other influence on his thinking was what most physicians of his day regarded as an old wives' tale. Dutch lore had it that rickets could be cured with cod liver oil. Putting these pieces together, Trousseau hypothesized that the disease was caused by an inadequate diet coupled with a lack of sunshine.[1]

A new scientific truth does not triumph by convincing its opponents and making them see the light but rather because a new generation grows up familiar with it. (Max Planck said that.) Trousseau's idea that rickets might be influenced by diet was simply unacceptable to the medical establishment of his time. His notion that sunlight might also be a factor was even more ludicrous. Never mind that in 1890, Theobald Palm, a British medical missionary, clearly demonstrated a world-wide correlation between lack of sunlight and rickets.[2] Never mind that Sir John Bland-Sutton in 1889 had cured rachitic lion cubs at the London Zoological Gardens by feeding them cod liver oil.[3] Diet and sunlight would have their day but it would come in the 20th century.

At the time that Edward Mellanby delivered a series of lectures at the Royal College of Surgeons of England in 1918 there were a number of hypotheses as to the cause of rickets. The domestication theory was that the disease resulted from the conditions associated with civilized life hence its prevalence in large cities. Another proposed the causes to be confinement in too small houses and imperfect parental care. In Glasgow, a city noted for a very high incidence of rickets, Leonard Findlay and Margaret Ferguson suggested the importance of fresh air and exercise.[4] Mellanby favored the dietetic hypothesis. By the time of his lectures, he had conducted experiments in more than 200 puppies. Fed a diet of bread and skim milk, they rapidly became rachitic. Supplementation with cod liver oil or other animal fats reversed the disease. Surprisingly, rickets was not prevented by providing more calcium in the diet. Mellanby's conclusion: "…the cause of rickets is a diminished intake of an anti-rachitic factor which is either fat-soluble A or has a similar distribution to fat-soluble A."[5]

But what of Jules Guerin's rachitic puppies raised in darkness? In the autumn of 1919, Harriette Chick, a 44-year-old British scientist, led a group from the Lister Institute of Preventive Medicine to the Children's Clinic at the University of Vienna. Dr. Chick was familiar with the most recent advances in nutrition and with the concept of accessory food factors or vitamins. In addition, she was aware of a recent publication by Kurt Huldschinsky, a Berlin pediatrician, entitled "The Treatment of Rickets by Ultraviolet Irradiation."[6] Over a period of three years, Dr. Chick's group found that rickets was cured equally well by cod liver oil, ultraviolet irradiation, and natural sunlight. Their results swept away the controversies of the preceding 80 years. On the one hand, the crucial difference between British farm children and city children was seen not to be diet but sunlight. On the other hand, the children of Greenland and other places as sunless as any city slum were protected by something in their diet's fish oils. The dietary hypothesis and the environmental hypothesis were each correct and were each incomplete.

If children in naturally sunless parts of the world are protected against rickets by a vitamin in fish oils and if the children exposed to sunlight have no need for these oils, might it be that sunlight causes children to manufacture that same antirachitic substance? In her 99th year, Dame Harriette Chick would recall that this was "an entirely new concept at the time."[7] But what a concept: the dual nature of the antirachitic substance was clearly seen. For humans exposed to adequate sunlight, it is a hormone produced in the skin and distributed about the body; no dietary source is needed. In a sunless environment, the antirachitic substance must come from food; it is then a vitamin.

While the British work went on in Vienna, investigators in the United States were not idle. Elmer McCollum of the School of Medicine and Public Hygiene of Johns Hopkins University had developed a rat model of human rickets. With it he and his associates confirmed the efficacy of ultraviolet light. Equally important, they were able to distinguish between vitamin A and the antirachitic substance. In 1922, McCollum, Nina Simmonds, and Ernestine Becker wrote that "the power of certain fats to initiate the healing of rickets depends on the presence in them of a substance that is distinct from fat-soluble A. These experiments clearly demonstrate the existence of a fourth vitamin whose specific property… is to regulate the metabolism of bones." For this fourth essential nutrient they proposed the name vitamin D.[8]

More than ninety years have passed since vitamin D got its name and its dual nature as vitamin and hormone was evident. Since then, much has been learned but, in the first decades of the 21st century, it is clear that much remains to be discovered. We now know that vitamin D undergoes two conversions in the body to reach its active form. The first occurs in the liver to what I will refer to as 25-OHD (calcidiol), the second in the kidney to $1,25(OH_2)D$ (calcitriol). It is 25-OHD that provides the best indication of your vitamin D status. In addition to facilitating the absorption of calcium from our foods, vitamin D is now recognized to influence the expression of several thousand genes with implications for multiple diseases. However, at this time, the only unassailable statement one can make is that vitamin D is required for the absorption of calcium; too little of the vitamin and the result will be rickets or osteomalacia.

What then are we to make of the claims that vitamin D plays a role in obesity, autism, schizophrenia, testosterone levels, athletic performance, falls and fractures, asthma, depression, cognitive impairment, cancer, rheumatoid arthritis, multiple sclerosis, diabetes, heart disease, autoimmune disorders, inflammation, and a variety of infectious diseases including influenza? A partial answer to that question comes in the recognition that there is a difference between correlation and causation. Many studies have identified a correlation between lower blood levels of 25-OHD and the presence of the conditions I have mentioned. But, if lower levels of vitamin D are causing a disease, we would expect supplementation to be beneficial. Regrettably, hundreds of studies have failed to demonstrate causation. Indeed, with the exception of rickets and osteomalacia, vitamin D has not been proven to prevent or effectively treat any of the diseases listed above. One intriguing hypothesis is that a decrease in blood 25-OHD is a natural reaction to disease rather than a cause; much as fever is a response to infection, not its cause.

Given the biological complexity of the actions of vitamin D and the often conflicting results of clinical trials, we turn to authoritative bodies for guidance. In 2010, the Institute of Medicine, the health arm of the National Academy of Sciences, recommended a daily intake of 600 International Units of vitamin D for adults up to age 70 with an increase to 800 IU after that.[9] These values assumed minimal exposure to the sun. A year earlier, the International Osteoporosis Foundation, a non-profit group based in Switzerland and representing more than twenty nations, had recommended that older adults have an intake of 800-1,000 IU.[10] Vitamin D enthusiasts in the medical and nutritional communities were not happy with the IOM recommendations. The Endocrine Society, a respected group devoted to research on hormones and the clinical practice of endocrinology, had issued a guideline calling for supplementation with 1,000 to 2,000 IU.[11] With respect to possible toxicity, the IOM set an upper limit of 4,000 IU but others said it should be 10,000 IU per day. It is obvious that, as regards optimal intake of vitamin D, consensus is hard to find. The situation is no more settled when it comes to recommending an optimal level of 25-OHD in our blood.

If you and your physician have decided to test your 25-OHD, what do you do with the results? The only point on which all agree is that a value less than 12 nanograms per milliliter (ng/ml) represents vitamin D deficiency and a high risk for osteomalacia or, in children, rickets. Supplementation is clearly in order. But what is an optimal level? The Institute of Medicine regards 20 ng/ml to be adequate[9] while the Endocrine Society Guidelines specify 30 ng/ml.[10] Robert P. Heaney, Professor of Medicine at Creighton University School of Medicine, has been for decades an advocate of increased intake of both vitamin D and calcium. Dr. Heaney suggests a range of 30-50 ng/ml.[12] Where lies the truth? We don't know.

Should everybody have their blood 25-OHD tested? The title of an article which appeared in 2012 in *The Lancet* by Naveed Sattar, Professor of Metabolic Medicine at the University of Glasgow, and his colleagues nicely expresses their answer: "Increasing requests for vitamin D measurement: Costly, confusing, and without credibility."[13] The authors cite the many uncertainties surrounding vitamin D and ask whether patient well-being is improved by such measurements. In Glasgow, requests for testing doubled in just two years based, Dr. Sattar believes, on media headlines casting vitamin D in the role of a miracle cure. In chapter 6.2 we met JoAnn E. Manson in connection with the ongoing trial she is leading to evaluate the effects of fish oil and vitamin D on the risk of heart disease or cancer. Writing in the *Journal of the American Medical Association* in 2014, Dr. Manson expressed her view that widespread screening of vitamin D levels represents "an unjustifiable health care cost of billions of dollars annually...more is not necessarily better..." Enthusiasts were not deterred; the aforementioned Dr. Heaney continues to recommend an annual test of 25-OHD.

Let us imagine that I have had my 25-OHD level tested and that it comes out to be 20 ng/ml. This is adequate by IOM standards but marginal by the Endocrine Society guidelines and grossly inadequate in Dr. Heaney's view. Is anything lost by my beginning to take a vitamin D supplement of, let's say, 2,000 IU a day? After all, vitamin D appears to be a very forgiving chemical; toxicity, including calcification of blood vessels, has been assumed to occur only at blood levels in excess of 200 ng/ml or in infants and children who carry a rare genetic defect. I would offer just one of several cautionary tales that might be told.

In 2012, nearly 40,000 Americans died of pancreatic cancer thus making it the fourth leading cause of cancer death. Usually not diagnosed until it is in an advanced state, three-quarters of patients die within one year and only five percent are alive after five years. What does this have to do with vitamin D? The answer starts in Finland with a study aimed at determining whether men aged 50 to 69 years who smoked and who received supplements of vitamin E or *beta*-carotene would alter their risk of lung cancer. As a part of that study, blood 25-OHD levels were measured. After 16 years, contrary to what was expected, men with pre-diagnostic levels of 25-OHD greater than 26 ng/ml had a three times greater risk of developing pancreatic cancer than did those with lower levels.[14]

At this point it is reasonable to ask whether results in smoking Finnish men are applicable to nonsmokers, women, or those of us living in another part of the world. A troubling answer was provided by a subsequent analysis of data from men and women of varying ethnicity in multiple geographic regions. After taking into account race, ethnicity, sex, smoking history, obesity, and diabetes, those with a 25-OHD level greater than 40 ng/ml doubled their risk of pancreatic cancer compared with those at 20-30 ng/ml. Dr. Rachael Stolzenberg-Solomon of the Nutritional Epidemiology Branch of the National Cancer Institute was a leading figure in both of the studies I have mentioned. In an admirably restrained statement, she said that "recommendations to increase vitamin D concentrations in healthy persons...seem premature."[15] In the meantime, it would be wise to wait for the results to appear in 2017 of Dr. Manson's VITAL trial which will assess the effects of vitamin D supplements on a variety of diseases including cancer.[16]

I hope that I have planted a seed of doubt in your mind as to the wisdom of extravagant use of vitamin D supplements. In doing so, it was not my intent to obscure the fact that there are those of us clearly in need of supplementation. A prime candidate would a house-bound elderly vegan.

Throughout the history of *Homo sapiens,* exposure of the skin to sunlight has generated more than adequate amounts of the vitamin. The house-bound are denied that source and the vitamin must come from the diet. Unfortunately, very few foods in their natural state contain significant amounts of vitamin D. The major exception of course is the fish oils which so nicely sustain those living in the Arctic and in other relatively sunless environments. A diet which contains no fish or eggs or fortified milk cannot substitute for exposure to sunlight. Finally, there are drugs commonly used in the elderly, especially anti-inflammatory agents, which interfere with the functions of vitamin D. Thus, much as I abhor supplements in general, an additional 400 IU of vitamin D, the amount found in a typical multivitamin, is a good idea for the elderly with an increase to 800 IU if fish and fortified foods such as milk and cereal are not regular parts of the diet.

NUTRITION

6.16 Vitamin E
A vitamin in search of a disease

Just after World War I when Herbert Evans began his research at the University of California at Berkeley, it was recognized that normal growth of adult rats required appropriate amounts of all four of the vitamins then known: A, B, C, and D. Evans wondered whether nutrient needs might be different during reproduction and, in the early 1920's, he and Katherine Bishop found that rats fed a rancid lard diet failed to maintain normal pregnancies. They also observed that lettuce was "spectacularly successful" in correcting whatever the deficiency might be.[1] The unknown dietary factor, designated X, was surely not the same as vitamin C because only the fatty component of the lettuce was effective.

The subsequent finding that wheat was as beneficial as lettuce led Evans to a flour mill in the town of Vallejo. In his own words:

I found there three great streams flowing from the milling of the wheat berry, the first constituted the outer cover or chaff, the second the endosperm, the white so-called flour, and the third, which came in flattened flakes stuck into such units by its oil content, the germ. Night had not fallen that day before all these components were fed to carefully prepared females...Single daily drops of the golden wheat germ oil were remedial. That an oil might enrich the embryo's dietary needs for vitamins A and D, the fat-soluble vitamins then known, was negated at once when we added the well-known source of vitamins A and D, cod liver oil, an addition that did not lessen but increased and made invariable our malady.[2]

When it thus became clear that crude materials such as wheat germ oil contain a substance essential for reproduction in the rat, factor X was assigned the next letter of the alphabet and re-designated vitamin E. Some years later the substance was purified by Oliver and Gladys Emerson together with Evans and given the name tocopherol from the Greek words *tocos*, childbirth, and *pherein*, to carry.[3]

Advertisements for vitamin E imply that we are all on the verge of deficiency if not already deficient. Like so many claims of the supplement industry, there is no evidence to support them. More than 60 years ago, Max K. Horwitt and his colleagues at the Elgin (Illinois) State Hospital tried for over six years to induce signs of deficiency in 19 of their patients.[4] (For ethical reasons, studies such as these would not be permitted today.) Dr. Horwitt was completely unsuccessful. Why then do we consider it a human vitamin at all? The fact is that the evidence for its essentiality has come entirely from persons who are unable to absorb it from the diet. For example, in cystic fibrosis, levels of the vitamin tend to be very low and there is a shortening of the life of red blood cells. In addition, there is some evidence that malabsorption of vitamin E is associated with deterioration of the nervous system very much like that seen in animals. However, these effects occur only in the presence of well-established diseases of the digestive system or in persons who have had large sections of the small intestine removed surgically. Vitamin E deficiency has never been detected in an otherwise normal human.

The first Recommended Dietary Allowance for vitamin E was set in 1968 at 25-30 International Units. Soon after, it was realized that a well-balanced American diet would provide far less than this and, by definition, nearly everyone in the country would be "deficient." Good news for the sellers of vitamins but obvious nonsense. Thus, in 1974, the value was reduced to 12-15 IU per day. In the most recent recommendation, the value is increased to 22.4 IU for all adults with the exception of nursing mothers for whom 28.4 IU are suggested.[5] (One sometimes sees the requirement expressed as "tocopherol equivalents" where 22.4 IU equals 15 TE expressed in milligrams.)

I mentioned earlier the unsuccessful attempts by Max Horwitt to induce vitamin E deficiency in patients at Elgin State Hospital. It is ironic that, Dr. Horwitt, who devoted much of his long career to studies of vitamin E, was a vocal critique of the RDA's for vitamin E set in the years 1968, 1974, 1989, and 2000 by the Food and Nutrition Board. Indeed, in 1961, on the occasion of his receiving the Osborne and Mendel Award of the American Society of Nutrition, he advised that no specific requirement for vitamin E be adopted. Dr. Horwitt's last scientific publication appeared in 2001, one year after his death at age 92. In it he expressed his opinion that setting the RDA at 22.4 IU "benefits only the commercial interests involved in the sale of vitamin E."[6]

Inasmuch as no normal human being has ever been found to be deficient in vitamin E, there seems little reason to specify foods rich in the substance. But, in the interests of further promoting diets of the Mediterranean and DASH variety to be discussed in chapters 7 and 8, I will mention that prime sources include vegetable oils, green leafy vegetables, almonds, peanuts, peanut butter, and whole grains. For those who simply can't resist a supplement, a typical multivitamin will provide 50 IU, more than twice the RDA.

Turning from vitamin E as an essential nutrient to the use of the vitamin as a drug to prevent or to treat disease, we enter an area of great and continuing controversy. A professor of medicine at the Mayo Clinic said that the list of conditions treated with vitamin E is limited only by one's imagination. Max Horwitt called it "a vitamin in search of a disease."[7] In various animal species, deficiency of vitamin E produces a bewildering array of pathologies, many of which resemble human diseases. Over the years, this has led to flurries of interest in the use of the vitamin in a variety of human conditions. As popularity has waned in one area, it has waxed in others.

When Evans in 1926 observed that male rats deprived of vitamin E suffered degeneration of the testicles and sterility, he gave birth to the myth that vitamin E is an anti-sterility, anti-impotence agent. Nearly ninety years after Evans' findings in rats, the myth abides. In 2014, one online advertisement read "Vitamin E is the sex hormone, sure to add spice to your sex life." Alas, there is no evidence that the vitamin influences impotence or sterility or libido in man.

A few years after the discovery of vitamin E, H.J. Metzger and W.A. Hogan of Cornell University reported "a queer degenerative process of voluntary muscle" in lambs. Because the condition was corrected by the addition of vitamin E to the diet, it was called "nutritional muscular dystrophy." One can imagine the hope engendered in persons afflicted with one of the several forms of muscular dystrophy. Alas, several subsequent studies in patients found the vitamin to be of no benefit.

The use of vitamin E in diseases of the heart and circulation has had great staying power. Shortly after World War II, *Time* magazine called vitamin E "a startling medical discovery (as) a treatment of heart disease." Within a decade, a dozen or more carefully conducted investigations refuted that claim. More recently, an international study conducted over a period of 12 years and reported in 2005 found that supplementation with 400 IU of vitamin E *increased* the risk of heart failure in persons with preexisting heart disease or diabetes.[8] That same year, combined analysis of 11 trials concluded that a daily supplement of 400 IU or more *increases* the risk of death.[9] Never mind, vitamin E continues to be promoted for heart disease and one-quarter of Americans over the age of 55 take a vitamin E supplement of 400 IU or more. The disparity between what the peddlers of vitamin E tell us and what medical science has found over the past 50 years is striking. Perhaps "striking" is the wrong word; "obscene" might be better since people's lives are at stake. An example: in 2014, a website called DoctorYourself tells us that "evidence supporting vitamin E's efficacy in preventing and reversing heart disease is overwhelming…extra vitamin E could save thousands of lives a month."

Just as in the preceding chapter on vitamin D in which high blood levels were associated with an increased risk of pancreatic cancer, a similar cautionary tale must be told for vitamin E. This time it is prostate cancer that concerns us. This disease kills about 30,000 American men each year. By the turn of the 21st century, a number of epidemiological studies had noted a connection between the consumption of diets high in vitamin E and a decreased risk of prostate cancer. Would supplements do the same? To help settle the issue, the Selenium and Vitamin E Cancer Prevention Trial (SELECT) was begun in 2001 headed by Eric Klein of the Cleveland Clinic. Nearly 35,000 men were divided into four groups to receive a selenium supplement, 400 IU of vitamin E, selenium plus vitamin E, or placebo. All men were 50 years of age or older and none had evidence of prostate cancer.

The study was meant to continue for eight years but was halted one year early because no benefit was apparent and there was a suggestion of harm. In 2011, it was reported that healthy men receiving the vitamin E supplement have a 17% *greater* risk of prostate cancer.[10] An extension of the study published in 2014 confirmed that finding and extended the warning to include selenium, a trace mineral with anti-oxidant properties.[11] Marc B. Garnick is a professor of medicine at Harvard Medical School who specializes in prostate cancer. In 2014 he said this about vitamin E: "I counsel all of my patients to absolutely avoid any dietary supplements that contain selenium or vitamin E, including multivitamins...supplements can cause real and tangible harm."[12]

NUTRITION

6.17 Vitamin K
A matter of balance

Although this book is primarily about aging and vitamin K is of definite interest to the elderly, I will begin with a story about a baby girl born in North Carolina a few years ago.[1] At 27 days of age, Mae began to bleed profusely from her umbilical stump. Attempts at her local hospital to stop the bleeding were unsuccessful and she was transferred to the neonatal intensive care unit of a regional medical center. A CT scan revealed a brain hemorrhage. Fortunately, three days after receiving a blood transfusion and the intra-muscular injection of vitamin K, Mae was able to go home, apparently fully recovered.

For more than half a century, the American Academy of Pediatrics has recommended that all newborns receive vitamin K to prevent what is now called vitamin K deficiency bleeding.[2] The condition was first described in 1894 but, prior to the discovery of vitamin K, no cause or treatment was known.[3] Despite the advice of the Pediatrics Academy, Mae's parents had refused vitamin K prophylaxis due to an unfounded fear that the vitamin is associated with an increased risk of leukemia, a now discredited suggestion made in the early 1990's in England.[4] Like so many other harmful myths, that fear is kept alive in large measure by numerous Web sites. In 2013, four infants born in Nashville suffered brain hemorrhages due VKDB. Only one recovered fully. In all four cases, vitamin K administration had been refused by the babies' parents. Similar refusal was found to occur in more than one-quarter of the births at a Nashville birthing center. Reasons given were fear of cancer, a desire to avoid "toxins", and the thought that vitamin K is simply unnecessary. In refusing vitamin K, parents expose their infants to an eightyfold increase in the risk of VKDB.[5]

The discovery of vitamin K follows a pattern we have seen earlier in which there is an observation of deficiency symptoms in man or animal, the reversal of these symptoms by certain foods, and the identification of a new vitamin responsible for that reversal. Also, as we have seen before, a novel discovery often is made when an inquisitive mind is applied to a quite unrelated question.

Beginning in the late 1920's, Henrik Dam, a biochemist at the University of Copenhagen, was studying cholesterol metabolism in young chickens. The suggestion had been made earlier that chicks, unlike humans, cannot synthesize this essential chemical. Professor Dam did not confirm that hypothesis but noted that chicks eating a diet devoid of cholesterol soon exhibited, in his words, "an unexpected symptom." The animals began to bleed under the skin, in their muscles, and in other organs. When tested, their blood showed delayed coagulation.[6] Similar hemorrhages are seen in scurvy but addition of vitamin C to the chicks' diets had no effect. Likewise, Canadian investigators failed to reverse the condition with vitamins A and D. By 1934, Dam was confident that the bleeding was due to the absence of "a hitherto unrecognized factor in the diet."[7] A year later, although the substance had not yet been isolated in pure form, it was given the name vitamin K. Again I quote Professor Dam: "The letter K was the first in the alphabet which had not...been used to designate other vitamins and it also happened to be the first letter in the word "koagulation" according to the Danish or German spelling."[8]

Pure vitamin K was first isolated from alfalfa by Edward Doisy, an American biochemist, and it was he and his colleagues who distinguished between two forms of the vitamin, K1 and K2.[9] Vitamin K1 is synthesized by plants where it plays an essential role in the process of photosynthesis. After eating these plants, our bodies convert K1 to K2, the form in which small amounts are stored. Utilizable vitamin K is also produced by bacteria residing in the gastrointestinal tract of man and animals. It is the absence of such bacteria in the gut of the newborn, coupled with low levels of the vitamin in breast milk, which explains babies' vitamin K deficiency bleeding. Fortunately, soon after birth we all develop a thriving microbiome based on the bacteria entering our bodies from our food and from the environment. (For their discoveries, Professors Doisy and Dam shared the Nobel Prize for Physiology or Medicine in 1943.)

It is obvious that an effective means of coagulation of the blood is essential for our survival. Without it, we would bleed to death following the most minor of injuries. But equally obvious is that a balance must be struck. Excessive formation of blood clots leads to heart attack and stroke. For those who already have suffered the consequences of such a clot or at high risk of developing clots, a means to decrease coagulation is needed. Today, millions are treated with just such a means. It is a drug called warfarin which is best known by its trade name Coumadin.

In the early years of the 20th century, sweet clover was introduced into the Dakotas and Canada as feed for cattle. Soon thereafter, it was observed that some cattle bled to death following minor cuts or a routine de-horning procedure. In 1922, Francis Schofield, a professor of bacteriology and pathology at Ontario Veterinary College, traced such events to a chemical produced by a fungus found in moldy clover.[10] The chemical was identified in 1939 as dicoumarol. Following World War II, a synthetic relative of dicoumarol was developed, given the name warfarin (from Wisconsin Alumni Research Foundation, holder of the patent), and sold as rat poison. By blocking the regeneration of vitamin K, warfarin produces vitamin K deficiency followed by uncontrolled bleeding and death in rats. Not a likely candidate for human use one might think.

We have talked elsewhere about the need to balance the benefits and the risks of any drug. Might a careful selection of the dose of warfarin avoid excessive bleeding yet produce a desired decrease in the formation of clots contributing to heart attack and stroke? In 1954, the Food and Drug Administration concluded that it might do just that and approved warfarin for human use under the trade name Coumadin. The next year, use of the drug increased dramatically after President Dwight Eisenhower was treated with warfarin following a heart attack.

In 2010, the Food and Drug Administration approved the use of warfarin to prevent strokes in those who experience atrial fibrillation a condition in which disorganized activity in the heart can lead to the formation of blood clots. This is of particular concern in those over age 75 when some 15% of the population is at risk and such clots account for one-third of all strokes. Similar risks are present for those of any age with high blood pressure or other factors contributing to vascular disease. In 2014, more than 30 million prescriptions for warfarin were written. Unfortunately, it is not an easy drug to use and it requires regular evaluation of the clotting status of the blood. On the other hand, with 60 years of experience with warfarin, many physicians are skilled in its use. In those instances when excessive warfarin has been used, vitamin K provides a ready antidote to correct the condition. As I said before, it is a delicate balance.

Those with vitamin K for sale, tell us that "everyone is deficient" and suggest you buy it for bone health, heart disease, varicose veins, leukemia, prostate, lung, and liver cancer, dementia, tooth decay, and infections including pneumonia. I would point out that all of these purported benefits are based on correlational studies in which it is found that those of us who eat a diet rich in green vegetables are less likely to suffer from these conditions. Unfortunately, over a period of more than three decades, interventional studies in which supplements of vitamin K have been given have failed to show benefit. Perhaps the most promising is a possible effect on bone, an action suggested by the discovery of receptors for vitamin K in that tissue. However, writing in 2014, Krupa Shaw and his colleagues at the Division of Geriatrics of the Washington University School of Medicine conclude that "...current evidence...is not strongly supportive of vitamin K supplementation in older adults for the intent of improving bone health."[11]

Vitamin K deficiency in all those who have a normal digestive tract, i.e., are able to absorb fat soluble vitamins, is very rare. Nonetheless, over the past 25 years, it has been suggested that our dietary intake of vitamin K should be somewhere between 60 and 120 micrograms per day.[12] Using 100 micrograms as a reasonable value, it is apparent that all who eat green vegetables readily obtain that much. For example, a half cup of kale provides five times that amount. For those with a taste for natto, fermented soybeans as found in traditional Japanese cooking, 3.5 ounces contain about 1,000 micrograms of vitamin K. Having said that, is there any risk that we will overdose with vitamin K and stimulate blood clots in all the wrong places. For the vast majority of us the answer is no. Nature does a wonderful job of regulating the amount held by our bodies.

Having said that food-derived vitamin K presents no risk for most of us, we should be aware that there is one group that must be particularly careful about avoiding excessive vitamin K in the diet. These are those millions I have mentioned who have been prescribed warfarin either because they are at high risk for developing a clot or have already experienced a heart attack, thrombotic stroke, or pulmonary embolism. The Mayo Clinic advises them to avoid large amounts of kale, spinach, brussels sprouts, broccoli, parsley, collard greens, mustard greens, chard, and green tea. It goes without saying that natto and vitamin K supplements should not be on their menu.

Earlier I mentioned the use of warfarin to diminish the risk of blood clots as a consequence of atrial fibrillation. For all those Americans with a functioning television set, atrial fibrillation has become about as familiar as erectile dysfunction (see chapter 9 for more on the latter condition). "Ask your doctor about A-Fib" is what the advertisements tell us. These are sales pitches for one of a new class of drugs which act to reduce clot formation in a way which differs from that of warfarin. Most heavily touted in my area is rivaroxaban (Xarelto) but you may also see ads for dabigatran (Pradaxa) and apixaban (Eliquis). They do have the virtue that they come with no vitamin K dietary restrictions and regular monitoring of the coagulability of the blood is not required. It remains to be seen if, in the long run, these drugs are superior to warfarin and, it should be noted that, in contrast with warfarin, there presently is no antidote available.[13] (In 2014, Boehringer Ingelheim, the maker of Pradaxa, paid $650 million to settle law suits alleging that patients and doctors had not adequately been told of the risk of bleeding and the absence of an antidote.[14] Personal injury lawyers have noted these risks and have begun to run advertisements seeking possible clients.) One other thing: the new drugs cost about fifteen times as much as warfarin.

NUTRITION

6.18 Calcium
A fallen star

We will begin this chapter by recalling a few things we learned about rickets in chapter 6.15. Given the fact that bones are made of calcium and the fact that rachitic children have too little bone, it required no great imagination to put these facts together to reach the conclusion that the disease would be cured by adding calcium to the diet. And it required no great effort to prove that conclusion wrong. The children of the smoky sunless cities of Europe were devastated by rickets not because there was too little calcium in the diet but, in the absence of sunlight-generated vitamin D, too little calcium was being absorbed from the food passing through their digestive systems. If adequate vitamin D is present, diets miserable by any standard provide enough calcium to avoid rickets. Conversely, no amount of dietary calcium is adequate if the body, because of the absence of vitamin D, is unable to absorb it.

In 1920 W. C. Sherman of Columbia University proposed that the human need for calcium is about 450 mg per day.[1] When the first edition of the Recommended Dietary Allowances appeared in 1943, 800 mg were called for with an increase to 1,200 mg during adolescence, the period of major skeletal growth. Some seventy years later little has changed: 1,100 mg per day during adolescence, 1,200 mg for women over the age of 50 and men over the age of 70, 1,000-1,300 mg for all others.[2] The relative stability of these values is deceptive; it masks a controversy over our need for calcium that has raged for nearly a century and shows no signs of ending.

On one side of the argument are those we might call the minimalists. Prominent among them were D. Mark Hegsted of the Harvard School of Public Health and Alexander R. P. Walker of the South African Institute for Medical Research in Johannesburg. In the late 1940's, Professor Hegsted was concerned about the low level of calcium in the diets of many of the people of South America. In most countries, dairy products and, to a lesser extent, green leafy vegetables, are the primary sources of calcium. For many in tropical and subtropical countries, especially the poor, these sources may be virtually absent from the diet.

Hegsted's subjects were ten male inmates of the Central Penitentiary of Lima, Peru. They had been in prison for two to twenty years and seemed well-adjusted to the food provided them.[3] Because of an almost total lack of foods rich in calcium, their intake of the mineral was estimated to be 100-200 mg, only a fraction of that now deemed necessary. In his experiments, Dr. Hegsted varied the amount of calcium in the diet and carefully measured the amount the men excreted. These data indicated an average requirement of 126 mg per day. Hegsted's conclusion was simple: "The minimum calcium requirement for adult males is so low that deficiency is unlikely on most normal diets." In his last scientific publication in 2002 at age 88, Dr. Hegsted asked this question: Why do populations who consume low-calcium diets have fewer fractures than do Western societies who consume high-calcium diets?[4] Today we have no certain answer to that question but some possibilities will be discussed in chapter 15.

Like Professor Hegsted, Alexander Walker began his studies of calcium in the 1940's. Earlier he had gained prominence as an advocate of increased fiber in the diet. The people of greatest interest to him were the natives of South and Central Africa, especially the South African Bantu. In comparison with Europeans living in South Africa, the Bantu intake of calcium was quite low. Walker estimated the range to be 175-475 mg per day. Despite these differences, rickets and osteomalacia were as uncommon in blacks as in whites. With respect to osteoporosis, elderly Bantu women suffer spontaneous fractures at a rate only one-tenth that of the Caucasians of South Africa. Dr. Walker's conclusion: "...there is no firm evidence that calcium deficiency exists in humans...it is questionable whether calcium merits a place in the tables of recommended allowances of nutrients."[5]

Now let's turn from the minimalists to the calcium maximalists; today their influence is far more in evidence both in government circles and in the popular media. Because it is so intuitively attractive to hypothesize that osteoporosis is the consequence of too little calcium in the diet, the idea suffered little from the work of people such as Hegsted and Walker. And, despite the suggestion in 1948 that estrogen was an important factor in osteoporosis, there was by the mid-1960's a move to increase calcium intake by all Americans but especially post-menopausal women, the population for whom osteoporosis is of greatest concern. Thus we moved in stages from the recommendation in 1962 by the World Health Association of 400-600 mg to today's 1,200 mg for men over the age of 70 and women of 50 years and older. I believe it futile to argue against the latter recommendation and will instead focus on two issues. The first is a consideration of how one might reach 1,200 mg of calcium from diet alone. The second addresses the use of calcium supplements.

Milk and milk products are a very convenient source of calcium. If you are not concerned about fat or calories in your diet, any milk product will do as far as calcium is concerned. But most of us do have such concerns so label reading is important. The 1,200 mg of calcium in a quart of fat-free milk carries with it only 360 calories. A quart of whole milk has no more calcium but more than twice the number of calories. Furthermore, the difference in caloric content is almost entirely in the form of saturated fat. My practice is to save whole milk for when strawberries are in season but make it a habit to drink at least a pint of skim milk every day including that which goes on my cereal in the morning. Though processed cheese, the kind that comes in single slices wrapped in plastic, is much derided for its fat and cholesterol content, a single slice provides nearly one-quarter of the daily need for calcium at a cost of just 70 calories.

Many Americans, particularly those of African descent, are intolerant of lactose, the sugar found in milk. For them, yogurt may provide a palatable alternative source of calcium. But a question comes immediately to mind: Why are those intolerant of milk able to eat yogurt, a milk product? It turns out that the bacteria essential for the production of yogurt, unlike many harmful bacteria, are able to survive the acidic conditions of the stomach. Upon reaching the friendlier environment of the small intestine, the bacteria are then able to digest the lactose of yogurt. Because some yogurts are heat-treated after fermentation, you should check for a brand carrying the Live & Active Cultures seal established by the National Yogurt Association.

Low fat and even no-fat yogurts are available if calories are of concern but, we must read the labels to know what we are getting. One other thing about yogurt: unlike milk, yogurt is usually not supplemented with vitamin D. As I suggested in chapter 6.15, a modest vitamin D supplement is not a bad idea for those of us who don't drink fortified milk, are habitually denied sunlight because of confinement indoors or by regular wearing of full body clothing for religious reasons or who live in a relatively sunless part of the country; pretty much anywhere above Northern Virginia is suspect. But do recall that extensive exposure to the sun for purposes of generating vitamin D is not a good idea.

With all this talk of dairy products as rich sources of calcium, we might think that deficiency is rampant among vegans, those who eat nothing at all derived from animals. In fact, adequate amounts of calcium can be provided by vegetables alone. The reason is that calcium is found in nearly all plants; cows, you may recall, don't drink milk. A study done some years ago in Sweden found that a group of vegans had an intake of calcium only 10% lower than that of persons eating a traditional Swedish diet.

Although all vegetables provide some calcium, only a few can be thought of as calcium-rich. These are dandelion, turnip, and mustard greens, kale, collard, rhubarb, beans, soy products, and several others. One should not conclude from what I have just said that any vegan diet will provide adequate calcium. When all dairy products are excluded, one must examine the diet carefully to insure adequate calcium intake especially for infants, children, adolescents, and pregnant or lactating women.[6]

Other than dairy products and the vegetables I've mentioned, not many foods can be regarded as reliable sources of calcium. Oysters and bony fish such as sardines and salmon are high in calcium but, because of cost or taste or availability, few of us eat them with regularity. Aside from skim milk, my favorite source of calcium is the almond. A cup of almonds provides about as much calcium as a cup of milk. The downside is that the cost of almonds per ounce is many times that of skim milk and provide about ten times the number of calories. Nonetheless, because of all the good things nuts in general and almonds in particular do for us, I have a dozen or so almonds with breakfast every morning and another dozen with my green salad in the evening. Many have the idea that red meat is a good source of calcium. This is not only not true, there is some evidence that excessive consumption of red meat impairs calcium balance.

With vitamin peddlers offering us supplements containing as much as 1,000 mg of calcium per tablet, it's not hard to imagine large numbers of people, especially post-menopausal women frightened by the specter of osteoporosis, consuming enormous amounts of calcium. Fortunately, most excess calcium simply goes down the toilet. However, a long recognized hazard is the formation of kidney stones. Certainly those with a history of stone formation should be wary of calcium supplements. The possibility of a still more ominous consequence of the use of calcium supplements has come to light more recently. A little background is needed.

About twenty-five years ago, correlational studies began to appear suggestive of a beneficial effect of increased calcium intake with respect to bone health, high blood pressure, colorectal cancer, osteoporosis, and a general decline in physical functioning with age. These results were highly publicized and, aided by relentless advertising by the supplement industry, we soon had on the order of 70% of postmenopausal women and 50% of men over the age of 50 taking a calcium supplement. In 2012, about a billion dollars was spent on calcium supplements in the United States.

Thomas Henry Huxley, a noted British biologist of the 19th century, said that "The great tragedy of science (is) the slaying of a beautiful hypothesis by an ugly fact." It is not fair to say that the beautiful hypotheses regarding calcium and the diseases I've mentioned have been slain but they certainly have been wounded by the results of subsequent investigations. The facts which have emerged call into question each of the purported benefits of calcium supplements and suggest the possibility that harm may be done.

The assault on the "more is better" campaign for calcium began with a study by Dr. Mark Bolland, Professor Ian Reid, and their colleagues at the School of Medicine of the University of Aukland and reported in the *British Medical Journal* in 2008.[7] A total of 1,471 post-menopausal women with a mean age of 74 years were randomly assigned to receive either placebo or a supplement of 1,000 mg of calcium citrate per day. Women were excluded from the study if they already took calcium supplements, had osteoporosis, or were deficient in vitamin D. After five years, it was found that the risk of heart attack *increased* by nearly 50%. This result stood in contrast with earlier studies in women which reported no effect or even decreased risk of heart disease in those with higher calcium intake. As would be expected, the study was immediately attacked by the supplement industry. More important, members of the scientific community pointed out weaknesses in the analysis. However, more was to come.

Over the next five years, reports of studies conducted in Finland, Germany, Sweden, and the United States over periods ranging from seven to fourteen years all pointed in the same direction: calcium supplements may harm the hearts of both men and women. This harm is manifest by an increased number of heart attacks and deaths related to heart disease. No study found harm associated with dietary calcium. Commenting on these findings in 2013, Dr. Susanna Larsson of the Karolinska Institute in Stockholm said this: "A safe alternative to calcium supplements is to consume calcium-rich foods, such as low-fat dairy foods, beans and green leafy vegetables, which contain not only calcium but also a cocktail of essential minerals and vitamins."[8] Amen to that.

CHAPTER 6

NUTRITION

6.19 Iron
Tonic or toxin?

Anemia is a condition in which the blood is unable to carry sufficient oxygen from the air we breathe to the tissues of our bodies. Among the possible consequences of anemia are pallor of the skin, shortness of breath, extreme weakness, heart palpitations, and death. In contrast, the symptoms of mild anemia may be so vague as to be ascribed to boredom or laziness.

The three nutritional factors most commonly associated with anemia are vitamin B_{12}, folic acid, and iron. Of the three, iron is numerically the most important. It often is said that anemia caused by lack of iron is the most common deficiency in the world. However, it must be added that in the United States iron deficiency is very uncommon in adult men and postmenopausal women.

Iron has a long history as a medicinal agent. Fifteen hundred years before the birth of Christ, the physician-priests of Egypt prescribed iron. However, it was not until quite recently that the central role of iron in the prevention of anemia was fully appreciated. Oddly enough, physicians over the centuries have been more likely to cause anemia than to prevent it. This was due to the widespread and longstanding practice by physicians of drawing the blood from sick people; John Burnum called them "medical vampires."[1]

Throughout this book we will see examples of plausible ideas which have turned out to be just plain wrong. Both the idea that we become

189

ill because of the bad things in our blood and the idea that we might become well by removing the bad blood certainly sound like common sense. George Washington reportedly had a quart of blood drained off on the day he died. On her deathbed three years earlier, the first thing done for Catherine the Great of Russia was to open a vein.

With a few notable exceptions, bloodletting is not much done these days. On the other hand, the curious notion that a mild degree of anemia may be good for some of us some has been with us for at least a half century. This idea has its roots in the observation that our bodies may protect us from invasion by bacteria and cancer cells by withholding iron from these culprits.[2] Whether excess iron in the diet can overwhelm these protective mechanisms remains to be established.[3]

Iron is essential for all forms of life. In the human body, most of the iron is found in the blood in the form of hemoglobin, the molecule that gives red blood cells their ability to carry oxygen. The barrier between the blood pumped through our lungs and the air we breathe is but a single layer of cells. Oxygen diffuses across that barrier, combines with hemoglobin, and the two are carried to all cells of the body where the oxygen is released.

Another gas with which hemoglobin combines is carbon monoxide. In fact, hemoglobin so much prefers carbon monoxide to oxygen that even a small amount of carbon monoxide in the air can cause oxygen deficiency in our tissues. Together with all the other hazards of their addiction, smokers of cigarettes are chronically exposed to low levels of carbon monoxide. The resulting deficiency of oxygen may be modest in degree and subtle in its consequences. If, on the other hand, I share a closed garage with a running automobile engine, carbon monoxide will quickly be lethal. Among many others, Anne Sexton, a Pulitzer prize-winning poet, chose that exit from life.

As I noted above, healthy adult males and postmenopausal females are the segments of the population least likely to suffer iron deficiency anemia. The reasons for this fact tell us much about the iron economy of the body. Mature men and postmenopausal women do not become pregnant, do not grow, and do not bleed on a regular basis. When their red blood cells become old at the age of 120 days or so, they are destroyed but the iron is saved, sent to the bone marrow, and made into the hemoglobin for new cells. Whatever tiny loses of iron that may occur are easily made up by absorption of iron from the diet. Anemia in post-menopausal women and adult men is most often a sign of hidden bleeding. Identification of the cause of the blood loss, for example, colorectal cancer, is far more important than the anemia that results.

When thinking about growth, things such as protein for muscle and calcium for bones come to mind. But when we grow, the volume of blood grows as well, and with it the need for iron. It is for this reason that iron deficiency anemia is of concern in children, unborn babies, and the women who carry them.

The lesser need of men and post-menopausal women for iron as compared with pregnant and menstruating women is reflected in the current recommendations for iron intake.[4] Thus, prior to menopause, women are advised to take in 18 mg of iron per day while for men the value throughout adulthood is just 8 mg. With the cessation of menses, 8 mg is recommended for all women as well. Reflecting a concern about excessive iron, these suggested intakes for men have fallen by 33% since 1980.

An obvious way to insure enough iron for our own blood is to drink the blood of other animals. As attractive as that prospect may be to Count Dracula, most of us prefer to be more subtle. We take our blood in the form of animal flesh. A mere 3.5 ounces of beef contain about 6 mg of iron. Furthermore, blood-iron or, as it is more formally called, heme iron, is very well absorbed by the human gut. As a further bonus, the presence of small amounts of meat or fish in the diet enhances the absorption of nonheme iron, the form found in grains, fruits, and vegetables. It is for these reasons that otherwise healthy people who consume animal flesh several times a week are assured an adequate supply of iron.

The fact that meat-eaters are well supplied with iron does not mean that even strict vegetarians need be anemic. Indeed, surveys of vegetarians who consume a variety of fruits, vegetables, and grains find no evidence of iron deficiency.[5] The single most important determinant of iron absorption from non-meat sources is vitamin C which enhances the uptake of nonheme iron. Thus, eating a serving of an iron-fortified cereal together with a few ounces of orange juice will provide an excellent start in the morning. Other vegetarian sources include nuts, beans, and, my favorite, dark chocolate.

Turning from iron as tonic to iron as toxin, we are again reminded that when it comes to vitamins and minerals, more is not always better. Iron poisoning takes place in two ways. The more readily understood is simple overdose. It is true that the normal human gut is able to reject large amounts of iron in the diet and thus protect most of us most of the time from being poisoned. But it is true as well that these barriers can be overwhelmed. A classic example it provided by the Bantu of South Africa.

Shortly after steel drums were introduced into South Africa by European settlers, the native Bantu began to use old drums as containers for brewing beer. Over a period of years, Bantu beer drinkers were found to have a very high incidence of cirrhosis of the liver, the condition that kills so many alcoholics. But the primary problem for the Bantu was not alcohol. It was an excess of iron leached from the drums during the brewing process.[6]

Given the vigorous promotion and availability of iron supplements in this country, it is remarkable that so little iron poisoning is reported. It appears that most of us can exceed the RDA for iron by several fold without causing obvious harm. This is not a recommendation for doing so. A recent advertisement from one of the national sellers of supplements proudly proclaims that just four of their iron pills provide 639% of the RDA for iron. A book on nutrition that I found online promises to tell us "How to pump up the iron content of your spaghetti sauce to *more than 8 times the RDA*" (their emphasis). No reasons for wishing to ingest a large excess of a potentially poisonous metal are given by either source.

Iron overdose would be a simple matter if it were dependent only upon iron intake. But, as is true for so many other aspects of our lives, genetic factors play a role as well. Ten percent of white Americans carry a gene that influences the absorption of iron; Victor Herbert called it the "iron-loading gene."[7] For the one in two hundred of us who receive the gene from both parents, iron poisoning is an ever present danger. The disease that results is called hemochromatosis. Ironically, hemochromatosis in its earliest stages is characterized by fatigue similar to that seen with iron deficiency. However, as hemochromatosis progresses, the functioning of the heart, liver, and pancreas are all affected. Its treatment, odd as it may seem, is periodic bleeding of the patient. The late William H. Crosby a pioneer in studies of anemia, said that "iron deficiency continues to be overplayed as a public health threat and hemochromatosis, a real threat, is played down."[8]

In all of this, the therapeutic principle is simple: Do not treat a disease, anemia, with a potentially toxic agent, iron, unless you know that the disease is present. Iron-deficiency anemia is readily diagnosed by laboratory tests. In the absence of anemia, the use of iron supplements in the form of pills or potions is generally a bad idea for men and post-menopausal women. With respect to the latter group, recent epidemiological findings are especially ominous.

The Iowa Women's Health Study was begun in 1986. A total of 38,772 women then age 55 to 69 years were followed for nineteen years. The express purpose of the study was to correlate the use of dietary supplements with a simple end point, death. During that period, just over 40% of the women died. With respect to iron supplements, I quote the lead author, Jaako Mursu of the School of Public Health of the University of Minnesota: "Of particular concern, supplemental iron was strongly and dose dependently associated with increased total mortality risk."[9] "Dose dependently" means that the more iron the women took, the worse the outcome.

The belief that dietary iron is essential if we are to avoid anemia is entirely valid. However, that belief is as well much too simple. It is now clear that iron is involved in a variety of biological functions only the most obvious of which are concerned with the blood. The recognition of this great complexity has forced rejection of the notion that more iron is better. Only for pregnant women can the assumption reasonably be made that supplemental iron is a good idea. For the rest of us, a diet in which modest amounts of meat and generous amounts of vitamin C are present will insure an adequate intake of iron. Worry or fatigue or athletic activity are not reasons to take an iron pill every day. Despite our desire to become independent in matters of our own health, anemia can only be diagnosed by appropriate laboratory tests. For the vast majority of us who are not anemic, the wisdom of iron supplements remains to be proven.

CHAPTER 7

OBESITY

I know it when I see it.

Sent to study planet earth, an extraterrestrial being might reach an odd conclusion about the diseases that afflict the citizens of the United States. To be sure, cancer and disorders of the heart kill most and AIDS, though now regarded as a chronic disease, causes great anxiety. But an analysis of the media together with a monitoring of the thoughts of American men and women would suggest that our major concern is the weight of our bodies. Our visitor would find that at any given moment, three-quarters of the females of the population regard themselves as too heavy and are "on a diet." The males are a little bit different; up until the age of 25 or so, many actively try to gain weight but then they too begin to diet, though seldom with the ferocity of the female of the species.

It is very hard to ignore obesity among us. The media are filled with images of fat people in bikini's and Speedo's, common folk in Walmart as well as celebrities in Malibu or on the Riviera. From the latter we may take some satisfaction from their sometimes less than svelte figures. On the other hand, the models seen on television and in the fashion magazines leave us with the impression that the American ideal can be achieved only with a starvation diet perhaps aided pharmacologically; the phrase "heroin chic" comes to mind. More serious places such as the Centers for Disease Control regularly tell us of an epidemic of obesity spreading through the nation and the world.

In many places at many times throughout human history, fatness was a goal to be achieved, a symbol of wealth and power; Henry VIII in his later years might serve as the poster boy. The most successful members of a society, those who had more than enough to eat, didn't drive a Bentley or a Lamborghini. Instead, they grew fat. Several factors have led us away from fat as a status symbol to a general desire for thinness. First of all, a status symbol that nearly everyone can have stops being a status symbol. In a society such as ours, where even the poorest can be fat and often are, fatness is now more often seen as a lack of discipline than a sign of prosperity. Thinness also has a medical rationale; it is widely accepted that being fat is unhealthy.

If we as a society are so concerned about our fatness, how do we explain the fact that, as a nation, we steadily have grown fatter? The percentage of Americans classified as obese has increased from 14% in 1976 to 35% in 2012 and still rising; that's a hundred million people give or take a few million.[1] There is particular concern about obesity among children; overweight children tend to become obese adults. Before considering possible reasons for these trends and what we as individuals might do about it, we need to define obesity and how best it is measured.

The most commonly used index of obesity is the Body Mass Index or BMI. The index expresses the relationship between height and weight. Let's use me as an example. Presently, I am six feet tall and weigh 178 pounds. My BMI in English units is arrived at by my weight in pounds times 704 divided by my height in inches squared.

$$(178 \times 704) \text{ divided by } (72 \times 72) = 24.2$$

If you prefer the metric system, it is my weight in kilos (178 lbs divided by 2.2 pounds per kilo = 80.9) divided by my height in meters (72 inches X 0.254 meters/inch = 1.83 meters) squared.

$$(80.9) \text{ divided by } (1.83 \times 1.83) = 24.2$$

The criteria from the Centers for Disease Control (CDC) are as follows.

BMI	classification
Below 18.5	underweight
18.5 to 24.9	healthy weight
25.0 to 29.9	overweight
30 or higher	obese

Is my present BMI of 24.2 OK? By the CDC criteria, the answer is just barely yes. However, at age 21, I was a very fit collegiate football player, 15 pounds heavier than today, with a BMI of 26.2, overweight by the criteria of the CDC. This brings us to a problem with the BMI, it does not apply equally well to all people. Consider marathon runners and professional football players. In a recent U.S. Olympic marathon trial, the athletes averaged 5 foot 10 inches and 147 pounds for a BMI of 21.1, well within the healthy weight classification. Meanwhile, at the 2014 Super Bowl, the Seattle Seahawks' interior offensive linemen had an average BMI of 36.1. Let's consider another athlete, Mike Tyson, former heavyweight boxing champion. At 5 foot 10 inches and 233 pounds he had, in his prime, a BMI of 33.5. Dave Powell writing in *The Economist* put it this way: I am not going to be the first in line to tell Mr. Tyson that he is morbidly obese.

Are we to conclude that marathoners are thin but healthy while professional football players and some boxers are dangerously obese? The answer is a most emphatic *no*. Instead we must conclude that the BMI may mislead us when applied to individuals. In 1943, Louis Dublin, chief Actuary of the Metropolitan Life Insurance Company and author of Proposed Range of Ideal Weights for Men and Women, said that "there is no one set of weights that can be called ideal and to which all of a given height should conform." The problem with BMI is that it doesn't tell us anything about body composition, the distribution of our weight between fat, muscle, and bone. And it is fat that interests us, for it is the proportion of our weight represented by fat that contributes to what has come to be called the metabolic syndrome. Nonetheless, BMI is still a reasonable guide and you may wish to calculate yours.

Despite widespread talk of the joys of the Golden Years, as far as health is concerned, not much good comes with the passing of the years. However, with respect to the BMI, a sliver of sunlight appeared in 2014. Like the CDC, the World Health Organization (WHO) defines a healthy body weight to be a BMI of 18.5 to 24.9. A somewhat different conclusion was reached by Professor Jane Winter (no relation to me) and her colleagues at Deakin University in Australia after examining data from nearly 200,000 individuals age 65 and over.[2] They found a U-shaped relationship between BMI and mortality; it was not healthy to be either too thin or too fat. At the fat end of the scale, mortality began to increase only after a BMI around 27.5; the WHO "healthy weight range" seems not to apply to older people.

An additional cost-free assessment of interest is your waist to hip ratio (WHR). The virtue of WHR compared to BMI is that it provides a better indication of the distribution of your fat. In general, pear-shaped is better than apple-shaped and sometimes WHR correlates better than does BMI with a variety of health risks. The recommended values for WHR vary depending upon who is giving the advice but, generally speaking, anything over 1.0, i.e., your waist is bigger than your hips, is not good. The CDC suggests healthy ratios of 0.8 for women and 0.9 for men. Those who ponder the role of evolution in shaping human behavior think that men are most attracted to women with a WHR even lower, around 0.7, e.g., a 22 inch waist above 32 inch hips. It is less clear what women find appealing; Will Durant expressed the view that women seek the best provider they can stomach.[3]

Useful as may be the BMI and WHR for epidemiological studies, it is you and I as individuals that concern us here. For that reason, I suggest two additional criteria. First is the *naked before the mirror test*. Obvious rolls of fat are unequivocal evidence of excess weight. Justice Potter Stewart's definition of pornography fits obesity as well: "I can't tell you what it is, but I know it when I see it."

As a scientist, I like to confirm my visual assessment in a more objective manner. My second test involves what I call the reference clothing, any one of a number of rather elderly pairs of trousers. They come from a time when I was much younger and reasonably happy with my body. Whatever else the passing years may do to me, so long as I can fit into the reference pants and so long as my full-length mirror image isn't too troubling, I am doing all right with respect to body fat. In my case, the reference pants and the mirror tell me the same thing: at my age I should weigh 15 pounds less than I did a half century or so ago hence my present target weight of 178 pounds. Male readers of a certain age will recognize what has happened to me; Calvin Trillin called it DTS, disappearing tush syndrome. As men age, there is a not very subtle shift in the areas where fat is deposited, from buttocks and upper leg to belly.

Let's consider the scary alternative to maintaining or even cutting back our weight as we age. Instead of losing seventeen pounds over the past 50 years what if I had increased my food intake by just 10 calories per day. That comes to 3,650 calories per year and a weight gain of 1 pound. A one pound weight gain per year would bring me today to 240 pounds and a BMI of 32.6; I would be obese and I certainly would not fit into my reference clothing. Did I mention that 10 calories are found in one (!) ounce of Coke or three (!) M&M's? Little things mean a lot. (If you are not into trousers, feel free to choose another item of clothing but remember that it should come from a time when you liked your body.) In the next chapter we will look more closely at the equation, 3,600 calories equals 1 pound weight gain or loss; like so many other things, it isn't that simple.

I have to warn you that there is a downside to never letting yourself get fat as the years go by. If you are as frugal as I, you may find yourself wearing some pretty old clothing. Years ago, partially in response to my wife's view that any item of clothing without the tags still on is old and ready for a charitable donation, I bought myself a very nice Brooks Brothers suit, wore it in 1985 to my elder daughter's graduation from The Culinary Institute of America, and, albeit a bit snugly, still can wear the suit today.

Imagine that you have failed in all respects: you can't fit into your old clothes, the mirror says you are fat, and your BMI and WHR are excessive? There are two reasons to lose weight: matters of health and matters of appearance. The latter we will leave to the next chapter. To settle the first you need simply visit your personal physician for a routine physical examination. (I realize that my assumption that you have a personal physician is optimistic in the extreme but I suspect that it is far more likely to be true for readers of this book than in the population as a whole.) The exam need not be fancy, no exotic tests or imaging, just a careful assessment of your medical history, your current physical state, and a little blood work. Even people who fall within an ideal weight range may benefit from a loss in body fat when conditions your doctor can easily identify are present. We now refer to these factors collectively as the metabolic syndrome. Components of the syndrome include an excess of abdominal fat, high blood pressure, diabetes, and elevated levels of cholesterol and triglycerides; each is a risk factor for heart disease and, in combination, they are especially lethal.

Many of us are intuitively if not explicitly aware that obesity is not smoothly distributed in the population. For example, in 2006, Leslie Schulz and her colleagues from the University of Wisconsin, on the basis of BMI measurements, observed that nearly 70% of the Pima Indians residing in Arizona met the CDC criterion for obesity.[4] In addition, these Native Americans have the highest prevalence of type 2 diabetes in the world. We might conclude that it must be in their genes and, indeed, there is a genetic component involved. However, as was astutely observed by Dr. Schulz, the Pima of Arizona share a very similar gene pool with the Pima Indians who reside in the Sierra Madre mountains of Mexico. In contrast with their American relatives, the Mexican Pima have a much lower prevalence of both diabetes and obesity. This being a book about aging and because it is known that for all of us age is an additional risk factor for diabetes, let us look at the older Pima in the study, those fifty-five or older. In Mexico the prevalence of diabetes in this group was 8.3% while in Arizona it was an astounding 82.2%. How do we explain these dramatic differences between genetically homogeneous peoples? Dr. Schulz concluded that the primary factors are diet and the level of physical activity; the Mexican Pima expend five times more energy in their daily lives. The Arizona Pima diet is high in fat, what some have called the Modern American Diet. In Mexico, the traditional diet is low in fat and high in carbohydrates provided by beans, potatoes, and tortillas made from wheat or corn flour. Even for the Pima, genes are not destiny.

For many others, income, race, nutrition, and culture are intertwined. Let's look at the states of Mississippi and Connecticut.[5] In terms of per capita income, Mississippi is the poorest and Connecticut the richest of the United States. Mississippi has the highest rates of heart disease, diabetes, and both childhood and adult obesity. Life expectancy in Mississippi is the lowest in the nation; a man in Mississippi can expect to live five years less than one in Connecticut. Mississippi is near the bottom with respect to physical activity and consumption of fruits and vegetables. The overall rate of obesity as measured by BMI in Connecticut is 21.8% compared to Mississippi's 34.4%. This contrast between the states of Connecticut and Mississippi together with the example drawn from the Pima Indians makes clear two things. First, multiple factors interact to shape our bodies. Second, obesity and all that goes with it are largely within our control whatever the hand dealt to us by our genetic endowment.

In the next chapter, we will consider some of the reasons why so many of us have to work so hard to lose weight and keep it off. We will consider a few diets, I will offer some advice, and will tell you what I do for myself. But before moving on I want to add just a bit more science with respect to why fat, especially abdominal fat, is medically bad for us; why obesity should be regarded as a life-threatening disease.

Syndrome is a term that has become familiar to all of us. It refers to a group of signs and symptoms that occur together to characterize a disease. For example, we now know that the Acquired Immunodeficiency Syndrome or AIDS is caused by a virus, our immune systems are compromised, and our ability to fight off infections diminished. Earlier in this chapter I mentioned another syndrome, the metabolic syndrome: excess abdominal fat, high blood pressure, diabetes, and disorders of cholesterol and triglycerides. A difference should be noted between classical diabetes and the type of diabetes embedded in the metabolic syndrome. Classical diabetes is an autoimmune disorder in which the cells of the pancreas responsible for the production of insulin are destroyed. It used to be called childhood-onset diabetes to distinguish it from adult-onset diabetes. However, it is now recognized that classical diabetes as studied by Frederick Banting and Charles Best, the discoverers of insulin in 1921, is fundamentally different from adult-onset diabetes. In the former, insulin is absent, in the latter we become insensitive to even increased levels of insulin hence the term insulin resistance. In addition, because it is now known that even obese children can develop insulin resistance, we refer to the condition as type 2 diabetes to distinguish it from the classical form or type 1 diabetes. The consequences of the two are equally bad.

If the human immunodeficiency virus, HIV, causes AIDS, might there be an analogous factor responsible for the metabolic syndrome? An answer to that question has begun to emerge only in the past decade and it is startling in its implications. It is now clear that our adipose tissue is not, as had long been thought, just a place to store energy. In addition to that role, our fat cells, the adipocytes, constitute a giant endocrine organ which secretes multiple factors to modulate a variety of functions. Although much remains to be learned, it is now clear that when the balance of these secretions is disturbed by the presence of obesity, a multitude of things happen, none of them good. I am inclined to agree with those who recently have hypothesized that obesity is not just an element of the metabolic syndrome; it is the cause of the syndrome. At its annual meeting in June 2013, the American Medical Association officially recognized obesity as a disease. In doing so, they followed the conclusion reached earlier by the American Association of Clinical Endocrinologists and the American College of Cardiology.

Not all are pleased with calling obesity a disease. For example, the National Association to Advance Fat Acceptance is dedicated to ending size discrimination and argues that the disease label stigmatizes the overweight and obese. Lindy West of *Jezebel* put it this way: "It's hard enough to be a fat kid without the government telling you you're an epidemic...there are a million different kinds of fat people in the world." Others suggest that labeling a condition such as obesity and various forms of addiction, including alcoholism, as diseases, contributes to a sense of helplessness among the victims.[6] That being said, it is my belief that more good than harm is done by the designation.

Perhaps the picture I have painted of the consequences of obesity is not sufficiently vivid or perhaps, happily, you are slender as a reed so you think obesity should be of little concern to you. Let me tell you about the economic consequences of just one facet of the disease. No taxpayer can avoid the costs of health care even when healthy and nowhere is this more evident than in how we, as a society, address chronic disease of the kidneys. These paired organs function to clear toxins and waste materials from the blood. When they begin to falter in that function, there are two options open to us, a kidney transplant or purification of the blood by a machine in a process called dialysis.

It has long been known from epidemiological studies that obesity, especially an elevated waist to hip ratio and diabetes are major risk factors for kidney failure. Presently there are about 600,000 Americans who regularly undergo renal dialysis and, thanks to a Federal program launched on July 1st, 1973, their costs are subsidized by our government. The End Stage Renal Disease program is a part of Medicare but open to patients of all ages. In 2011, the program cost us taxpayers approximately twenty-seven billion dollars, fully six percent of all Medicare spending. Returning to science for a moment, there is increasing evidence that a very significant portion of all renal failure is related to obesity, the underlying disorder is inflammation, and the mediator of that inflammation is adiponectin and related pro- and anti-inflammatory secretions of our adipocytes.[7]

In speaking of the epidemic of obesity, many have simply thrown up their hands and said that there is no way to get people to decrease their energy intake by eating less and to increase their energy expenditure by exercising more. Some authorities have even given us a free pass. For example, Sir David King, chief scientific advisor to the British prime ministers Tony Blair and Gordon Brown, writing in *The Lancet* in 2011 expressed the opinion that "…the present epidemic of obesity is not really (due) to laziness or overeating but that our biology has stepped out of kilter with society."[8] Or Boyd Swinburn, a noted Australian authority, also in *The Lancet*: "Obesity is the result of people responding normally to the obesogenic environments they find themselves in."[9] As to what we can do about it, we find statements such as "moderation doesn't work", "measures to increase consumption of healthy food are unlikely to be effective", "assumptions about speed and sustainability of weight loss are wrong", and (Professor Swinburn again) "…there are no exemplar populations in which the obesity epidemic has been reversed by public health measures…"

I prefer to believe that recognition of obesity as a preventable disease with dire consequences both for the individual and for our society is but one step of many to be taken. The contrasts I have noted between the states of Mississippi and Connecticut make clear the influence of poverty, education, and social acceptance on the prevalence of the condition. An educational campaign similar to that applied to smoking holds out great hope. The central message of the program would be that obesity is a preventable disease, a disease with terrible consequences. As with smoking, these consequences can be graphically illustrated in multiple ways: a patient on dialysis, a diabetic amputee, and so on. Because the adverse effects of obesity are magnified as we age, it is especially important that we recognize obesity as a chronic disease while still young, long before the consequences are irreversible.

The role of government in controlling obesity is a contentious issue. Phrases such as "the nanny state" and "food Nazis" are common. Should the government tell us what to eat? Again, tobacco provides a useful model. When smoking was banned in restaurants in New York City, it was said that the industry would be destroyed. It was not and we non-smokers can now breathe easier while dining. Unfortunately, Mayor Michael Bloomberg's campaign against super-sized sugary drinks was less successful. Ever increasing taxes on cigarettes appear to have contributed to a steady decline in this most dangerous addiction. Application of similar taxes on sugary drinks can be expected to meet serious opposition from makers of the drinks. For example, in 2012, the city of Richmond, California moved to impose a soda tax. The beverage industry spent $2.8 million in opposing the measure; that's $27 for every man, woman, and child in the city.[10] The tax was defeated. How our society's war on obesity should best proceed is uncertain but this book is about me and you as individuals and, in the next chapter, I will tell you what you and I can do for ourselves.

CHAPTER 8

WEIGHT LOSS AND MAINTENANCE

Never say diet.

In 1961, a book appeared called *Calories Don't Count.*[1] The author was Herman Taller, described by *Time* magazine as a Romanian-born physician who lived and practiced obstetrics in Brooklyn. The book in several editions ultimately sold more than two million copies. Dr. Taller's premise was that we become obese because of an evil by-product of carbohydrate metabolism. His answer was a high-fat, low carbohydrate diet supplemented with daily capsules containing safflower oil. In 1961, the Food and Drug Administration had sharper teeth than it does today; this was long before passage of the Dietary Supplement Health and Education Act discussed in chapter 2. Shortly after the publication of Taller's book, the FDA Commissioner condemned it as full of false ideas. For his promotion of safflower capsules, Taller was found guilty of postal fraud, fined, and put on probation. The book is now out of print and the author is long dead but his theme lives on. *Calories Don't Count* is the dream of many a dieter and the promise of many a diet book. It is utter nonsense.

In the previous chapter I touched on some of the economic, educational, and cultural factors that influence the incidence of obesity in any given segment of our society. Without diminishing the role of factors such as these, we must acknowledge something even more fundamental: our genetic endowment. For a woman born with the genes of a Russian shot-putter to covet the jeans of a Bolshoi ballerina is to invite frustration and failure. This fact of life has been the basis for many pessimistic statements regarding weight loss and, too often, a ready excuse for those who have failed to conquer obesity. Let's consider more closely the differences between us.

On May 24, 1990, a report appeared in the *New England Journal of Medicine* with the provocative title "The Response to Long-term Overfeeding in Identical Twins."[2] Claude Bouchard and his colleagues at Laval University in Canada sought to determine whether our genes are important in how much weight we gain. Their subjects were twelve sets of identical twins, pairs of persons whose genetic makeup is the same. Over a period of 100 days, the twins were fed a total of 84,000 calories in excess of their energy needs.

Our simple formula, 3,600 calories equals one pound of weight gain, predicts that all of the subjects will gain 23.3 pounds in body weight. In fact, the average weight gain was 17.8 pounds, 24% less than predicted. However, there was a broad range in the individual values. By the end of the overfeeding, one person had gained only 9.5 pounds, almost 40% less than expected, while another's body weight increased by 29.3 pounds, 26% more than our formula predicts. Equally remarkable was the observation that there was very little variation in weight gain or distribution of body fat within twin pairs, those sharing identical genetic factors. In contrast, the differences between pairs was much greater.

Dr. Bouchard's group reached the obvious conclusion: our genes play a significant role in how we respond to overfeeding. They went on to suggest that genetic factors might influence our resting energy expenditure or basal metabolic rate (BMR). In a sedentary adult, the BMR may account for as much as 70% of total energy use. It is ironic that a low BMR is advantageous to humans in a setting of food scarcity but predisposes to obesity in those for whom food is abundant, the situation in which most of us find ourselves today.

Whatever the differences between us with respect to BMR, weight loss still would be rather straightforward if we could plan on having the same rate while gaining or losing weight. Make no such plans; BMR responds to caloric intake. With a sustained reduction in our intake of food, our bodies become more efficient in its use of energy; the BMR decreases and the initial rate of loss declines. A study done in the Netherlands by Dr. Janna de Boer and her colleagues is illustrative.[3]

Fourteen women with an average weight of 206 pounds were put on a 1,000 calorie per day diet for eight weeks. There average weight loss was 22 pounds. However, over the course the diet, BMR was found to decrease by 15%. The practical consequence of this change is that these women would have to continue indefinitely to eat less than before simply to maintain their weight loss.

The fact that the BMR plays an important role in determining energy needs together with the observation that the rate changes in response to an excess or deficiency of food have led to something called the set point theory. The thought is that perhaps body weight is regulated in the same way as body temperature or the level of carbon dioxide in the blood. Thus, each of us would have a pre-determined adult body weight. Movements above or below the set point would call into action compensatory mechanisms, changes in BMR for example. Those we call obese would simply be those whose natural set point clashes with what current fashion calls attractive or contemporary medicine thinks to be healthy.

Some, including a few overweight professionals, have used set point theory as an excuse not to lose weight. They say that some of us are naturally obese and some are naturally lean and there's nothing to be done about it. The weight of scientific evidence does not support this position. Though we may accept as fact the existence of physiological mechanisms that function to conserve body fat and as fact that there are genetically-determined individual differences in the level of body fat which triggers those mechanisms, there is no reason to conclude that weight loss is impossible for anyone. The fortunate few will find it an easy task but with the practice of patience and discipline, virtually all of us are capable of achieving a desired body weight.

The program I want to suggest to you for weight loss and maintenance rests upon two unshakable principles:

(1) Calories count and

(2) Exercise is an essential component.

In the simplest terms, if your food intake exceeds the energy requirements of your body, you will gain weight and if your food intake does not
meet the energy requirements of your body, you will lose weight.

Why is the subtitle of this chapter *Never Say Diet?* After all, diet is
a perfectly proper word derived from the Greek *diaeta* meaning "manner of living." In the English language it can refer to the "food and
drink regularly consumed." Unfortunately, today it most often is used
in connection with weight loss as in "I am dieting" or "I am on a diet."
Some such as the DASH and Mediterranean diets discussed below are
soundly based on current nutritional principles but many more are what
I referred to in another place as *Tales of the Supernatural.* The authors of
the latter, like Dr. Taller before them, promise to reveal heretofore undis-
covered secrets of nutrition and guarantee weight loss without sacrifice
or effort on your part.

I most definitely do not want to put you on a "diet." Instead, I want
you to adjust your "manner of living" such that excess weight is reduced
and maintained at a healthy level. The adjustments are to be life-long
but not of a constant character; our tactics must adapt to ever-changing
circumstances: travel, a wedding, a holiday, a celebration, illness, or any
of the many adjustments needed as we age. Nonetheless, the principles
regarding energy intake and expenditure are as written in stone. Until
someone comes up with a better word, let's just say that we will change
our manner of living from now until the end of our days.

Why is there a constant stream of "diet" books? Have not the principles of weight loss been known for decades? The simple answer is that
for most people most of the time the diets don't work in the long run.
And, after all, it is the long run that interests us. Whether or not I have
lost a few pounds prior to a wedding or class reunion is of only transient
importance. Our real goal is to maintain an acceptable weight for a
lifetime. To accomplish that requires a manner of living and eating that

enhances rather than disrupts our lives. Put me on an ultra-low fat diet such as is offered by the late Nathan Pritikin or Dean Ornish and I will be obliged to stop sharing meals with my family or eating in my favorite restaurants. This is no way to begin.

I am going to tell you of a very simple, life-long manner of living to control your weight and to insure optimal nutrition. (Actually, no one knows what is truly optimal but we can come close.) Before giving you my suggestions, let us consider for a moment what is out there already. At a wonderful internet site called *WebMD* you can find critiques of 90 (!) different diet plans, all written by Kathleen Zelman, a Registered Dietician and Master of Public Health, who is director of nutrition for *WebMD*. For each, she describes the plan, quotes the thoughts of various mainstream authorities, and then gives her candid opinion. I should note that while 90 may seem a large number, Ms. Zelman could have added many more including some of my old favorites such as *The Beverly Hills* Diet, *The Last Chance Diet,* and *The Drinking Man's Diet*; these are representatives of the *Tales of the Supernatural* to which I referred earlier. For a diet junkie, it makes for great reading. For those not so inclined, we will consider just two before settling on our own plan.

Stripped down to their essentials, virtually all diet plans can be classified as (a) high fat, (b) high carbohydrate, (c) balanced, or, to use a technical term, (d) just plain crazy. I will largely ignore category (d) except to say that they usually are based upon some bizarre, untested, and scientifically unsound principle of nutrition of which establishment nutritionists are strangely unaware. They promise that a particular food from a strange land or a way of combining foods or a revolutionary metabolic principle recently discovered by a Bulgarian chiropractor or a newly unearthed secret of the ancients will allow you to eat all you want while losing fat. Such plans often are promoted with lines such as "Your doctor didn't learn this in medical school but for just $29.95 plus S&H we are going to share our secret with you."

We have earlier considered the elements of nutrition in chapter 6. There we learned that only fat, carbohydrate, and protein, the macronutrients, need concern us with respect to body weight. Two factors which are worth thinking about are (1) the distribution of our energy intake between the macronutrients and (2) the identity of the foods within each macronutrient, i.e., what fats, what carbohydrates, and what proteins are best for us. With respect to the proportion of calories represented by fat, carbohydrate, and protein, the acceptable values cover a broad range. The two excellent nutritional plans we will consider in detail below are a Mediterranean-type diet where as much as 50% of the caloric intake is in the form of fat and the DASH (Dietary Approaches to Stop Hypertension) diet with only about 25% fat. More important is the choice of foods within each category of macronutrient. Thus, both diets emphasize a reduction in saturated fat, the primary source of which is animal products, and an increase in mono- and polyunsaturated fats as found in vegetable oils, fish, nuts, and vegetables. Both are excellent in terms of nutrition and weight control. The one you choose or the variant of the one you choose is that which best suits your present dietary patterns or cultural heritage. Many a plan has been self-anointed as being "revolutionary." We are not interested in revolution; it is evolution of your present manner of living and eating that we seek.

Let us begin with a high fat diet. You might think that no one would recommend such a thing for weight loss or maintenance. Has not Pierre Dukan of the *The Dukan Diet* said that "Fats are the absolute enemy of anyone trying to be slim?" Have not many condemned what is perhaps the most famous of the high fat diets, *The Atkins Diet Revolution*? But Atkin's is not the high fat diet to which I refer. Instead we want to consider what is called the Mediterranean diet or more properly the Mediterranean diets as there are multiple forms in a region stretching from Spain in the West to Syria in the East. What we now regard as the prototypical Mediterranean diet is based on studies done following World War II on the Greek island of Crete by a Rockefeller Foundation epidemiologist named Leland Allbaugh.[4] He found that the principal source of fat in the Cretan diet is olive oil. As was noted in chapter 6, olive oil, like canola oil, is mono-unsaturated and, unlike saturated fat, is heart-protective. The person generally credited with bringing the Mediterranean diets to their current prominence is Ancel Keys, an American physiologist who was struck by the low incidence of heart disease especially in Southern Italy where, as on Crete, olive oil was a mainstay of the diet. (The "K" in K rations may well have been taken from Keys, who developed these military rations during World War II.)

Among its many virtues, the diminished role of meat, especially red meat, in the Mediterranean diets will reduce your risk of colorectal and breast cancers (see chapter 13 for details). However, the Mediterranean diets are far removed from that advocated by those such as Dean Ornish who advises the avoidance of meat of all kinds including fish, vegetable oils, nuts, and seeds. The Ornish diet provides less than 10% of total calories as fat. In contrast, the fat content of the Mediterranean diets may approach 50%. Keys described for us the 1950's diet of what he called "the common folk" of Naples: "...homemade minestrone...pasta in endless variety...served with tomato sauce and a sprinkle of cheese, only occasionally enriched with some bits of meat or served with a little local sea food...a hearty dish of beans and short lengths of macaroni...lots of bread only a few hours from the oven and never served with any kind of spread; great quantities of fresh vegetables; a modest portion of meat or fish perhaps twice a week; red wine...always fresh fruit for dessert..." The high fat content of the Mediterranean diet comes largely from extra-virgin olive oil and the poly-unsaturated fats found in a variety of vegetables. We might also note that it includes pasta and "lots of bread", items condemned by those who advocate the avoidance of carbohydrates.

In 1959, Ancel Keys and his wife, Margaret, wrote a book entitled *Eat Well and Stay Well.*[5] In it they gave this nutritional advice: restrict saturated fats; prefer vegetable oils to solid fats; favor fresh vegetables, fruits, and non-fat dairy products; avoid heavy use of salt and refined sugar. Since the time of Allbaugh and Keys, many excellent studies have concluded that a Mediterranean diet is beneficial in terms of extending life and avoiding heart disease, obesity, type 2 diabetes, and some forms of cancer. Indeed, there is suggestive evidence that this manner of eating may reduce the likelihood of cognitive decline[6] and perhaps even Alzheimer's disease.[7] The role of inflammation in each of these diseases is uncertain but I would note that the "anti-inflammatory diet" described by the estimable Andrew Weil in his multiple books, has all the elements of a Mediterranean diet.

The features of a Mediterranean diet are simple and require no great culinary skills. However, for those who love to cook, a number of excellent compilations of advice and recipes are available. Amazon Books alone lists nearly 150. Of recent vintage, we have *The Everything Mediterranean Diet Book* by Connie Diekman and Sam Sotiropoulos published in 2010 and, from 2008, *The New Mediterranean Diet Cookbook* by Nancy Harmon Jenkins and Marion Nestle. I would note that Ms. Diekman of Washington University in St. Louis is past president of the American Dietetic Association and that Dr. Nestle is Professor of Nutrition, Food Studies, and Public Health at New York University; amateurs they are not. However, I must add that I have no culinary skills and have not personally used either book. As I am often reminded by my elder daughter, replicating a recipe in your own kitchen is the ultimate test.

In 1995, Frank Sacks and his colleagues described a study designed to assess the influence of dietary patterns on blood pressure. It was to be called the "Dietary Approaches to Stop Hypertension Trial" or DASH for short.[8] Sponsored by the National Heart Lung and Blood Institute the trial was to be conducted at a number of leading medical institutions in the United States and involved a total of 459 adults. The intent was to determine the effects on blood pressure not of individual nutrients but of their combined effects.

Three diets were compared. The first or control diet was low in fruits, vegetables, and dairy products; fat represented 36% of calories. The second diet added fruits and vegetables but the fat content remained at 36%. With addition of fruits and vegetables, the potassium and calcium content of the diet was significantly increased. The third or combination diet also was rich in fruits and vegetables but included low-fat dairy products and reduced intake of beef, pork, and ham with an increase in poultry and fish. As a result, the fat content of the combination diet was reduced to 26% of calories with compensatory increases in carbohydrates, fiber, and protein. Salt, i.e., sodium chloride, a factor often invoked with respect to elevated blood pressure, was virtually identical in the three diets, about 2,900 mg of sodium per day. (High blood pressure will be discussed in detail in chapter 14.)

Results of the DASH trial were reported in the *New England Journal of Medicine* in 1997.[9] Addition of fruits and vegetables to the control diet significantly reduced blood pressure. Still more effective was the combination diet: rich in fruits, vegetables, and low-fat dairy products with reduced saturated and total fat. In a subsequent study, it was found that by reducing the salt content of the combination diet by about one-third, the beneficial effects on blood pressure were even further enhanced. Even more important than the absolute amount of sodium is the ratio of potassium to sodium; potassium counteracts the adverse effects of sodium. Fortunately, the fresh fruits and vegetables of the DASH diet provide potassium in abundance.

Despite the fact that the DASH trial lasted but 11 weeks, it has been influential in shaping the Department of Agriculture's *Dietary Guidelines for Americans* ever since. Subsequent to the 1997 report, many studies have demonstrated benefit for the DASH diet not only for reduction of blood pressure but also in type 2 diabetes, an effect attributed to the anti-inflammatory effects of the diet, in prevention of obesity in adolescent girls, and a decreased incidence of colorectal cancer. As is true for the Mediterranean diet, there are countless books which provide recipes for use in following a DASH diet. An excellent recent addition is *The DASH Action Diet Plan* by Marla Heller, a Registered Dietician who has promoted the diet for many years. Free of charge are the DASH recipes found at the Mayo Clinic web site. Once again I endorse only the science; I have not tried the recipes.

The beauty of the Mediterranean and DASH diets is that both are palatable, both depend on ordinary foods, neither demands drastic alterations in our eating patterns, and both have been proven to be beneficial in preventing or ameliorating a variety of diseases. Both are characterized by abundant fruits and vegetables, whole grains, low-fat and non-fat dairy products, lean meats, fish, beans, and nuts. Their primary difference is in the fat content with the Mediterranean emphasis on extra-virgin olive oil as a staple of cooking. Neither involves the use of supplements such as protein, fiber, magnesium, potassium, or calcium. Indeed, studies of nutrients in isolation have generally been disappointing with respect to either weight loss or health benefits.

Earlier I mentioned the excellent evaluation of 90 different diet plans by Kathleen Zelman on the internet site called *WebMD*. In addition, the magazine, *U.S. News and World Report*, loves to rank lots of things, diets included. Their "panel of health experts" recently listed 32 plans for overall quality. Not surprisingly, at number one was the DASH with a Mediterranean plan and one from the Mayo Clinic not far behind. All are excellent. Not so satisfying to me is that U.S. News' ranking of "weight loss" plans fails to list *Dr. Winter's Chocolate Cake and Ice Cream Diet*, something I proposed in my earlier book on nutrition and exercise. Eat all the cake and ice cream you want up to a daily limit of 1,200 calories. Over a two week period, I guarantee weight and fat loss equal to that of the Dukan Diet or any other plan you wish to choose. The "secret" is in limiting yourself to 1,200 calories; unfortunately, it is not good nutrition. (If not satisfied with the *Chocolate Cake and Ice Cream Diet*, return all uneaten ice cream and cake to me for a full refund minus shipping and handling.)

With the DASH and Mediterranean diets as background, let us consider my personal six-step program for weight loss and maintenance. You will wish to formulate your own plan and develop your own tricks while maintaining the essential elements of nutrition and the daily monitoring of weight. I include my personal practices merely as illustrations.

(1) Begin your fitness plan as outlined in chapter 5. After you are exercising regularly and have settled into a routine, move to step 2.

(2) Determine whether you need to lose weight or simply to maintain your present weight. With the previous chapter as a guide, measure

your body mass index (BMI) and waist to hip ratio (WHR) and conduct the naked before the mirror and reference clothing tests.

(3) Assess your current nutritional manner of living by maintaining a journal for one normal week; not around Christmas or Hanukkah or a family reunion, not while on vacation. Record everything that you eat and drink together with approximate quantities. This may seem silly to you; do we not all know already what we drink and eat? Often we do not.

(4) On the basis of your one-week journal, begin to shift your eating pattern toward that of a DASH or Mediterranean style of eating, with emphasis on fruits and vegetables, whole grains, low-fat dairy products, lean meats preferably non-red, fish, beans, and nuts. If you need further guidance or like to try new recipes, go on line or buy one of the books I've suggested.

(5) On the basis of your one-week journal, begin to decrease your consumption of the following items. I emphasize the word *decrease*; I am not at all attracted to the notion of absolute elimination; food is not poison; food is to be enjoyed. Nonetheless, decrease your intake of (a) sugar-sweetened drinks such as Coke and Pepsi and the multitude of sugar-laden "fruit" drinks out there (plain water, filtered if you prefer, is always the fluid of choice at meals and in between), (b) deep-fried foods; the primary culprit for many is French fries, (c) processed snack foods, and (d) red meat. (Full disclosure: In New York City, there is a restaurant called The Palm, a classic steak house specializing in red meat. Perhaps three times a year I go to The Palm with members of my family and have an 8-ounce fillet mignon with baked potato and butter; I love it. As I have said, food is not poison; food is to be enjoyed. But, I must confess that I probably would be better off with The Palm's crab cakes, equally delicious.)

(6) After you have modified your eating habits in steps (4) and (5), it is time to think about weight maintenance or loss. It is only at this point that a mechanical aid is required: a reliable bathroom scale.

(a) At a fixed time each day weigh yourself; I do it first thing in the morning before I have exercised. Decide what your desired weight should be. On any morning that you weigh more than your desired weight, reduce your caloric intake for that day and for as long as it takes to reach your target weight. This reduction does not take the form of eliminating healthy items or by modifying your overall plan of eating but simply by decreasing quantity.

Only a fortunate few will achieve a desirable weight without reducing caloric intake. On the other hand, most of us will have obvious places to cut back. Let's use me as an example. I told you in the last chapter that I have decided that my desired weight is 178 pounds. If this morning I weighed more than that, I would cut back slightly on the quantity of food I have for breakfast, lunch, and dinner; I do not eliminate items but simply decrease their quantity; perhaps substitute more fruit for that piece of cake I might normally eat. But let us imagine that I have been away from home for a week, have had no access to a scale, and, upon my return, I find myself at 182.3 pounds (it is a digital scale). More drastic steps are needed: As before, I decrease my intake of all foods but in addition, I eliminate my daily beer ration until I return to 178. Do I miss my beer? Absolutely I do. But it is a reminder that any deviation from my desired weight will be addressed immediately not mañana. Not a beer-drinker? Eliminating desert or cookies or a snack will do as well. If for some reason I fall a pound or two below my target weight, I have the wonderful opportunity to gain it back by indulging in more of what I normally eat or even a few of those sinful foods I love so much. Intentionally getting a few pounds below your target weight is a nice thing to do when coming into a holiday season.

(b) If your desired weight is significantly higher than your actual weight, say 20 pounds higher, the principles remain the same but the time frame lengthens out; you did not get into your present state in a week and you should not expect to get out of it in a week. Most nutritionists think that a loss of 2 pounds per week is healthy and doable. If that strikes you as too little, recall that it amounts to 20 pounds in 10 weeks. Again, your pattern of eating, whether it be DASH or Mediterranean, does not change. Only the quantity of foods is decreased. A simple measure is to cut your caloric intake at dinner by about 50% by the simple measure of never filling your plate a second time. Eliminate desert or cut it too in half. Reduce the number of snack foods in your pantry, things like cookies, cupcakes, potato chips, cheese doodles, etc. You don't need the temptation; recall that Trappist monks do not surround themselves with dancing girls. Be patient; it may be hard at times but it will work. You may also wish to increase your duration of exercise. The program outlined in chapter 5 begins with exercise three times a week. As you become comfortable with exercise, you may wish to increase its frequency. (I try to engage in aerobic exercise, running, every day of the week with the addition of strength training on alternate days.) However, we should not overestimate the role of exercise in weight loss. Unless I am an ultra-marathoner or a North Woods logger before the advent of power saws, I can always out-eat my exercise. Caloric restriction remains the key to weight loss.

What about the diet plans which promise quick weight loss? The basis for most of them is the virtual elimination of carbohydrates and the substitution of fat and protein, things such as eggs, cheese, and meat in abundance. To understand what happens next we need to recall that we store energy in two forms, fat and glycogen. The latter, also called animal starch, is a polysaccharide composed of many units of glucose and stored largely in the liver with lesser amounts in muscle. When we drastically reduce our intake of carbohydrates, it is to glycogen that the body turns for energy.As glycogen is used up, large amounts of water are excreted and there is the illusion of rapid fat loss; you might lose ten pounds in ten days but little of it is fat.

But what if we combine the virtual elimination of carbohydrates with a reduction of caloric intake below our energy needs? This is when real fat loss can begin in a phenomenon called ketosis. After our store of glycogen is exhausted the body converts fat and protein to a utilizable source of energy called ketone bodies. This conversion of fat and protein to energy is done with reluctance. Our body may signal its displeasure with bad breath, fatigue, nausea, loss of appetite, and a general lousy feeling. Of course, proponents of low-carbohydrate diets use these side effects of ketone bodies as a selling point and tell you that you will no longer think about food. (I am reminded of *Mad* magazine's "Gross Out Diet" in which interest in food is diminished by eating spaghetti with a can of live worms on the table or an open diaper pail beneath it.) A young woman of my acquaintance used a high-fat diet for a time and it worked quite well in terms of weight loss. However, her conclusion was that "to be on the Atkin's diet is to have an eating disorder" and she has now moved on to be a lacto-ovo-piscine vegetarian, not far from the DASH and Mediterranean diets described above. (My apologies to any vegan readers who might object to calling anyone who eats milk, eggs, and fish a vegetarian.)

Earlier I cited William Manchester as "a man who usually prefers his own company, finding contentment in solitude" and went on to tell you that I am a solitary exerciser. Likewise, you can maintain an appropriate body weight on your own and that is what I do. But, just as is true for exercise, many will benefit from the support of others in weight loss plans such as those offered by Jenny Craig, Weight Watchers, and Nutrisystem. Indeed, in a much publicized study reported in 2011 by Susan Jebb and her colleagues in England, Germany, and Australia, it was observed that Weight Watchers, with its program of regular weighing, advice about diet and physical activity, motivation, and group support was superior to once a month consultation with a primary care physician.[10] This finding will not deter the creation of physician-based weight loss programs encouraged by the decision by Medicare in January of 2012 to reimburse physicians for this service. However, Dr. Jebb's study strongly suggests that weight loss need not be medicalized.

A feature of the commercial weight loss programs is that many sell you prepared meals. I am not a great fan of you spending any money at all to lose weight but, at least for some, a financial investment will provide a useful incentive to continue with the program. For those with truly excessive money to devote to the project, various residential programs are available costing as much as $8,000 per week. It is your responsibility to decide what works best for you. Some experimentation may be needed. Most will find the six-step program I outlined above to be more than adequate and devoid of expense.

Science is iconoclastic; it moves forward by tearing down what has come before. A persistent nutritional icon, drummed into our heads for more than forty years, is that "low-fat is good." However, we have seen illustrated in the Mediterranean diets the fact that high fat, when those fats are of the mono- and polyunsaturated variety, can be very good indeed. Furthermore, it has become increasingly clear from studies based on hundreds of thousands of individuals that fat, even saturated fat, is less of an evil than we have supposed. Indeed, as Walter Willett and his colleagues of the Harvard University School of Public Health have forcefully pointed out, replacement of saturated fat by sugar and refined carbohydrates is bad nutrition and may well be a major factor in the rise of obesity.[11] This is not to say, as is made clear in the DASH and Mediterranean diets, that we should not reduce our intake of red and processed meats. It does mean that the compensatory fat calories should come from vegetable oils, fish, and nuts.

What I have proposed to you is an all-natural approach to a healthy weight. But does it not require self-discipline and even a modest degree of hunger at various times during the day? It does indeed. (By the way, there is a proverb in many cultures which tells us that "hunger is the best sauce"; do not come to any meal without a touch of it; your pleasure will be enhanced.) Many think there must be an easier way and they are encouraged in that belief by countless advertisements on line, in the print media, and on television for products that offer, for example, "a pill that can reshape your entire body in 30 days" or "weight loss without diet or exercise." They are fantasy; ignore them all.

I began this chapter with Herman Taller and his 1961 book *Calories Don't Count*. For his promotion of safflower oil he was convicted of postal fraud. Lest you think that Alexander Pope was wrong to say that "Hope springs eternal in the human breast", I invite you to consider the March 12, 2012 cover of *Woman's World*, a publication I found at my supermarket check-out. In bold red letters we are promised that "Dr. Oz reveals the oil that SHRINKS BELLY FAT! Lose 6 lbs and 5" a week without dieting or working out!" (*Woman's World* is big on exclamation points and capital letters should you miss the import of their words.) The "secret" is safflower oil. "Dr. Oz" is Mehmet Oz, professor of surgery at Columbia University's College of Physicians and Surgeons, and host of *The Dr. Oz Show* which twice has won Daytime Emmy-awards. Unlike Dr. Taller, Dr. Oz need not fear prosecution; the Dietary Supplement Health and Education Act of 1994 that we discussed in chapter 2 has taken care of that threat.

CHAPTER 9

ENHANCEMENT OF PERFORMANCE

Athletic, cognitive, sexual

The idea that drugs, perhaps even certain foods, might enhance athletic performance has been with us for a very long time.[1] There is convincing evidence that participants in the games at Olympia in 776 BC were already exploring the advantages that might be gained from a variety of crude materials which we now know contained alcohol, caffeine, strychnine, and even opium. With the rebirth of the Olympic Games in Athens in 1896 and continuing to 2012 in London, allegations of and, all too often, proof of seeking advantage through chemical means have been quadrennial events. As the medical sciences have advanced so too have the options open to athletes. Human growth hormone and anabolic steroids to increase muscle mass, erythropoietin (EPO) to expand the oxygen carrying capacity of the blood, and stimulants of all kinds are part of a continuing contest between aspiring cheaters and those charged with detecting the cheats. The future promises to be even more complex. Alterations of gene expression and even of genes themselves by the methods of molecular biology seem a likely possibility.

But what do competitive athletes in the prime of their lives have to do with successful aging? The answer is that, unlike athletic events, pharmacological intervention to enhance performance is, in many instances, both ethical and desirable. Furthermore, much as we might learn from the experience of athletes, potential enhancement extends beyond the physical to include the functioning of the nervous system, an issue of direct interest to me and my aging brain.

I will begin with amphetamine, a drug first synthesized in the 1920's. A proud achievement but Mother Nature had beaten the medicinal chemists to performance enhancing substances by countless millennia. When one of our ancestors was confronted by a lion or tiger or perhaps a nasty human carrying a club, that branch of the nervous system called the sympathetic was activated. The messengers of the system are adrenaline and noradrenaline. (American pharmacologists call them epinephrine and norepinephrine.) Acting at multiple sites, these chemicals increase heart rate and the volume of blood pumped, more air flows through the lungs and more blood is directed to our muscles. Just as we would be today, the sympathetic nervous system made our ancestor ready either to flee or to stand his ground. Drugs like amphetamine (now known to many as Adderall, a mixture of amphetamines), which replicate these effects, are called sympathomimetics. Other prominent members of the family are methamphetamine, methylphenidate (Ritalin), and cocaine.

Sympathomimetic drugs also act directly upon the brain. If sleepy, we become alert. If fatigued, we become energized. The most significant mediator of these effects is an increase in levels of dopamine, a brain chemical closely related to adrenaline. Brain circuits in which dopamine serves as the neurotransmitter are intimately involved in all manner of pleasure: food, drugs, sex, Rock and Roll, you name it, all trigger release of dopamine. In chemically mimicking these naturally occurring pleasurable events, sympathomimetics such as cocaine can induce euphoria, a major contributor to their addictive properties

The ability of sympathomimetic drugs to counter fatigue and increase endurance did not go unnoticed by the military. During Germany's *Blitzkrieg* of 1939-40 in which Poland, the Netherlands, Belgium, and France were overrun, it is estimated that 35 million tablets of methamphetamine, known to the Germans as Pervitin, were issued to ground troops and pilots.[2]

After conducting a series of laboratory and field tests with amphetamine purchased from Smith Kline & French, an American pharmaceutical house, Britain's Royal Air Force began in 1942 to issue the drug to crews of Bomber Command. Bernard Montgomery, famed for his defeat of Erwin Rommel in tank battles at El Alamein, was a particular advocate of amphetamine use and issued it to all in his Middle East group.

Following experiments by Andrew Ivy in medical students at Northwestern University, the United States military made amphetamine available to all theater commanders in early 1943. General Dwight Eisenhower, then Supreme Commander of the North African Theater of Operations, requested three million tablets. Stimulant use by the US military has continued to this day, in war and in peace. (Richard Friedman, professor of psychiatry at Weill Cornell Medical School, has hypothesized that the recent use of stimulants by soldiers in Iraq and Afghanistan increases the likelihood of post-traumatic stress disorder.)

Despite the acceptance of stimulants by the military, there remained uncertainty as to exactly what the drugs were doing. Many regarded them only as a means to elevate soldiers' mood and to boost morale. However, in a series of experiments conducted in the late 1950's by Henry K. Beecher, professor of anesthesiology at Harvard Medical School, it was clearly shown that performance by collegiate swimmers could be improved by 1 to 2% by modest doses of amphetamine.[3] Not much, you might say, but recall that the difference between winning and losing in elite competition can be very slight indeed. For example, at the 2012 London Olympics, swimmer Nathan Adrian of the United States won the men's 100 meter freestyle event by one one-hundredth of a second over James Mannussen of Australia. That's a difference of 0.02%. The fourth place finisher's time was only 0.7% slower than the winner. Given the promise of even a slight gain in performance and given the very significant financial rewards to be had, it is not difficult to understand why a sport such as professional cycling could be plagued with instances of stimulant use.

What about a role for sympathomimetics in improving the functioning of my aging brain? Might an age-related memory impairment be improved? Might I better remember the name of the person I was introduced to this morning or the star of the movie I saw just yesterday but can't recall? In contrast with physical activities, the answer is a bit murkier. When Henry Beecher tested the effects of amphetamine on performance in calculus, no improvement was seen.[4] (I didn't mention earlier that his subjects were students at the Massachusetts Institute of Technology. At M.I.T. calculus is a second language known to all.) But the story doesn't end there. Despite remaining uncertainties about the effects of stimulants on mental processes, we today have millions of children being treated with sympathomimetic drugs to improve their school performance and countless adults seeking a boost to their careers.

What we now call attention deficit hyperactivity disorder or simply ADHD had its origins in 1937 in a residential school for unruly children, mostly boys.[5] There it was observed that amphetamine had a seemingly paradoxical calming influence accompanied by increased attentiveness to school work. In the United States in 2013, 3.5 million children, age 17 or younger, were treated with stimulants following a diagnosis of ADHD. Indeed, many parents actively seek the ADHD label for their teenagers in the hope that test scores, including those on the SAT, will improve. Some well-intended physicians prescribe the drugs for poor children in the hope that they will compensate for the multiple adverse effects that poverty has on learning. An additional 1.5 million older Americans are treated for the adult version of ADHD. Professional athletes may receive that diagnosis and with it ready access to amphetamines or methylphenidate.

As was noted in chapter 3, depressed mood is a common accompaniment of old age and is the frequent target of pharmacological intervention. Might the acknowledged mood enhancing effects of sympathomimetics be useful? More than a century ago, Sigmund Freud said this of coca, the natural source of cocaine: "In my last severe depression, I took coca again and a small dose lifted me to the heights in a wonderful fashion...I expect it will win its place in therapeutics by the side of morphine and superior to it." Indeed, before the discovery of the drugs presently used to treat depression, amphetamines were widely prescribed for that purpose. In the late 1940's, an advertisement for Dexedrine (*dextro*-amphetamine) showed a smiling housewife running her vacuum cleaner together with the words "for proved antidepressant effect---both rapid and prolonged." To this day, respected textbooks of geriatric medicine often suggest the use of methylphenidate for mild depression in the elderly. In 2013 the United Nations Convention on Narcotic Drugs legitimized the chewing of coca leaves in Bolivia, a practice begun several millennia ago.[7] The United States was one of the minority of nations to object.

It sounds good to this point: increased physical performance, improved concentration, elevated mood. Are septuagenarians, and those even older, candidates for stimulant treatment? Should every old person get a trial with an amphetamine? To answer that question we need to consider what is called the benefit-risk ratio. The potential benefits I have listed. Now we must consider the potential risks.

We have all heard stories of persons, often elderly, who have dropped dead of a heart attack or stroke upon being confronted by an intruder or upon greeting a long lost relative. Is there such a thing as dying of fright or happiness? Recall that one of the effects of stimulation of the sympathetic nervous system is to increase the rate of beating and force of contraction of the heart. Accompanying those desired actions, blood pressure is elevated and, particularly, in the elderly, the risk of stroke increases. In addition, a rapidly beating heart is more likely to experience arrhythmia, a disordered pattern of beating which may lead to cardiac standstill and death. Sympathomimetic drugs can produce similar effects and are of particular concern in the aged heart.

I have already noted Freud's endorsement of cocaine as a means to elevate mood. But one need not be depressed to experience such effects. In describing his first use of methamphetamine, the American writer Nick Sheff said "My God, this is what I have been missing my entire life."[8] These euphorigenic properties of cocaine and the amphetamines are a major factor in their potential for addiction. Addiction, the behavioral state of compulsive, uncontrollable drug craving and seeking, was discussed more fully in chapter 1. Suffice to say that it is a condition best avoided. It is for this reason that the prescription of amphetamines for their appetite-suppressing properties is banned in New York State and elsewhere. The risk of abuse simply outweighs the potential benefit of weight loss.

Countless studies over many decades have concluded that benefits may be derived from the use of cocaine and amphetamines in the aged, whether for improving physical performance, elevating mood, or stimulating mental activity. However, these desired effects are generally outweighed by concerns about adverse cardiac events and the risk of compulsive use. However, with increasing acceptance of the use of stimulants for adult ADHD, apparently with minimal adverse effects, we may soon have a reexamination of their use in the elderly. In the meantime, we have other drugs to consider.

Narcolepsy is a condition in which a person may have a sudden onset of sleep sometimes accompanied by hallucinations. Amphetamines have been used extensively in the treatment of narcolepsy but, as with all other uses of these drugs, there is concern about adverse effects including addiction. Michel Jouvet, now Emeritus Professor of Experimental Medicine at Claude Bernard University in Lyon, France, has devoted his professional life to the study of sleep and its disorders and has published a number of popular books on the subject. It was thus not surprising that an alternative stimulant, modafinil, would be brought to his attention by its French discoverers. In the mid-1980's, Professor Jouvet reported that modafinil was effective in narcolepsy.[9] The United States Food and Drug Administration approved the drug for that condition in 1998 to be sold by Cephalon, an American pharmaceutical house, with the name Provigil. Later the FDA allowed its prescription for night shift workers and for excessive sleepiness associated with obstructive sleep apnea. In 2009, with the patent protection running out on Provigil, Cephalon introduced a closely related drug, armodafinil, under the trade name Nuvigil. A third member of the family is adrafinil, sold on line with the name Olmifon.

Modafinil remains a bit of an enigma in terms of its mechanism of action. Initially it was thought to act in a fashion distinct from that of cocaine and the amphetamines. However, more recent studies suggest that it, like the amphetamines and cocaine, increases levels of dopamine and norepinephrine, the neurotransmitters intimately involved with pleasure, addiction, and alertness. In 2009, Nora Volkow, Director of the National Institute on Drug Abuse, and her colleagues at Brookhaven National Laboratory, provided evidence in human subjects that modafinil acts in a fashion much more like cocaine and the amphetamines than had been suspected. She went on to call for "heightened awareness for potential abuse and dependence…in vulnerable populations."[10]

Although the use of modafinil is now widespread, there are few reports of adverse effects and little to suggest that it is cocaine-like in it abuse liability. The Drug Enforcement Administration has placed it in schedule IV meaning that it has accepted medical uses and a low potential for abuse. Many in the military believe that it provides a reasonable alternative to the amphetamines in sustaining alertness. Suggestions for the use of modafinil range from attention deficit disorder to schizophrenia to the treatment of stimulant abuse. Efficacy in none of these conditions has been proven. Nonetheless, I look forward to careful studies in aged populations particularly with respect to age-related memory impairment.

Richard Ben Cramer won the Pulitzer Prize for international reporting in 1979. His obituary in the *New York Times* in 2013 was written by Margalit Fox.[11] In it she says that "he ritually began his day with five cups of coffee, purchased en masse from the (*Baltimore Sun*) cafeteria, lined up on his desk and drunk in quick caffeinated succession." Caffeine is the most widely consumed stimulant drug in the world and I feel safe in saying that nearly every reader of these words has consumed caffeine today in the form of tea, coffee, chocolate or a soft drink. Making consumption of caffeine even more likely is the rise of "sports", "performance", and "energy" drinks. Most of these are witches' brews of sugar, B vitamins, and various exotic ingredients. But make no mistake, Red Bull, Rockstar Energy, Monster Energy, 5-Hour Energy and virtually all the rest depend on caffeine for any significant effects. No-Doz and Vivarin are just plain caffeine and much cheaper.

More than a century ago, March 16, 1912 to be exact, a brief item in the *Journal of the American Medical Association* summarized studies of caffeine on "mental and motor efficiency."[12] One of the tasks employed was typewriting; both speed and accuracy were improved. Similar beneficial effects were observed in other mental and physical tasks and, with the exception of a slight decrement in holding the outstretched hand steady, no adverse effects were noted.

What have we learned about caffeine in the last 100 years? Well, we now talk with confidence about its mechanism of action. In chapter 1, I introduced you to the concept of the drug receptor. Caffeine acts primarily on the adenosine receptors of the brain. These systems exert a generally suppressive effect on nervous activity and are thought to play a major role in sleep. The ability of caffeine to counter fatigue and prolong wakefulness is thus due to a blockade of elements of the adenosine system. In addition, there is convincing evidence that caffeine, again acting via adenosine, enhances the release of dopamine, one of the neurotransmitters via which cocaine and the amphetamines act.

Having mentioned the amphetamines in the same sentence with caffeine, it is important that we compare and contrast them. With respect to performance enhancing and anti-fatigue effects, the World War II studies that I mentioned earlier often found them to be quite comparable in improving the ability of a fatigued subject to maintain attention to a task. For these purposes, caffeine is a remarkably effective drug.

In chapter 1, I described the related phenomena of drug tolerance, physical dependence, and addiction. Do those who regularly ingest caffeine become tolerant to the effects of the drug? Yes, to a moderate degree. No harm is done. Does physical dependence accompany this tolerance? Yes. The classic withdrawal symptom for caffeine is headache often accompanied by irritability. Is it appropriate to speak of caffeine addicts? My answer to that question is a tentative yes. For example, coffee drinkers familiar to me do appear to engage in compulsive drug craving and seeking, a part of our definition of addiction. However, it appears that cocaine or amphetamine-induced addiction is far more compelling. But what really sets caffeine apart as a stimulant is the response of our society to it. Unlike cocaine and the amphetamines, we do not put people in jail for the use or sale of caffeine.

Beginning in 2006, there began to appear scattered accounts of fatalities in Canada and the United States related to caffeine ingestion in the form of energy drinks. By the end of 2012, the Food and Drug Administration had received reports of about two dozen deaths associated with the use of drinks such as 5-Hour Energy, Red Bull, and Rockstar Energy Drink. The number of emergency room visits involving energy drinks doubled between 2007 and 2011. In about half of these, alcohol or another drug was taken in combination with the energy drink.

The complex interaction between drugs and underlying disease is illustrated by the death in 2011 of Anais Fournier, a 14-year-old Maryland girl.[13] She consumed about 48 ounces of Monster Energy Drink over a two day period. The medical examiner attributed her death to the toxic effects of caffeine on her heart. That much Monster Energy Drink contains about 500 mg of caffeine, roughly the amount in Richard Ben Cramer's five cups of coffee. However, unlike Mr. Cramer, Anais suffered from a genetic disorder in which connective tissue is defective. Science cannot decide the respective roles in her death of that disease, the caffeine, or their combination. The lesson for all of us is that the heart, especially an aged heart, is not an organ to be trifled with.

A recent basis for optimism regarding coffee drinking comes from a huge study conducted under the auspices of the National Institutes of Health and the AARP.[14] After excluding persons with pre-existing cancer or heart disease or who had previously suffered a stroke, the investigators ended up with 402,260 men and women age 50 to 71. A questionnaire was completed and the participants were then followed for 14 years. During that period, there were 52,515 deaths (13%).

First the bad news: coffee drinkers, both men and women, were more likely to die. However, coffee drinkers were also more likely to smoke cigarettes, less likely to exercise, and ate fewer fruits and vegetables. Now the good news: when the role of smoking, exercise, and diet were excluded by statistical methods, coffee drinkers had a reduced risk of death due to heart or lung disease, stroke, diabetes, and infection; incidence of cancer was unchanged. About one-third of the subjects drank decaffeinated coffee and were equally well protected thus suggesting that the essential factor in coffee may be other than caffeine. In concluding their 2012 report in the *New England Journal of Medicine,* Neal Freedman and his colleagues said this: "Our results provide reassurance with respect to the concern that coffee drinking might adversely affect health."

Amphetamine, methylphenidate, cocaine, modafinil, caffeine: each of these drugs can, under appropriate circumstances, improve physical and mental performance, alleviate fatigue, and brighten mood. Their future role in medicine, geriatric medicine in particular, and in everyday life remains to be established. But what of all those wonderful-sounding things promoted in the print and television media and available via the internet? A full page advertisement in USA Today is typical: "Memory pill does for the brain what prescription glasses do for the eyes…restore up to 15 years of lost memory power in as little as 30 days!…Revitalizes tired sluggish brain cells…reenergize your brain and restore its health."

You will notice a subtle difference in this approach. The advertised potion is not, like caffeine or modafinil or amphetamine, simply enhancing performance of a normal brain. Instead, we are being told that our brains have deteriorated and need to be restored. This being the message, it is not surprising that many such products contain vitamins, most often the B vitamins we talked about earlier. In addition, there usually will be a variety of botanical materials, often with exotic names and histories in some ancient medical practice. One such product contains 22 separate ingredients. The claims made for these products neatly elude any meaningful control thanks to the Dietary Supplement Health and Education Act of 1994 discussed in chapter 2. Despite their extravagant advertising and unsubstantiated promises of efficacy, no benefit will be derived from such "brain supplements." However, be assured that your brain, like your heart, will benefit from a nutritious diet and physical exercise.

If I were designing a potion to be sold as a brain restorer, I would follow the pattern of all those snake oil salesmen who have come before me. But, to a complex mix of botanicals and vitamins, I would add one more thing: lots of caffeine. Indeed, if I were really adventuresome, and had my plane ticket to a country with no extradition treaty with the United States in hand, I would add a significant amount of modafinil or amphetamine or cocaine. It is drugs such as caffeine and the amphetamines which have proven efficacy rather than any concoction of vitamins and herbal materials.

I mentioned the possibility of "dying of fright" due to overstimulation of the sympathetic nervous system. Another phrase, "trembling with excitement", also a consequence of sympathetic stimulation, reminds us that our performance might sometimes be enhanced by dampening our excitation. Indeed, millions of Americans take a drug every day to do just that as a part of a drug cocktail to treat high blood pressure. The drugs used are called *beta*-adrenoceptor antagonists or simply *beta* blockers. One member of this drug family familiar to many is metoprolol under the trade names of Toprol and Lopressor.

Imagine that you are about to shoot a pistol in Olympic competition or are walking across the stage of Carnegie Hall for your solo violin debut. Your heart is racing and your hands tremble with excitement. Might metoprolol improve your performance by slowing your heart and abolishing the tremor? That question was answered decades ago in the affirmative in carefully designed experiments in competitive shooters[15] and professional musicians.[16] The effect on rifle and pistol accuracy is significant enough that *beta*-blockers are banned in Olympic shooting competitions. No such ban is imposed on musicians or others encountering stage freight for any reason.

In chapters 4 and 5, I went on at some length regarding the virtues of regular physical exercise of both the aerobic and anaerobic kind. But what about exercise of the brain itself? Well, we do it all the time; it's called cognitive activity: thinking, planning, solving problems, laying down memories, experiencing the people, the places, the things which surround us. Numerous studies have found a correlation between life-long brain activity and a diminished probability of dementia in old age. However, life-long brain activity is also correlated with education, socio-economic status, obesity, illicit drug use, smoking, nutrition, and a variety of other factors. The relative contributions of these elements to the aging of the brain have not yet been teased out. But what about improving my brain function right now, perhaps even increasing my IQ?

The basic functional unit of the brain is the neuron. We all have a lot of them. A recent estimate puts the number at about 86 billion.[17] Were that not sufficient complexity, there are as well many billion supporting cells. Furthermore, each neuron may communicate with several thousand other neurons. The nature of this communication is both electrical and chemical. An electrical signal moves from a neuron down its axon, the wire if you will, to connect with another neuron. But the connection is not direct. Instead, from the end of the axon, a chemical is released which then moves to the receptive neuron at a junction called the synapse, hence the term synaptic transmission. When an advertisement tells you that you may have a "chemical imbalance", it is referring to one or another of these neurotransmitters. Much mentioned today are neurochemicals such as serotonin and dopamine.

Until relatively recently, the prevailing view was that we are born with all the brain cells we will ever have, that we will progressively lose these cells as we age, and that connections between neurons is unchanging over time. However, beginning in the early decades of the 20th century, a series of findings, including the demonstration that we constantly form new neurons, has led us to the concept of neuroplasticity. This is the idea that not only is our brain undergoing constant remodeling but also that we can influence this remodeling by what we do and the drugs we take. For example, a currently popular conception of drug addiction is that the brain is physically altered. David Wilcox, a musician, not a neuroscientist, put it nicely: "My old addiction changed the wiring in my brain."

In 2008, a group led by Martin Buschkuehl and Suzanne Jaeggi of the University of Bern in Switzerland and the University of Michigan reported that their memory training program could produce lasting improvements in problem solving, stave off age-related memory impairment, and even increase intelligence.[18] Despite the inability of others to replicate their findings, a minor industry was born. As of this writing, there are nearly two dozen training programs which offer to improve the functioning of our brains. They carry names such as Brain Spa ("exercise your brain and stimulate mental fitness"), HAPPYneuron ("stimulate your cognitive function"), Cogmed ("a solution for attention problems"), and Brain Age ("train your brain in minutes a day"). Such programs were said to bring in more than $1 billion in 2012 with rapid growth expected. Just five years after the reports by Buschkuehl and Jaeggi, a similar program under the trade name Lumosity advertised that it had 50 million users.

Although skeptics remain and there is little doubt that claims for the programs are influenced by the financial interests of their sellers, a study sponsored by the National Institute on Aging and reported in 2014 gives modest support.[19] Begun in 1998, it was called Advanced Cognitive Training for Independent and Vital Elderly (ACTIVE). Participants numbered 2,832 with an average age of 74 years. All were free of physical or cognitive impairments and were living in the community. They were assigned to one of three training programs focused on memory, reasoning, or speed-of-processing. A fourth group served as a no-contact control. Training consisted of ten 60-75 minute training sessions conducted over a period of 5 to 6 weeks. As expected, all training groups showed immediate improvement in their assigned cognitive tasks. More remarkable was the observation that improvement in the reasoning and speed of processing was retained 10 years later. Unfortunately, no significant retention was seen in the memory group and only very modest improvements in daily functioning were observed. Nonetheless, the results of ACTIVE provide the first unbiased evidence that such training may produce lasting benefit. What is yet to be determined is whether a formal program of training is superior to simple, pleasurable activities of the mind. (My insurance company has already offered me something called Drivesharp™ Online Training designed to improve my attention to hazards on the road.)

As I noted above, it is now an accepted fact that, in a process called neurogenesis, new neurons are constantly being created in our brains. At the present time, we don't know how to influence that process but I would note that, at least in rodents, physical exercise promotes neurogenesis. Once again, there is every reason to believe that what is good for your heart is good for your brain.

Earlier, in speaking of obesity and ways to lose weight, I said that an extraterrestrial might think these to be the most important health issues facing us. However, after exposure to prime time television, our visitor could be inclined to place erectile dysfunction, or ED as the ads like to call it, close behind. Virtually every household in the country has been exposed to exhortations to "be ready when she is" and the problem of "an erection lasting more than four hours." Blame pharmacological science. More about that in a moment.

Impotence, the inability to attain or maintain a penile erection sufficient for successful vaginal intercourse, is not a new condition; it is mentioned in the Ebers Papyrus which tells us much about medicine in Egypt some 4,000 years ago. Contemporary writers speak of it often, sometimes subtly as with John Updike's "when the apparatus fails", sometimes not so subtly; Philip Roth's laments on aging and the "spigot of wrinkled flesh" come to mind.

Erectile dysfunction is relatively uncommon in men younger than 40 years but then steadily increases until, beyond age 70, it is seen in three-quarters or more. While age is the most common risk factor, ED, especially in younger men, can be a result of high blood pressure, type 2 diabetes, or obesity. Many now regard ED in young men as a marker for heart disease. Numerous studies have found treatment of these factors to improve ED together with many other benefits.

For some men and their partners, impotence in advanced age comes as a relief while others regard it as a major health problem. Over the centuries, many have sought and many have claimed to have found true aphrodisiacs, substances to arouse sexual desire. Most are fanciful; to this day, items such as powdered horn of the rhinoceros are sold in teahouses from Queens to Beijing. In a charming book published in 2014 called *Plants with Benefits*, Helen Yoest tells us of the many fruits and vegetables and other foods reputed to be aphrodisiacal.[20] Her prescription for a pre-sex meal is champagne, almond soup, quinoa salad, and chocolate. I can't testify to the efficacy of the prescription but it hard to argue with any of the ingredients. Anything to increase the intake of fruits and vegetables with a little alcohol and chocolate thrown in can't be bad.

Agents to increase sexual desire are one thing but what shall we do when the mind is willing but, to use Updike's phrase, "the equipment fails." This brings us back to pharmacology and male physiology. Imagine the penis to be an air mattress but, instead of air being pumped in, it is blood that causes it to inflate. In fact, the external male urethra is surrounded by two columns of spongy tissue called the corpora cavernosa. When excited by sight or touch or thought, blood flows into the corpora, exit of the blood is blocked by compression of the veins of the penis, and an erection results.

Blood flow in our arteries is under the control of the smooth muscle which lines these vessels. Between the smooth muscle and the blood is a second layer of cells, the endothelium. In the late 1970's, Robert Furchgott, a professor of pharmacology at the Downstate Medical Center in Brooklyn, identified a chemical released from the endothelium which is able to relax the arterial muscle leading to increased blood flow.[21] Because its composition was unknown, it was simply called EDRF, endothelium-derived relaxing factor. In the decade which followed, it was shown that EDRF is in fact nitric oxide, the chemical responsible for the relaxation of coronary blood vessels by nitroglycerin in the treatment of angina pectoris. Furthermore, it was shown that nitric oxide acts to relax arterial muscle via a second messenger whose activity is limited by the enzyme, phosphodiesterase, responsible for its breakdown. Inhibit that enzyme and levels of the second messenger are maintained and arterial relaxation continues. (For their discoveries,

Furchgott, together with the Americans Ferid Murad and Louis Ignarro, received the Nobel Prize for Physiology or Medicine in 1998.)

These findings did not go unnoticed by the pharmaceutical industry. In the hope that they might find a phosphodiesterase inhibitor that would be useful in relaxing blood vessels in the treatment of conditions such as high blood pressure and angina pectoris, chemists at the British research laboratories of Pfizer synthesized a series of drugs. One of these, sildenafil, produced disappointing results with respect to angina but it was noted by the investigators that penile erections often occurred in their subjects. This predictable but nonetheless remarkable property was first brought to the attention of the medical community in 1996 and sildenafil was approved by the Food and Drug Administration on March 27, 1998 with the name Viagra. An obvious advantage of Viagra is that it can be taken by mouth; a previous treatment for ED required penile injection, a squirm-inducing thought for most men. Viagra was soon followed in the marketplace by drugs acting in the same fashion. These now include vardenafil (Levitra), tadalafil (Cialus), and, most recently approved, avanafil (Stendra). Prescription sales of these drugs in the United States exceeded $4 billion in 2014 in addition to a vigorous black market.

So far, Viagra and its relatives appear to be quite safe though the advertisements ask that you make sure that "your heart is healthy enough for sexual activity." Exactly how that is to be determined is unclear and there certainly have been deaths due to heart attack associated with the use of these drugs. A fatalist might suggest that the men died happy but the victims are not available for comment. The contribution which ED treatments have made to an increase in sexually transmitted disease in those over the age of 50 is uncertain but there is a significant correlation between the number of prescriptions for these drugs and the incidence of HIV/AIDS, syphilis, and gonorrhea in this population.[22] A probable contributor is that, freed of concerns about pregnancy, condom use is less common than in younger men. It would appear that sex education should not be reserved for adolescents and young adults.

CHAPTER 10

STEROIDS

From Dog testicles to "Is It Low T?"

Sequarine: The medicine of the future. The mere fact that scientists are now able to transfer the energy from one animal body to another is sufficient to rouse enthusiasm among Doctors. Sequarine is being used with astonishing success in treating nervousness, arthritis, sciatica, diabetes, kidney and liver disease, general weakness, and a variety of other disorders.

I didn't find that description of Sequarine on the internet though it may look familiar to those who read 21st century ads online, in magazines, or on television. No, it comes from an advertisement published in 1912 for extracts prepared from the testicles of dogs. Not mentioned are the purported effects of Sequarine on your sex life; that would be too racy for the reader of that time. Sequarine took its name from Charles-Edouard Brown-Sequard. A physician and scientist, he held prestigious academic posts in France, England, and in the United States at the Harvard Medical School before finally settling in Paris as professor of experimental medicine in the *College de France*. It was April in Paris in 1889 when, at the age of 72, Brown-Sequard stood before the *Societie de Biology* and told of injecting himself with testicular extracts which, in his words, "have taken 30 years off my life."[1] (For those keeping score, Brown-Sequard died five years later.)

The notion that a person with a malfunctioning organ might benefit from consuming the same organ taken from an animal is both plausible and ancient. Prescriptions such as rabbit brain for mental disorders and lung of the fox for problems of breathing can be found in the earliest medical writings. However, a scientific basis for this idea did not come until the mid-19th century. Arnold Berthold, a professor of physiology at the University of Gottingen, proposed that the testes are necessary for the development of male characteristics. This was not a new idea, three hundred years before the birth of Christ, Aristotle said that "All animals when castrated change over to the female state." But Professor Berthold did more than hypothesize. He observed that young castrated male chickens fail to develop into roosters but instead are smaller, less aggressive, and have little interest in mating. Remarkably, Berthold found that replacement of the testes by implantation in the abdomen reversed these deficits. He correctly concluded that the testes must be secreting a substance responsible for these effects.[2] Though Berthold's work was largely ignored at the time and Brown-Sequard's testicular extracts were widely ridiculed, they laid the groundwork for endocrinology, that branch of medical science concerned with the internal secretions we now call hormones

Endocrinology began, not with testes, but with another gland, the thyroid. Myxedema is the name given to the disease resulting from an underactive thyroid. Signs and symptoms vary with the severity of the deficiency but commonly include fatigue, depression, hair loss, and, less commonly, a peculiar psychosis called myxedema madness. A hypothyroid woman may give birth to a cretin, a child who suffers severe mental and physical retardation. In 1891, an English physician, George Murray, successfully treated myxedema with injections of an extract from the thyroid of a sheep. Twenty-four years later the American chemist, Edward C. Kendall, isolated the active principle, later to be named thyroxine, from three tons of hog thyroid glands.[3] Thyroxine is still used today to treat hypothyroidism.

The progression from a crude glandular preparation to the isolation of a pure active principle such as thyroxine was later repeated with testosterone. This time however, the raw material was 40 pounds of bull testicles obtained from the Chicago stockyards by Fred C. Koch, professor of physiological chemistry at the University of Chicago. In 1927, Koch demonstrated that his bull extract could restore male sexual characteristics to castrated animals. Eight years later, the active principle of Koch's extract was identified, the name testosterone given to it, and chemical synthesis became possible.[4] The availability of pure testosterone triggered a remarkable growth in human research during the decades surrounding World War II.

We know much about the effects of testosterone deprivation, hypogonadism, because men have been castrating other men and boys for thousands of years. The reasons for doing so have been varied, sometimes subjugation or punishment, in other instances with the thought that eunuchs could serve in a sultan's harem without temptation. The pure soprano singing voice of pre-pubertal boys can be preserved only by removal of the testes. For more than three hundred years, the Catholic Church sanctioned the castration of boys at age seven or eight for that purpose. These castrati served most famously in the choir of the Sistine Chapel in Rome into the early years of the 20th century.

Soon after Koch's isolation of testosterone, his University of Chicago colleague, Allan Kenyon, found that treatment with testosterone in hypogonadal men and women not only enhanced, to varying degrees, sexual characteristics and libido appropriate to the gender but also caused a gain in body weight with the suggestion that a portion of this gain was due to increased muscle mass.[5] If it strikes you as odd that female eunuchs might benefit sexually from testosterone, it turns out that women derive some of the same sexual consequences, so called androgenic effects, as do men. In addition, it was later learned that testosterone is converted by both men and women into estrogen.

Testosterone is a member of a family of chemicals, the steroids, which includes cholesterol, well-known in terms of heart disease but also the source of my body's testosterone. The muscle-promoting ability of testosterone, termed anabolic effects, did not go unnoticed by athletes of all kinds. Indeed, the use of anabolic steroids is now well known to even the casual reader of the sports pages. It became clear in the latter part of the 20th century that countless amateur and professional athletes used anabolic steroids, usually in conjunction with weight training, to enhance muscle mass and strength. To the sports aficionado the names are familiar: Ben Johnson and Marion Jones in track, Andy Pettit, Roger Clemons, and Alex Rodriguez of the New York Yankees, in cycling, Floyd Landis and Lance Armstrong; the list is long indeed.

Quite aside from the ethical issues involved, we must be concerned that, as with every drug we know, adverse effects emerge as doses are increased in an attempt to achieve even greater benefits. Barry Bonds, the noted baseball player, might serve as a poster boy. His long-time mistress testified in court that, as a result of his use of anabolic steroids, Bonds suffered from acne, diminished sexual interest and performance, and shrunken testicles.[6] Because of the partial conversion of testosterone to estrogen, gynecomastia, enlargement of the male breast, is not uncommon with pharmacological doses of anabolic steroids. In women, the most notable effects are virilism; women become more manlike with an increase in muscle mass but accompanied by a deepening of the voice and growth of hair in all the wrong places. The most dramatic demonstrations of virilism were provided by the state-sponsored track and field and swimming programs in the Soviet Union and East Germany during the 1970's.[7] It should be noted that these programs contributed to remarkable athletic performances, an outcome not lost on many aspiring young and not so young athletes.

No sports organization in the world advocates the use of testosterone or other performance-enhancing drugs. Indeed most now conduct regular tests designed to detect their use. However, a far more subtle and in many ways more appealing promotion of the use of testosterone for both androgenic and anabolic effects is presently underway. To quote a recent advertisement: "Sluggish? Low energy? No sexual drive? Low testosterone? Attack the nasty symptoms of male menopause and make yourself strong, sexy, and virile again." In 2012, more than $100 million was spent to bring this message to the men of the United States. Money well spent: this campaign resulted in sales of more than $2 billion.[8]

Testosterone levels in the male fluctuate markedly during fetal development and in the first three months after birth. Precise regulation of testosterone during this period is essential for appropriate sexual development. Testosterone then falls to very low levels only to rise again with the onset of puberty. The peak is reached at about age eighteen and is maintained into the mid-twenties. Testosterone then begins a long slow decline until, at age 80, the level of free testosterone is perhaps 50% of that in a healthy young male.[9] Might it be that this decline of testosterone with age accounts for common accompaniments of aging: decreased muscle mass and bone density, increased fat around the middle, and diminished sexual interest and performance? Might it be that all men can remain functional 20-somethings, a kind of perpetual youth, if only there is enough testosterone? If women can have hormone replacement therapy, why not men?

In recent years there has grown up a minor medical industry devoted to promoting the idea that all men need supplemental testosterone. Prominent in the industry is an American physician, Jeffrey Life, a partner in the Cenegenics Medical Institute located in Las Vegas. Dr. Life was the subject of a 2011 feature article by Catherine Mayer in *Time* Magazine.[10] There we learned that the program includes "nutrition, exercise, and hormone optimization." Ms. Mayer was offered testosterone and DHEA, short for dihydroepiandrosterone, a hormone secreted by the adrenal glands in both men and women. Like testosterone, DHEA has anabolic effects and, like testosterone, levels decline with age. In the body, DHEA is converted into androstenedione, the drug used by Mark McGwire while breaking major league baseball's record for home runs in 1998. If you should decide that the Life program is for you, Ms. Mayer tells us that the initial consultation and tests cost $3,400 and maintenance runs about $1,000 a month. Testosterone levels in women are typically only 5-10% those of the male but, as in men, there is a decrease with age and, as was the case for Ms. Mayer, augmentation is suggested for the same reasons, including a waning sex life. I should add that Dr. Life is hardly alone in this endeavor. In a website called *isitlowT.com*, you will find numerous pharmaceutical houses touting their testosterone products and urging you to "talk to your doctor" about "increasing your sexual power."

The rationale for testosterone replacement therapy in aging men and women is so clear and so appealing one might think that medical groups around the world would endorse it. They do not. The major concern centers on cancer. A consensus statement prepared for the International Society of Andrology and the International Society for the Study of the Aging Male says this: "Testosterone administration is absolutely contraindicated in men suspected of or having carcinoma of the prostate or breast."[11] Not a problem you might say. Why not just rule out those cancers and get on with the restoration of my virility and all those other good things? To answer that question we need to talk a bit about the prostate.

Most men begin to take note of their prostate gland in early middle age. It is at this time that the prostate begins to enlarge, an almost universal condition called benign prostatic hyperplasia or hypertrophy, BPH for short. The enlarged prostate may compress the urethra leading, in most cases, to nothing more than the inconvenience of getting up in the middle of the night to urinate. Cancer of the prostate is another matter entirely. In the United States alone, about 200,000 new cases are diagnosed each year and it kills more American men than any other cancer with the exception of that of the lung.[12]

We no longer castrate boys to maintain their singing voices. Nonetheless, this year in the United States and Canada alone, about 60,000 men will be castrated either surgically or chemically. The reason is that just as certain forms of breast cancer are stimulated by estrogen, the prostate itself and cancer of the prostate are stimulated by testosterone. The treatment of choice for locally advanced or high-risk non-metastatic prostate cancer is called androgen deprivation therapy and it is achieved either by removal of the testes or by chemical suppression of testosterone production. Does this fact plant a seed of doubt in your mind regarding the wisdom of contravening nature to restore in old age my testosterone level to that of a hormone-driven teenager? "But wait", you reply, "that caution applies only if I have prostate cancer." And that brings us to another fact regarding the disease.

Numerous studies which began in 1935 have shown that as men age there is an increasing probability that cancer cells will be present in the prostate. At age 60, this will be true for half of all men and by age 80 two-thirds or more will be affected. The vast majority of these men will die of causes other than prostate cancer. Indeed, barring an autopsy, none will have been aware of the cancer. I will quote from just one recent study. In 2010, Isaac Powell and his colleagues at the Wayne State University School of Medicine in Detroit reported that autopsies on 1,056 men aged 20 to 79 *who had died of causes other than prostate cancer,* revealed its presence in 45%.[13] There was a steady increase with age until, in the 70 to 79 year-old group, it reached 72%. Observations such as these have led to the conclusion that, beyond a certain age, we are better off not knowing about these cells. Use of a screening device such as a test for prostate specific antigen (PSA) is not recommended at all in most European countries and, in this country, the National Comprehensive Cancer Network recommends that it stop at age 75. The risks of treatment simply outweigh the benefits to be derived.

It is likely then that during my life I, together with a majority of men will, in fact, have cancerous cells in my prostate. Will these cells spread or will they lie quiescent until another cause of death overtakes me? Might lifelong maintenance of a testosterone level appropriate for a young adult stimulate these cells to progress to a life-threatening disease? We presently have no answers to these questions. They might be provided by something akin to the Women's Health Initiative. Enroll perhaps 100,000 men, assign them to testosterone supplementation or placebo, wait 10 or 20 years for the consequences to be known, and hope for the best. Alas, I may not be here to learn the results of that study, if indeed it is ever undertaken. But, for now, I say "No, thank you." For those who do choose to supplement with testosterone, my advice is to keep in touch with a urologist who in turn will keep in touch with your prostate.

A second and more ominous cloud has recently appeared on the horizon of those who would sell us testosterone. A study led by Shehzad Basaria of the Boston University School of Medicine and funded by the National Institute on Aging set out to determine if testosterone supplementation would be helpful in older mean with limited mobility; most earlier studies had been conducted in healthy men.[14] Dr. Basaria's patients were all age 65 or older with an average age of 74. In the group there was a high prevalence of high blood pressure, type 2 diabetes, elevated cholesterol, and obesity. As the study progressed, it was clear that those receiving testosterone had greater improvements in strength, a well-established and much coveted effect of testosterone. Nonetheless, in December 2009, the trial was stopped because the board monitoring its safety determined that testosterone treatment was associated with adverse cardiovascular events.

Note much note was taken of the Basaria study; the numbers were small and the trial had not been carried out to its conclusion. However, in November 2013, a group led by Rebecca Vigen of the Southwestern Medical Center in Dallas reported the results of testosterone therapy in 1,223 men treated in the Veterans Administration health care system.[15] They found an increase of 6% in the rate of death, heart attack, and stroke following testosterone supplementation. Reaction to this finding was swift with five letters appearing in the *Journal of the American Medical Association*. All were critical of the conclusions drawn by Dr. Vigen and her colleagues. Interestingly, four of the letters were from physicians with commercial ties to the testosterone industry. Indeed, two of the writers were affiliated with the aforementioned Cenegenics Medical Institute of Las Vegas.[16]

In an attempt to bring closure to the issue of whether testosterone supplementation is bad for the heart, a review of all published studies was undertaken by Lin Xu of the School of Public Health of the University of Hong Kong and her colleagues.[17] They identified 27 trials that met their criteria for inclusion with a total of 2,994 mainly older men. Cardiovascular-related events were recorded. These included heart attack, unstable angina, congestive heart failure, and several other indices of heart disease. Testosterone treatment increased the risk of these events by 54 percent averaged across all of the 27 studies. Remarkably, but not surprisingly, the thirteen trials funded by the testosterone industry found a statistically non-significant benefit while in the fourteen independent studies, risk of adverse effects was more than doubled. I am inclined to put my money on the latter particularly in view of the results of another large study reported in January 2014 which concluded that, in younger men with heart disease and in all men age 65 and older, testosterone treatment increases the risk of heart attack.[18]

As of this writing, it is unclear when, if ever, these questions surrounding testosterone supplements and the risk of prostate cancer or heart attack will definitively be answered. Currently the Food and Drug Administration is evaluating the risk of stroke, heart attack, and possible death in those taking testosterone products and in June 2014 the FDA issued additional warnings about the risk of blood clots. The good news is that if you or a loved one suffer a heart attack or other adverse effect while using testosterone, there will be a lawyer close at hand. For example, a Baltimore firm advertises that they "are reviewing potential lawsuits for testosterone replacement therapy users who have suffered serious health problems from Androgel, Androderm, Axiron, Testim or other testosterone treatments."[19]

My view of testosterone supplements was nicely expressed in a commentary which appeared in the June 2013 issue of the journal *JAMA Internal Medicine*. The authors were Lisa Schwartz and Steven Woloshin of the Veterans Affairs Medical Center in White River Junction, VT. The title they chose was "Low T as in Template *How to sell disease.*"[20]

> …there is a strong analogy between the marketing of testosterone therapy for men and estrogen therapy for women. Ignoring the lessons of estrogen therapy is scandalous. Before anyone makes millions of men aware of Low T, they should be required to do a large-scale randomized trial to demonstrate that testosterone therapy for healthy aging men does more good than harm.

CHAPTER 11

PAIN

A more terrible lord of mankind than even death

The words of Albert Schweitzer provide the title for this chapter. Writing in 1931, Dr. Schweitzer went on to acknowledge that "We must all die but if I can save a person from days of torture, that is what I feel is my great and ever new privilege."[1] Indeed, most of us fear pain and strive to avoid it. Why then does Paul Brand refer to pain as "a gift?"[2] This apparent contradiction provides an introduction to the complexity of pain, its functions, and its relief.

Paul Brand, son of missionary parents, was trained as a surgeon in England but spent his career serving the needs of lepers, first in India and later, beginning in 1966, at the National Leprosarium of the United States in Carville, Louisiana. Leprosy is also called Hansen's disease in honor of the Norwegian physician, Gerhard Armauer Hansen, who in 1874 identified the responsible bacillus, *Mycobacterium leprae*.[3] Known to man for several millennia, the Bible makes multiple references to lepers as "the unclean." Marked by lesions of the face and by suppurating wounds to the hands and feet, lepers have long been rejected by the societies in which they live. It was Dr. Brand who called attention to the nerve damage and loss of sensory function characteristic of the disease. It was this absence of the warning system provided by pain that allowed minor injuries to progress until soft tissue and even bone was lost. In what he called "a terrible irony", Brand "found painlessness to be the single most destructive aspect of this dread disease."

With the exception of those who suffer a rare genetic disorder rendering them insensitive to pain or who have pathological loss of pain sensation as occurs in leprosy, none of us need worry about an absence of pain. We have fully functioning systems which carry painful sensations from the skin and other parts of our bodies via peripheral nerves to the spinal cord whence they rise to the level of consciousness. Indeed, these protective circuits can respond even without conscious intervention. Touch a hot stove and my hand is immediately withdrawn. Only later, as the pain signal moves from the spinal cord to the higher centers of my brain, do I grasp the nature of the painful stimulus. The protective function of pain has served me well: my hand is withdrawn even before I am consciously aware of the hazard and tissue damage is thus minimized. In addition, pain provides the physician an invaluable guide to the diagnosis of disease. It is a cardinal rule of diagnostics not to mask pain before its origin is determined.

Unfortunately, the vast majority of pain afflicting mankind serves no diagnostic or protective purpose. It is that pain we strive to relieve. The most desirable means is the elimination of the disease or condition causing the pain. For example, simply relieving the inflammatory pain caused by a bacterial infection rather than using an appropriate antibiotic is foolish indeed. In most cases, however, immediate removal of the source of pain is not possible and symptomatic relief is then highly desirable.

We may interact with the pain-sensing circuits at any level, from a nerve ending to the spinal cord to those areas of the brain responsible for the perception of pain and our responses to it. At one end of the spectrum is what we now call local anesthesia and, at the other, general anesthesia. Each has its virtues, each its drawbacks.

Fanny Burney, English novelist and playwright, while living in France with her husband received a diagnosis of breast cancer. On September 30th 1811 she underwent a mastectomy. Later, in a letter to her sister, she described her experience.[4]

I mounted therefore, unbidden, the bedstead – and Dr. Dubois placed me upon the mattress, and spread a fine linen handkerchief upon my face. It was transparent, however, and I saw, through it, that the bedstead was instantly surrounded by seven men and my nurse. I refused to be held; but when, bright through the cambric, I saw the glitter of polished steel – I closed my eyes. I would not trust to convulsive fear the sight of the terrible incision. Yet – when the dreadful steel was plunged into the breast – cutting through veins – arteries – flesh – nerves – I needed no injunctions not to restrain my cries. I began a scream that lasted unintermittingly during the whole time of the incision – and I almost marvel that it rings not in my ears still, so excruciating was the agony. When the wound was made, and the instrument was withdrawn, the pain seemed undiminished…I concluded the operation was over – Oh no! presently the terrible cutting was renewed – and worse than ever, to separate the bottom, the foundation of this dreadful gland from the parts to which it adhered – Again all description would be baffled – yet again all was not over…I then felt the knife rackling against the breast bone – scraping it.

Had Fanny Burney's operation taken place just 36 years later, she could have been spared her torment. On October 16th, 1846, a heretofore obscure dentist named William Morton, by means of a simple chemical, rendered Edward Abbott unconscious so that a neck tumor could be removed without pain. The public demonstration by Dr. Morton was sponsored by and the surgery performed by John Collins Warren, a distinguished Harvard Medical School surgeon. The discovery was announced to the world on November 3rd in a paper read before the American Academy of Arts and Sciences by Henry J. Bigelow, then a junior surgeon at Harvard.[5] The chemical used was diethyl ether, a volatile liquid which boils at just 95 degrees Fahrenheit. News of what had transpired quickly spread around the world. In December of that same year, Robert Liston, a renowned surgeon at London's University College Hospital, performed the first operation in Europe under ether anesthesia.[6] The era of general anesthesia had begun. The site of Morton's demonstration, now called the Ether Dome, remains in use today as a part of the Massachusetts General Hospital.

Ether and several other chemicals including nitrous oxide and chloroform had been known to the medical profession for decades but, quite remarkably, had remained curiosities. Indeed, in 1800 Sir Humphry Davy, had made the explicit suggestion that nitrous oxide be used in surgical operations.[7] However, like Ecstasy and the designer drugs of today, these chemicals were largely used by students for recreational purposes. Their ability at low doses to induce a largely happy, drunken state was recognized both in Europe and the United States. One participant in what came to be called "ether frolics" was Crawford Long, a country doctor in Jefferson, Georgia. He noted that he and his friends "received falls and blows" but "did not feel the least pain from these accidents." On March 30th, 1842, fully four years before the ether dome, Long removed a tumor from a patient who "did not experience the slightest degree of pain."[8] However, it was only several years after learning of Morton's demonstration that he published his findings. Thus, it is to Morton that, as a contemporary writer put it, "the chief glory goes."

Despite the rapid adoption of general anesthesia in this country and around the world, not all were pleased with medicine's newly found ability to abolish pain. Objections were usually based on religious grounds especially with regard to childbirth. In 1847, James Young Simpson, professor of obstetrics at Scotland's University of Edinburgh, wrote the following.[9]

Not a few medical men...have refused to relieve their patient from the agonies of childbirth on the allegation that they believed that their employment of suitable anesthetic means for such a purpose would be unscriptural and irreligious. And I am informed that, in another medical school, my conduct in introducing and advocating anesthesia in labor has been publically denounced *ex cathedra* as an attempt to contravene the arrangements and decrees of Providence, hence being reprehensible and heretical in its character, and anxiously to be avoided and eschewed by all properly principled students and practitioners.

Simpson's critics were of course referring to the curse placed upon Adam and Eve which included, in Simpson's bible, the words "I will greatly multiply the sorrow of thy conception; and in sorrow thou shalt bring forth children." A recent translation of the bible is more explicit: "I will make your pains in childbearing very severe; with painful labor you will give birth to children."

Simpson's answered his critics by questioning the implication that "sorrow" means "physical and bodily *pain*". In addressing the issue more broadly he wrote the following.[9]

>...those that urge, on a kind of religious ground, that an artificial or anesthetic state of unconsciousness should not be induced merely to save frail humanity from the miseries and tortures of bodily pain, forget that we have the greatest of all examples set before us for following out this very principle of practice. I allude to that most significant description of the preliminaries and details of the first surgical operation ever performed on man, which is contained in Genesis II.21: "And the Lord God caused a deep sleep to fall upon Adam; and he slept; and He took one of his ribs, and closed up the flesh thereof."...John Calvin, in his commentary on this verse, noted that "Adam was sunk into a profound sleep, in order that he might feel no pain."

For many years I traveled to a medical school in northeastern Ohio to give a series of lectures on the drug treatment of pain. After my talk on opiates, a student approached me and expressed his view that pain is an ennobling experience not to be blunted by artificial means. He went on to quote several biblical passages in support of this idea. Following our exchange, my unexpressed hope was that this young man would not continue on his path to a career in medicine. And I most certainly would not wish to come under his care at some future date. Returning for a moment to the pain of childbirth, Queen Victoria did much to further the judicious use of drugs when she received chloroform during the births of Prince Leopold and Princess Beatrice in 1853 and 1857, respectively.[9] For purposes of our further discussion, I will assume that relief of pain, once it has served its protective and diagnostic purposes, is good, everywhere and always, a basic human kindness.

The obliteration of consciousness in general anesthesia is of immense value to mankind but equally clearly it can be a dangerous undertaking. One anesthesiologist expressed it this way: "the patient is suspended between life and death." By contrast, in local anesthesia, the transmission of pain signals from a discrete area of the body is blocked while full consciousness is maintained.

The natives of the Andes Mountains of South America discovered many centuries ago that chewing the leaves of the coca plant allowed one to work longer and harder even at high altitude. However, it was only with the rise of organic chemistry in Germany in the 19th century that the active principle of these leaves was isolated by Albert Niemann who gave to it the name so familiar to us today: cocaine.[10] Niemann described the drug as having a bitter taste and he observed that, when applied to the tongue, it caused a kind of numbness. In a classic example of missed opportunity, more than two decades would pass before medical use was made of this property. In 1884, just two years after completing his medical training in Vienna, Carl Koller reported to the German Ophthalmological Society that cocaine applied to the eye causes complete anesthesia.[11] He had observed this phenomenon first in animals, then in himself, and finally in patients on whom he performed surgery. Before the close of the century, cocaine was in use in dentistry and the efficacy of direct application to the spinal cord had been demonstrated for regional anesthesia. Today, cocaine has been almost totally supplanted by newer drugs. The most familiar of these is lidocaine, a drug introduced in 1904, still in use today, and known to many as Novocaine. Few who enter a dentist's office do not experience the benefit of such drugs.

Lying between the numbing of a relatively small area of the body in spinal or local anesthesia and obliteration of all sensation by general anesthesia is the use of drugs to dull the sense of pain. Throughout man's recorded history, attempts have been made to identify plants which might provide pain relief. *The Odyssey* by Homer provides a mythic account of the use of one such agent.[12]

> Then Helen, daughter of Zeus, took other counsel. Straightaway she cast into the wine of which they were drinking a drug to quit all pain and strife, and bring forgetfulness of every ill. Whoso should drink this down, when it is mingled in the bowl, would not in the course of that day let a tear fall down over his cheeks, no, not though his mother and father should lie there dead... Such cunning drugs had the daughter of Zeus, drugs of healing, which Polydamna, the wife of Thor, had given her, a woman of Egypt, for there the earth, the giver of grain, bears the greatest store of drugs...

More than a century ago, it was suggested by Oswald Schmiedeberg, a German scientist regarded by many as the father of modern pharmacology, that the drug to which Homer refers is opium: "no other natural product on the whole earth calls forth in man such a psychical blunting as the one described."[13] Virginia Berridge, in her elegant history of opium in England, tells us that the effects of opium on the human mind have probably been known for about 6,000 years and that opium had an honored place in Greek, Roman, and Arabic medicine.[14] Thomas Sydenham, a British physician of the 18th century, described opium this way: "Among the remedies it has pleased Almighty God to give to man to relieve his sufferings, none is so universal and so efficacious."[15]

When today, in the fields of Afghanistan or Turkey or India, the seed capsule of the opium poppy, *Papaver somniferum,* is pierced, a milky fluid oozes from it which, when dried, is opium. It is from this crude material that, early in the 19th century, a German chemist named Friedrich

Serturner isolated a chemical to which, after observing that the drug caused sleep in dogs, he gave the name morphine from the god of dreams, Morpheus.[16] Serturner's subsequent experiments to demonstrate the effects of morphine in man would in the 21st century shock the regulatory authorities and no doubt put him in prison for a very long time: "To obtain a reliable assessment of morphine's action, I myself acted as a subject and asked others to do the same…I persuaded three people under the age of seventeen to join me in taking morphine…" Opium remains in American medicine only in the form of paregoric, camphorated tincture of opium. Many a parent has witnessed relief of their child's diarrhea without knowing the origins of this remedy. Other babies, born of heroin-dependent mothers, have had their withdrawal eased by paregoric.

Just as was true in the 19th century when William Osler referred to morphine as "God's own medicine", it is the standard against which all other drugs are measured for the relief of severe pain. But morphine's sword is double-edged. Heroin, its close chemical cousin, is used in England to relieve pain but in this country and elsewhere it is a major element in the illicit drug market. Other drugs such as oxycodone, hydrocodone, and methadone, which mimic the actions of morphine, are widely prescribed, widely diverted to illicit use, and have become significant instruments of death in overdose, causing nearly 17,000 fatalities in the United States in 2010.[17] But, as I will explain more fully below, no person suffering severe pain should be denied relief because of an irrational fear of addiction or overdose.

It has long been known that opiates and opioids, the general terms applied to morphine-like drugs, can dull pain and relieve suffering without affecting consciousness. Based on this observation it was long assumed that opiates act only on higher centers of the brain. However, with the discovery of the opiate receptor, it was soon recognized that these receptors are distributed widely in the body. For example, ingenious devices have been invented to deliver small amounts of morphine directly to opiate receptors in the spinal cord for the control of cancer pain without risk of more general effects.

In addition to the inherent pain-relieving properties of opium and morphine, two other factors encouraged the very widespread use of these drugs in both the United States and Great Britain. First was the fact that in neither country were there any legal restrictions on their sale in any drugstore without prescription until the late 19th and early 20th centuries. Second was the absence of any alternative drug treatments for pain. This situation changed in 1899 with the introduction of acetyl salicylic acid, aspirin.

We hear much these days about "steroids" in connection with their use as aids to athletic performance as we have seen in chapter 9. These are the anabolic steroids related to the adrenal hormone, testosterone, which are able, like testosterone, to increase muscle mass. But our adrenal glands secrete other steroids in addition to testosterone. Among them is hydrocortisone which is valued for its ability to suppress inflammation. However, steroidal anti-inflammatory drugs carry with them a wide range of adverse effects not the least of which is suppression of the immune system with an increase in the risk of infection of all kinds. For this reason, the use of steroids to fight inflammation is usually limited to brief durations of treatment under strict medical supervision. Nonsteroidal anti-inflammatory drugs (NSAIDs) offer an alternative.

I have already given you in chapter 6.2 a brief account of aspirin and how it's anti-fever, anti-pain, and anti-blood clotting effects all were explained on the basis of the inhibition of synthesis of several members of the prostaglandin family. Beginning in the 1960's a series of drugs with effects similar to those of aspirin were brought to market. Like aspirin they successfully treat pain and fever as well as inflammation. An exception is acetaminophen (best known by the trade name Tylenol) which has only modest anti-inflammatory effects and is not properly classified as an NSAID. Extensive print and television promotion of these drugs has made many of them familiar under the trade names Celebrex (celecoxib), Motrin/Advil (ibuprofen), Indocin (indomethacin), and Aleve (naproxen). In contrast with the opioids, of whose lethal properties we are often reminded, the toxicity of acetaminophen and NSAIDs is the subject of much less scrutiny. No good data are available for the number of deaths attributable to these drugs but some think they rival the opioids in this respect. For the NSAIDs the primary culprit is bleeding in the stomach. Acetaminophen is primarily a liver toxin and the FDA has recently added a caution about rare but serious skin reactions.

Today, NSAIDs and the opiates remain our primary weapons against pain. However, they are now complimented by a number of other drugs and procedures for those all too common instances where neither opiates nor NSADs provide satisfactory relief. Writing in the *British Medical Journal*, Andrew Moore and his colleagues, specialists in pain treatment at the University of Oxford, entitled their article "Expect analgesic failure; pursue analgesic success."[18] The principles they elaborated include recognition that the responses of individual patients vary greatly, that switching drugs may be necessary, and that the failure of initial attempts should not discourage continued pursuit of more effective treatment.

As is already obvious, pain comes in many forms and precise categorization is difficult. We will consider three types: acute pain, cancer pain, and chronic non-cancer pain. The pain following surgery is an example of acute pain. A clear causative factor is present and we expect the pain to be limited in time. Despite this relative simplicity, the under-treatment of postoperative pain is widely recognized. In unveiling standards for management of pain at the turn of the 21st century, the Joint Commission on Healthcare Organizations estimated that in the United States only one in four surgical patients received adequate relief of acute pain.[19] There are no data which suggest that the situation has since improved. Indeed, further efforts, led by the Drug Enforcement Administration, to restrict the use of opiates in medical practice can only be expected to further exacerbate the situation.

If you or a loved one must confront postsurgical pain, my hope is that you will be served by physicians familiar with the most recent guidelines regarding the use of NSAID's, opiates, patient-controlled analgesia (PCA), and a variety of others measures currently available. PCA refers to a programmable device which permits the patient to administer an opiate in controlled amounts as needed. Studies have repeatedly shown that allowing patients to control their analgesia leads to superior pain relief with lesser amounts of opiate being used. PCA stands in contrast with p.r.n. orders. With respect to a physician's drug order, the Latin phrase *pro re nata*, as matters stand, is taken to mean "as needed." Unfortunately, this often places a patient in an adversarial position with a nurse or other care giver who is too busy to provide more analgesia as needed or who has been schooled to minimize the use of opiates. In either case, the patient suffers needlessly.

Except in unusual circumstances where acute post-surgical pain evolves into a chronic condition, the passage of time can be expected to bring relief whatever the adequacy or inadequacy of medical intervention. The same is not often true for cancer pain. Indeed, in the absence of treatment, it can be expected that the severity of pain will increase as the disease progresses.

Over the past three decades, many treatment guidelines have been issued to aide physicians in the treatment of cancer pain. When closely adhered to, most patients will experience satisfactory relief. Unfortunately, it has been estimated that more than four in ten cancer patients in the United States receive less than optimal care for pain.[20] In many other parts of the world the situation is much worse. The International Narcotics Control Board estimates that access to morphine is virtually non-existent in 150 countries.[21] Perhaps most ironic is the case of India, one of the world's largest producers of opium, where it is estimated that less than five percent of patients suffering moderate to severe pain due to advanced cancer receive morphine.[22]

The most influential and enduring guideline for the treatment of cancer pain was first issued by the World Health Organization in 1986 and revised in 1997.[23] With it was introduced the idea of an "analgesic ladder" in which one progresses from non-opioids such as acetaminophen (Tylenol) and NSAID's to codeine and finally to morphine. At the third step, NSAID's and an opiate are used in combination to achieve what is called multi-modal analgesia.

The analgesic ladder incorporates five simple principles. (1) An assessment of the level of pain is provided by the patient. The medical staff's perception of the patient's pain is not a factor in that assessment. (2) Drugs should be administered by mouth whenever possible. (3) Drugs are to be given at regular intervals around the clock. *Pro re nata* orders are discouraged, i.e., pain should be suppressed continuously. (4) There are no standardized doses of drugs. The correct dose is that which relieves pain in the individual patient. (5) There should be a written personal program provided to the patient, the patient's family, and to the medical staff.

Over the years, the WHO ladder has been criticized and modified but its principles remain. Foremost among these is that opioids are the mainstay of the treatment of cancer pain. With the recognition that codeine, which the body converts into morphine, is subject to widely different rates of metabolism, use of the drug has fallen into disfavor with some recommending the elimination of the second step of the ladder or the substitution of a low dose of morphine or oxycodone. For the relief of breakthrough pain, i.e., a sudden and transient increase in the level of pain, a rapidly acting opioid such as fentanyl can be used. The drug, sometimes in the form of a lollypop, can be quickly absorbed from the mouth. At the time the analgesic ladder was introduced, the use of adjuvant drugs such as antidepressants and anticonvulsants was much more limited than it is today. These will be discussed in the context of chronic non-cancer pain but are applicable to cancer pain as well. Some have suggested the addition of a fourth step to the ladder to incorporate a variety of neurosurgical procedures and techniques such as nerve blocks.

Patients with ready access to the internet often prove to be a curse on today's physician. All aspects of care are interpreted against the background of the information and, too often, the misinformation the patient has gathered from relentless web searches. As we saw in chapter 1 with the story of Fervid Trimble, such challenges can serve a useful and essential function but often these assaults on the physician's wisdom lead to a worsening of the doctor-patient relationship. I do not wish to contribute to that deterioration. It is instead my hope that these details of the analgesic ladder will provide a basis for insuring that you or a loved one do not become one of the many who receive inadequate relief of cancer pain.

In chapter 1, I defined drug-induced physical dependence and contrasted it with addiction. I told you that physical dependence upon an opiate such as morphine will develop in every person treated with significant doses for an extended period of time. It is a fundamental pharmacological phenomenon, neither more nor less. Physical dependence is expected to occur in every patient treated for chronic cancer pain. Physical dependence is not addiction. The latter is defined in various ways with my preference being that addiction is the behavioral state of compulsive, uncontrollable drug craving and seeking. It is irrelevant to the treatment of cancer pain.

One of the enduring concerns about opiates in the minds of patients and their caregivers, perhaps second only to addiction, is the idea that in deadening the pain of cancer these drugs invariably cloud consciousness. Tennessee Williams provides a fictional illustration in *Cat on a Hot Tin Roof.* In the film version, Big Daddy Pollitt, the head of a prosperous Mississippi family, is suffering from terminal cancer and is in severe pain. His physician has left a supply of morphine and his son offers an injection saying "It will kill the pain, that's all." Big Daddy responds "It'll kill the senses too. When you got pain at least you know you're still alive…I don't want to stupefy myself with that stuff."

The late Cicely Saunders would beg to differ with Big Daddy and his thoughts on the effects of opiates. First trained as a nurse during World War II and later as a physician, she had a lifelong interest in the treatment of pain and suffering particularly at the end of life. In 1967, she founded St. Christopher's Hospice in southwest London. It soon became a model for similar institutions around the world. She had this to say about drugs used at St. Christopher's.[24]

We find that for severe pain nothing can replace the opiates… We know that nothing else will so fully ease physical and mental distress, or help the patient who feels isolated in the meaningless

endurance of severe chronic pain...we use heroin almost exclusively...Although other opiates may relieve pain just as effectively, only heroin will do so with so few side effects or leave the
patient so alert and serene...

The St. Christopher's pain-relieving mixture is composed of heroin,
cocaine, gin, and an anti-nausea drug. Unfortunately, heroin is not available for medical use in the United States. Nonetheless, judicious use of
opiates following the guidelines provided by the analgesic ladder of the
World Health Organization can be expected to provide very significant
relief of pain while leaving the patient, in Dame Cicely's words, "alert and
serene." (Cicely Saunders died at St. Christopher's of breast cancer at age
87.)

The challenges presented by post-surgical pain and cancer pain are
relatively simple compared with those encountered in the treatment of
chronic non-cancer pain. A part of this complexity is due to its multiple
origins. One of two broad categories is nociceptive pain, which arises
from pain receptors localized in an area of tissue damage as, for example,
an arthritic joint. The second is neuropathic pain due to damage to
the central or peripheral nervous system. Examples include the pain
accompanying nerve damage due to diabetes and post-stroke pain. An
especially common form of neuropathic pain is chronic low back pain.
In conditions such as fibromyalgia there is widespread pain of uncertain
origin. Were these multiple forms not sufficiently complex, we must recognize that long-lasting pain does not occur in isolation. Chronic pain
may interact with emotional, cognitive, and personal factors to cause
what is best called suffering.

Given the complexity of chronic non-cancer pain, we should first
seek every possible means to avoid it. Foremost among preventive measures is the lifelong maintenance of a healthy body weight. There is a
clear relationship between obesity and the neuropathic pain of type 2
diabetes. In addition, obesity contributes to the wear and tear on the
joints leading to the nociceptive pain of osteoarthritis. Another form

of neuropathic pain arises in shingles, a viral infection caused by reactivation of the chickenpox virus. Shingles can largely be prevented by a simple vaccination after age 50. Much low back pain can be avoided by a lifetime of appropriate aerobic and anaerobic exercise.

When prevention fails and we experience chronic non-cancer pain, we must face the sobering fact that no single treatment or drug is universally successful. Professor Dennis Turk and his colleagues of the Department of Anesthesiology and Pain Medicine at the University of Washington writing in 2011 reached the following conclusion. "...the best evidence for pain reduction averages roughly 30% in about half of the treated patients...none of the most commonly prescribed treatment regimens are, by themselves, sufficient to eliminate pain and to have a major effect on physical and emotional function in most patients with chronic pain."[25] But, to paraphrase the words of Andrew Moore, although we should expect analgesic failure, we should continue to pursue analgesic success.

When, as is the case for much of chronic pain, no completely effective remedy is available, several bad things can happen. Countless quacks, hucksters, and charlatans will rush in to fill the therapeutic void with unproven methods which do no good, may do harm, and distract us from finding effective measures. A variety of witch's brews, including vitamin supplements and "natural" remedies, are peddled online. The medical establishment is not without fault. For example, extensive imaging, spinal injections, and surgery may be employed for neuropathic back pain before more conservative and far less costly approaches, including physical therapy, are tried. The use of opiates to treat chronic pain illustrates the dangers of assuming that all forms of pain respond similarly to a given drug or treatment.

Opiophobia is the term applied by John Morgan in 1985 to describe the inadequate treatment of severe pain "based on an irrational and undocumented fear that appropriate use will lead patients to become addicts."[26] Opiophobia is of particular concern in the treatment of acute pain and chronic cancer pain.

In recent decades, influenced in large measure by Cicely Saunders, much progress has been made to reduce opiophobia and permit the effective use of these agents. There is however a darker side to this story. As was previously noted, data from the Centers for Disease Control and Prevention for 2010 indicate that there has been a dramatic rise in deaths from overdose of opioids since 1999. For women the upward slope was especially steep with a four-fold increase. In 2010 more women died from prescription opioids than from automobile accidents or from cocaine and heroin combined. There are multiple reasons for this increase but a significant factor is the over-use of opiates for the treatment of chronic non-cancer pain.

I would not diminish the role that opioids have to play in severe pain of all kinds. Earlier I told you of my personal use of hydrocodone for sciatica. This opioid permitted me to function while the passage of time and physical therapy relieved the condition. However, the simple fact is that opioids don't work very well for most forms of chronic non-cancer pain and, used indiscriminately, carry with them the very real risk of fatal overdose. Indeed, national and international guidelines only rarely recommend opioids as a first line treatment for chronic non-cancer pain.

If NSAID's and opioids are relatively ineffective in conditions such as the neuropathic pain of diabetes or the generalized pain of fibromyalgia, what more can be done? As I noted earlier, drugs from other pharmacological classes are often employed. Most prominent among these are antidepressant agents such as amitriptyline (Elavil) and duloxetine (Cymbalta) and the anticonvulsant agents, gabapentin (Neurontin) and pregabalin (Lyrica). The mechanisms by which these drugs diminish pain are uncertain but a reasonable body of evidence supports their use. Thus, duloxetine is considered by many to be a first-line treatment for fibromyalgia and neuropathic pain and it is widely advertised for those conditions.

Given the fact that at present we have no fully satisfactory pharmacological or interventional means to relieve any of the multiple forms of chronic non-cancer pain, it is understandable that many would turn to alternative or complementary medicine. The list of possibilities is long. Among them are meditation and other forms of relaxation therapy, acupuncture, physical therapy, spinal manipulation, yoga, massage, and counseling of various kinds. Evidence of the efficacy of any of these approaches is meager but each has its advocates. As a component of a multimodal approach to chronic pain, each may be of value. However, before considering any of these, I would try to get myself to one of the great medical centers of the country, perhaps the clinics of Mayo or Cleveland, for a thorough evaluation by those who specialize in the diagnosis and treatment of chronic non-cancer pain.

David Livingston, a Scotsman, rose from poverty to fame in Victorian England as a medical missionary and explorer in Africa. Dr. Livingston told of how he had once been seized by a lion and was saved from death only by a lucky shot from the gun of a companion. He escaped with a broken arm. Later, in pondering the experience, he recalled how calm he had been and he imagined "an endogenous physiological system, switched on at the point of death, carrying us through in a haze of tranquility."[27]

A physiological basis for Livingston's observation was provided in the 1970's by the discovery of a family of naturally occurring chemicals in the brain which have many of the properties of opioids. These chemicals are now collectively called endorphins. They are the transmitters in our bodies own analgesic system. Morphine and other opiates merely mimic the action of these endogenous substances but in a very powerful way.

In pop psychology, release of endorphins is commonly invoked to explain the joy of sex, exercise, food, and other pleasurable human activities. A "runner's high" is sought by many but experienced by few. But, to borrow a word from Dr. Livingston, runner's *tranquility* is not uncommon. In the context of chronic non-cancer pain, it may be that practices as disparate as meditation, behavioral therapy, physical exercise, and acupuncture all act via activation of endorphins. While it is clear that this physiological system is inadequate to suppress all pain, it is plausible that some non-pharmacological approaches may augment the analgesic effects of drugs. Only by a systematic and individualized plan can the best combination against chronic pain be discovered.

CHAPTER 12

DEMENTIA

Auguste Deter and Dr. Alzheimer

On November 25, 1901, a 51 year old woman named Auguste Deter was admitted to the Frankfort Hospital for the Mentally Ill. The following day she was examined by Aloys Alzheimer, a 37-year-old staff psychiatrist. Dr. Alzheimer's notes from that meeting will appear familiar to any who have cared for a loved one suffering from the disease which now carries his name.

> She sits on the bed with a helpless expression. What is your name? *Auguste.* What is your last name? *Auguste.* What is your husband's name. *Auguste, I think.* Your husband? *Ah, my husband.* She looks as if she didn't understand the question. Are you married? *To Auguste.* Mrs. Deter? *Yes, yes, Auguste.* How long have you been here? She seems to be trying to remember. *Three weeks.* (She was admitted the previous day.) What is this? I show her a pencil. *A pen.* At lunch she eats cauliflower and pork. Asked what she is eating she answers *spinach.* Asked to write "Auguste", she tries to write Mrs. and forgets the rest…[1]

Later Alzheimer would learn that Auguste's symptoms began with changes in her behavior. She became suspicious of her husband and unpredictable in her interactions with others, sometimes agitated, sometimes fearful, sometimes hearing voices. Soon thereafter Auguste showed rapidly increasing memory impairments and difficulties in expressing herself.

Although Dr. Alzheimer would move from Frankfurt, first to Heidelberg and then to the Royal Psychiatric Clinic in Munich, he continued to follow Auguste until her death on April 8, 1906. At that time, he asked that her brain be sent to him so that he might study the neuropathological features of her disease. Alzheimer was particularly suited for these studies because, complementing his clinical skills in conducting autopsies, he had a long-term interest in establishing a possible physical basis for mental disorders; he once said that he "wanted to help psychiatry with the microscope." In addition, it was his good fortune to have had Franz Nissl as a colleague in Frankfort. Nissl's name is now known to all who study medicine. While still a student, he developed novel methods for the staining of microscopic preparations of the brain.

With his microscope and the techniques of Nissl, Alzheimer set out to examine the brain of Auguste D. Seven months after her death he presented a lecture to a meeting of psychiatrists in Tubingen.

> In the center of an almost normal cell there stands out one or several fibrils...numerous small miliary foci are found in the superior layers. They are determined by the storage of a peculiar material in the cortex...all in all we face a peculiar disease process....[2]

The peculiar materials described by Alzheimer in the brain of Auguste Deter are now universally referred to as neurofibrillary tangles and plaques. To this day, their presence provides the definitive diagnosis of Alzheimer's disease. Until recently the presence of tangles and plaques could be determined only after death but imaging techniques now promise their identification in living brain thus offering the possibility of early diagnosis. It is thought that these structures account for the ravages of the disease and that they arise from the abnormal accumulation and aggregation of specific cellular proteins called *beta*-amyloid and *tau*. For an unfortunate few, perhaps 1%-2% of all persons afflicted, the condition is the result of the presence of an altered gene called *APOE-epsilon4*. In these individuals, deterioration of memory may be manifest as early as the third decade of life. For all others, age is the primary risk factor with more than 95% of its victims age 65 or older. In March 2014, it was estimated by the Alzheimer's Association of America that the disease affects 5.2 million Americans. Barring the discovery of a means to prevent or reverse the disease, that number is expected to rise to 16 million by 2050.

Alzheimer's disease accounts for fully 80% of all dementia. Given its intractable nature, it is essential that preventable or correctable causes of other forms be considered. Foremost among these is a condition called multi-infarct dementia. Although its signs and symptoms closely parallel those of Alzheimer's disease, its origins are different and, most important, it is largely preventable. An infarct is an area of dead tissue arising from blockage of the blood supply to that tissue. When the blockage is in the heart, it is called a myocardial infarction or heart attack. In the brain, the result is called a stroke. (In a recent campaign to raise awareness of stroke, neurologists began to refer to strokes as "brain attacks.") Most of us are at least vaguely familiar with the effects of a major stroke leading to loss of speech or paralysis or death. In contrast, multi-infarct dementia arises from a series of mini-strokes, each being largely undetectable by either patient or physician but the cumulative effect of many tiny infarcts is dementia.

The risk factors for heart attack and cardiovascular disease are identical to those for cerebrovascular disease and stroke. If you have high blood pressure, smoke, are obese or diabetic, your odds of suffering either multi-infarct dementia or a heart attack are increased significantly. If more than one of these risk factors is present, your future is even more precarious. As we have seen in chapter 7, type II diabetes is closely tied to obesity and obesity can successfully be attacked by a combination of diet and exercise. These also will reduce blood pressure but, if exercise and diet are insufficient, a combination of inexpensive drugs is very effective. If you smoke…what can I say?

Those who view television on a regular basis may have been surprised by my earlier statement that we presently have no means to alter the course of Alzheimer's disease. Have I not seen the cheery advertisements for one or another of the prescription drugs promising to "help dad to be more like himself?" The drugs of which I speak go by the trade names Aricept, Razadyne, Exelon, and Namenda. All of them interact with neurotransmitters, the chemical messengers in our brains. The first three of these drugs increase the levels of acetylcholine, a neurochemical long associated with memory. Block the sites at which it acts and a drug-induced dementia results. Might it be that cholinergic activity is diminished in Alzheimer's disease and might we improve the situation by increasing the amount of acetylcholine available? The last drug of the group, Namenda, acts differently; it blocks the actions of glutamate, an excitatory neurotransmitter. It is thought that excess glutamate released at the time a stroke or mini-stroke occurs might lead to further damage to the brain. Both hypotheses are plausible and all four of the drugs were approved by the Food and Drug Administration for use in moderate to severe Alzheimer's disease largely on the basis of studies sponsored by the drug companies wishing to sell them. Unfortunately, subsequent investigations have provided little evidence that they produce significant improvement in Alzheimer's patients. In 2009, the situation was put into perspective by no less an authority than Richard J. Hodes, Director of the National Institute on Aging: "No drug prevents or slows progression once present." (I thank Susan Jacoby for bringing Dr. Hodes' comment to my attention in her lovely book, *Never Say Die*.[4])

Would I deny any patient the hope offered by the drugs presently available? I would not but I would also caution caregivers and patients to be modest in their expectations. These drugs most certainly are not curative agents and, as do most drugs, they carry with them a variety of undesired effects. Just as with the use of antipsychotic drugs to control behavioral changes in the later stages of dementia, constant vigilance is needed to insure that drugs intended to comfort the patient do not, in fact, make matters worse.

Instead of treating the symptoms of Alzheimer's disease, why not go after its cause? Unfortunately, although the plaques and tangles described by Dr. Alzheimer are now known to be formed from amyloid-*beta* and *tau* proteins, respectively, there is no consensus regarding which of the two is causative.[5] Some have even suggested that formation of amyloid-*beta* is a protective response to the disease much as fever is to inflammation. At the present time, vaccines against *tau* proteins, the basis of neurofibrillary tangles, are under development but proof of their safety and efficacy are years away.

More fully developed are attempts either to decrease the formation of amyloid-*beta* or to remove established plaques. Regarding formation, it is known that inhibition of an enzyme called *beta*-secretase will diminish the cleaving of amyloid precursor protein to amyloid-*beta*. Hope that such an approach might be successful was encouraged by a remarkable observation reported in 2012.[6] Thorlakur Jonsson and his colleagues in Reykjavik, Iceland, observed that persons carrying a rare mutation that leads to inhibition of *beta*-secretase had very low levels of amyloid-*beta*. Still more remarkable, persons with the secretase mutation who also carried two copies of the *APOE-epsilon4* gene and thus were at very high risk, were protected from Alzheimer's disease. Unfortunately, the initial attempt to apply this approach was unsuccessful. When a secretase inhibitor called semagacestat was administered to 1,537 patients with probable Alzheimer's disease, cognitive function was not improved, functional ability worsened, and there was an increase in skin cancer and infections. The trial was terminated earlier than planned.[7]

As an alternative to blocking the formation of amyloid-*beta*, a form of immunotherapy has been employed. Just as our immune system meets foreign invaders with antibodies, drugs have been designed to attack and remove amyloid-*beta*. The reports in 2014 of trials in Alzheimer's disease patients of three such agents were disappointing: no meaningful improvement was observed either in terms of progression of the disease or in the functions of daily living.[8, 9] Some viewed this as the end of the amyloid-*beta* hypothesis of Alzheimer's disease. Others argued that amyloid plaques probably begin to form twenty to twenty-five years before signs of the disease are evident.[10] Might it be that early intervention, before signs of the disease appear, would be successful? By 2013, funds had been committed to the testing of that hypothesis in persons at high risk of developing Alzheimer's disease. The same drugs that failed to correct the disease once established will be used. Unfortunately, definitive results will be a long time in coming.[11]

In the absence of a truly effective treatment from the pharmaceutical industry and with the prospect that means to prevent or cure the disease remain somewhere in the perhaps distant future, we should not be surprised that many have turned for hope to alternative sources. In their desperation, what caregiver or patient would not respond to a headline reading "Daily pill that halts Alzheimer's disease is hailed the 'biggest breakthrough against disease in 100 years." This claim comes to us from Patrick Holford, founder of the Institute for Optimal Nutrition in London, author of 34 books, and advocate of a nutritional approach to AIDS and autism as well to Alzheimer's disease. The *breakthrough* takes the form of vitamins, specifically the B vitamins, pyridoxine (B_6), cobalamin (B_{12}), and folic acid. These vitamins together with other components of the diet are often referred to as anti-oxidants. Oxidation is the process by which iron rusts, butter turns rancid, and, in Mr. Holford's view, we become demented.

But what of Holford's "daily pill that halts Alzheimer's disease?" Are B vitamins the answer? Were it true, we would have no need to spend hundreds of millions of dollars developing exotic drugs. Given the devastating nature of the disease and the absence of effective treatment, the B vitamin hypothesis had to be tested and tested it was.[12] In 2008, Paul Aisen of the University of California at San Diego, and his colleagues provided their answer based on 409 individuals suffering from mild to moderate Alzheimer's disease. For eighteen months, 245 of them received each day 5 milligrams of folate, 25 milligrams of vitamin B_6, and 1 milligram of vitamin B_{12}; the rest received an identical placebo containing no vitamins. Patients, caregivers, and physicians were unaware of who was in the placebo and vitamin treatment groups. Memory was examined every three months using standard tests widely used to assess Alzheimer's patients. When the study was completed and the code was broken, it was found that the vitamin treatment had produced no beneficial effect whatsoever. Dr. Aisen's study was later included in an overall analysis of 11 large trials involving more than 22,000 persons with Alzheimer's disease treated with B vitamins. The conclusion drawn from that overall analysis and reported in 2014 by Dr. Robert Clarke of the Nuffield Department of Clinical Medicine, Trinity College, University of Oxford, was simple: despite lowering homocysteine levels, B vitamins had no effect on mental performance or on progression of the disease.[13]

Regrettably, as witnessed by today's Internet, these results will not deter those who would sell you vitamins, usually at much inflated prices, for the treatment of dementia. Lewis Thomas once said that vitamins have replaced prayer. For Alzheimer's disease, prayer is the better bet.

So far I have offered precious little hope for those of us destined to develop Alzheimer's disease. Is there nothing we can do to reduce our risk? Do we have no clues as to how it might be prevented? Most of what can be suggested comes from studies of correlation. For example, the risk of Alzheimer's disease is correlated with the level of education one achieves, the higher the level, the lower the risk. But, as we have seen before, correlation is not causation. With respect to education and Alzheimer's disease, it is likely that a high level is simply a marker for a variety of other factors which may have some causal role. Thus, for example, obesity, diabetes, high cholesterol, and smoking are all risk factors for dementia and all are more common in the less-educated. Social engagement and mental activity, sort of exercise for the brain, are often suggested to be protective. It appears that all the things that are good for our bodies, exercise in particular, are also good for our brains.[14, 15, 16] So, do all the right things and, if you are so inclined, pray that some scientist soon will solve the puzzle of Dr. Alzheimer's disease.

CANCER

What is the Optimal Lifestyle for Prevention?

We most often use the singular form in speaking of cancer; we shouldn't. Cancer is not one disease but a whole family of diseases, perhaps 100 or more in number, each with its own peculiarities of origin and course. For this reason, the potential means to avoid cancer are varied and often seem unrelated. We must ever keep in mind that our present understanding of the diseases called cancer is woefully inadequate; much of the advice and treatment of today will inevitably be shown to be bad advice and bad treatment. Finally, despite the pessimistic sound of the preceding, there is overwhelming evidence that the risks of some forms of cancer can be reduced significantly.

Cancer is a disease that has afflicted humans for as long as we can remember. Five thousand years ago an Egyptian papyrus said of the disease "There is no treatment."[1] Ancient Greeks called it *karkinoma*, which became the Latin word cancer with the dual meaning of a crab or an ulcer that moves crablike from one spot to another. Cancer is characterized by uncontrolled growth of cells and a tendency to spread from the site of origin to new places in the body, a phenomenon now called metastasis. In the United States in 2010, there were more than1.5 million new cases of cancer[2] and, with the aging of the population, that number will continue to grow.[3] Treatment will cost about $125 billion with an ever increasing number of patients unable to afford that which is available. Without insurance coverage, it will bankrupt most. An example: in March 2011, the Food and Drug Administration approved the use of a drug called ipilimubab for the treatment of melanoma, an especially lethal form of skin cancer; four treatments cost $120,000. But how can we put a price on a cure? Unfortunately, in the case of ipilimubab, it is not a cure of which we speak. A subsequent study of the drug found that median survival time after treatment was just six months.[4]

We have come to expect that modern medical science, given enough time and money, can find a remedy for every disease. That expectation justifies the War on Cancer and the billions of dollars lavished on cancer investigators. But many have suggested that the war on cancer, focusing as it does on the cure of disease once established, is not being won. Since President Richard Nixon signed the National Cancer Act in 1971, an event marking the beginning of the war, the mortality rate from cancer has changed little despite advances in some areas. Indeed, the absolute number of deaths in the United States from cancer has increased 74% since 1970 largely due to a growing and aging population.[5] The promise of molecular biology and of personalized medicine made possible by genomic sequencing is great but presently unfulfilled. Many argue that greater emphasis on prevention is what is needed.

There is no question that prevention is far preferable to cure. But, given cancer's roots in antiquity, what stretch of the imagination leads us to believe that it can be prevented? The answer lies in a simple observation: The incidence of specific cancers is quite different from place to place and from group to group. For example, in 2003, American women were twice as likely to die of breast cancer as were women in Japan[6] whereas stomach cancer developed in Japanese men eight times as often as in their American counterparts.[7] Does this mean that Japanese women have a genetically determined resistance to breast cancer while Japanese men have an inherent susceptibility to stomach cancer? It does not: Move the Japanese to America and in two generations they will develop cancer as Americans do.

International comparisons of cancer incidence suggest that external factors markedly alter the probability of occurrence of many forms of the disease. But there has been much confusion about the nature of these "external factors." Influenced in large measure by a flood of information and misinformation on the subject, many people have decided that "everything causes cancer" so there is no point in worrying about anything. Others have come to believe, wishfully perhaps, that a little more fiber or a vitamin supplement or avoiding food additives will reduce the risk of cancer to the vanishing point. The truth, as best we know it today, lies somewhere between these two extremes.

In 1952, John Higginson, an Irish physician and scientist, concluded that two-thirds of all cancer is environmentally determined and thus preventable.[8] Later, as the founding director of the World Health Organization's International Agency for Research on Cancer, Dr. Higginson did much to educate the world about the preventability of cancer. Unfortunately, his message was often misunderstood and sometimes willfully distorted. The problem centers on the diverse meanings given such words as "environment", "behavior", and, one of today's favorites, "life style."

Higginson defined environment as "what surrounds people and impinges on them"; not far from my dictionary's definition as "the total circumstances surrounding us." Environment, as Higginson intended it, includes virtually all factors in human life other than genetic endowment; and it is now recognized that even genes can be altered by environmental factors; that is what epigenetics is about. Professional and amateur environmentalists have tended to focus on clean air and pure water---important items but hardly the whole story. For the Higginson environment, we must add sunlight, cosmic rays, radon from the earth, sexual practices, age at menstruation, number of children, lifetime habits of exercise, history of viral and bacterial infection, every element of the diet, medical treatment, tobacco, alcohol, and, no doubt, a whole lot of things not yet discovered.

But it is not enough simply to list every factor ever associated with cancer. To bring order to this chaotic array, we need a point of reference; something of known cancer-inducing efficiency against which to measure everything else. Tobacco provides that point of reference.

In 1912, Irving Adler apologized to his readers for writing at such great length about a disease as uncommon as lung cancer. One hundred years later, lung cancer is the leading cause of death from cancer in both men and women in the United States. Five years after diagnosis, 85% of its victims are dead and 160,000 Americans die of the disease each year, more than the sum of those dying from cancer of the breast, colon, and prostate, combined.

The *British Medical Journal* for December 13, 1952 included an article by Richard Doll and A. Bradford Hill entitled "A Study of the Etiology of Carcinoma of the Lung."[9] Based on interviews with 1,488 patients with lung cancer and an equal number of persons without the disease, they concluded that "the association between smoking and carcinoma of the lung is real." In 1957, the Medical Research Council of Great Britain went further: "the relationship (between smoking and cancer) is one of direct cause and effect." Seven years later even the Surgeon General of the United States was ready to act: "The magnitude of the effect of cigarette smoking (on lung cancer) far outweighs all other factors." In 1979: "Cigarette smoking is the single most important preventable environmental factor contributing to illness, disability, and death in the United States."

Today it is estimated that 90% of all lung cancer results from the smoking of tobacco products. Add in the contribution of tobacco to cancer of the mouth, tongue, larynx, esophagus, and bladder, to heart disease, and to a variety of chronic obstructive diseases of the lungs, and we do indeed have a towering point of reference, one un-approached by any other environmental factor. The best current approximation is that tobacco causes 20% of all new cancers.

We have come a long way in the decades since Doll and Hill first convincingly made the connection between smoking and lung cancer. Those of my vintage will recall the 1950's image of a white-coated, avuncular physician together with the words "More Doctors Smoke CAMELS than any other cigarette!" By 1971, less than twenty years after Doll and Hill, all advertising of cigarettes had been banned on television and radio in the United States. We no longer have before us pictures of happy, healthy, beautiful people in advertisements for cigarettes. Nonetheless, the addictive powers of nicotine rival that of heroin and the allure of smoking remains strong especially among the young. Youthful rebellion is one element and the glamour of Hollywood films, past and present, continues to work its wonders. No lover of classic movies can forget Paul Henreid in *Now, Voyager* as he puts two cigarettes to his lips, lights both, and hands one to Bette Davis. Perhaps we should be reminded that smoking-related cancer took the lives of many of the stars of those films; Gary Cooper, Yul Brynner, and John Wayne readily come to mind. Their average age was just 65; Humphrey Bogart was 58 at the time of his death from cancer of the esophagus. It is estimated that smokers on average lose more than a decade of life. The good news is that those who stop before age 40 cut their risk by 90 percent. Richard Doll began his studies of smoking and lung cancer in 1949. That same year, at the age of 37, he stopped smoking. Sir Richard was 92 at the time of his death.

All right, we have our reference point; tobacco is without question the single most important risk factor for lung cancer, as is well known, but in addition an element in cancer at many other sites including the oral cavity, pancreas, bladder, and kidney. Tony Gwynn, a member of the Baseball Hall of Fame and one of the greatest hitters in the history of the game, died in 2014 at age 58 from cancer of the mouth and salivary glands. He attributed his disease to his long time use of chewing tobacco. The practice has now been banned at all lower levels but Major League Baseball has not yet summoned the courage to do so. Currently, nearly 20 percent of Americans continue to smoke. That rate is admittedly a great improvement over previous years when more than 40% of Americans did so but it obscures the fact that smoking has been driven into those segments of the population whose health is most precarious to begin with. Fifty-five percent of smokers in this country have a high school education or less. It is estimated that three quarters of homeless adults are smokers. My sentiments regarding tobacco were nicely expressed by an anonymous author in *The Lancet* who wrote that "Renewed effort…is needed to put tobacco where it belongs: in the history books, as a sad and strange episode in the story of human health."[10]

It is now time to turn to all of those other carcinogens in our environment in order to answer our question, "What is the Optimal Lifestyle for Prevention?" Be prepared for a bumpy ride; estimates are widely variable and are subject to regular change as more evidence is gathered.

In the April 1975 issue of the *International Journal of Cancer* was an article entitled "Environmental factors and cancer incidence and mortality in different countries with special reference to dietary practices."[11] Its authors were Bruce Armstrong and Richard Doll who earlier had sounded the alarm with respect to smoking and lung cancer. By this time Doll was Sir Richard, and Regius Professor of Medicine, Radcliff Infirmary, Oxford University. Their article is long and complex and filled with statistical jargon but its conclusions are admirably simple and modest and provocative.

Armstrong and Doll correlated incidence rates for 27 cancers in 32 countries with a wide range of dietary factors. In their words "the strongest points to emerge from these analyses are the suggestions of associations between cancers of the colon, rectum, and breast and dietary variables—particularly meat (or animal protein) and total fat consumption...it is clear that these and other correlations should be taken only as suggestions for further research and not as evidence of causation or as bases for preventive action...(however), it is possible that diet may have an effect on many cancers...the subject warrants more attention"

In the United States that attention took the form of a study commissioned by the Division of Cancer Cause and Prevention of the National Cancer Institute. On June 16, 1982, the National Academy of Sciences issued a 550-page report simply entitled Diet, Nutrition, and Cancer.[12] The conclusions and suggestions for dietary modifications were the following.

(1) Reduce the amount of fat consumed (the effects of different types of fat were not noted).
(2) Increase the intake of fruits, vegetables, and whole grains.
(3) Drink alcoholic beverages only in moderation.

(4) Minimize consumption of foods preserved by salt-curing and smoking.

Evidence was not considered to be adequate to permit recommendations with respect to the intake of protein, fiber, carbohydrates, cholesterol, most minerals, vitamin E, the B vitamins, and, most significantly, total caloric intake. (The possibility that supplements *beta*-carotene or vitamins D or E may be hazardous with respect to cancer was addressed above in sections 6.5, 6.15, and 6.16, respectively. These cautions do not apply to dietary sources.)

In summing up Diet, Nutrition, and Cancer, Clifford Grobstein, the chairman of the committee, put it this way: "Certainly we have no ideal cancer-preventing diet to announce." Indeed, there were critics of even the modest recommendations made. Not surprisingly, the American Meat Institute and the National Meat Association, who saw any anti-fat advice as being anti-meat, characterized the report as "a simplistic approach to a very complex question" and as "misleading advice which does no service to the public." Some pointed out that just two years earlier, the Food and Nutrition Board of the National Academy of Sciences in a publication called Toward Healthful Diets had noted that there was no basis for recommendations to modify the proportion of fat consumed by Americans.

John R. Block, the Secretary of Agriculture, was "not so sure that government should be telling people what they should or shouldn't eat." (How quaint that sounds today. I am reminded that 100 years ago it was argued that banning child labor was an unjustified intrusion by the government.) But, taken as written, few objected strongly to the report; consumption of less fat and alcohol and eating more fruits, grains, and vegetables makes sense for reasons quite unrelated to cancer. In fact, the advice has elements of the DASH and Mediterranean diets we talked about in chapter 8 with respect to weight loss.

The report was not always "taken as written." Predictably, every charlatan in the country who had ever advocated a change in diet as a means to prevent disease saw *Diet, Nutrition, and Cancer* as vindication of "natural healing." The prize for audacity perhaps should go to Mishio

Kushi. Just a year after the appearance of the committee report, Kushi, a lawyer by training, published a book called *The Cancer Prevention Diet.*[13] This is what he had to say about lung cancer. "To prevent and *heal* (my emphasis) lung cancer, first, all extreme foods from the yang category are to be avoided or minimized including meat, poultry, eggs, dairy products, and seafood as well as baked flour products. It is also necessary to avoid foods and beverages from the yin category, including sugar and all other sweets, fruits and juices, spices and stimulants, alcohol and drugs, as well as all artificial, chemicalized (*sic*), and refined food." Kushi's claims were not burdened by any supporting evidence.

All of us wish for a simple, inexpensive, truly effective way to avoid cancer and an alternative to today's surgery, radiation, and chemotherapy. Wishing does not make it so but, fortunately, there are things that we can do to reduce our risk.

More than three decades have passed since the appearance of Diet, Nutrition, and Cancer. Long enough, one might think, to get these matters sorted out. Regretfully, that is not the case. Despite the results of thousands of epidemiological studies involving many millions of people, much uncertainty remains. Advice given to the public with great confidence has been muted. Words like "convincing" became "probable" and "probable" morphed into "possible." In 1984, a book called *The Doctor's Anti-Breast Cancer Diet* promised a 50% reduction in the risk of breast cancer.[14] At about the same time, the august *Harvard Medical School Health Letter* stated that "the association of breast cancer with a diet high in animal fat is real." Today, a specific role for dietary fat remains unproven and it is now thought that obesity rather than any specific component of the diet is the real culprit with respect to breast cancer.[15] The best current estimate of the contribution of all aspects of lifestyle to the risk of breast cancer is 27%. Unfortunately, this scientific vacillation has led some to believe that there is nothing we can do to reduce the incidence of cancer.

The most recent and, to my mind, the most successful attempt to summarize all that we know about the prevention of cancer appeared in 2011 as a supplement to the *British Journal of Cancer*. A series of reports was entitled The Fraction of Cancer Attributable to Lifestyle and Environmental Factors.[16] The senior author was Professor D. M. Parkin of the Center for Cancer Prevention, Wolfson Institute of Preventive Medicine, Queen Mary University of London. Although their research applied explicitly to the United Kingdom, there is no doubt that it is broadly relevant to the citizens of the United States and other developed countries. Their reports provided no new data but instead brought together the results of hundreds of, in their words, "high-quality epidemiological studies." Put another way, this is the best evidence we have today.

Let me provide a quick summary of Parkin's recommendations to reduce risk. We will then consider the individual items in somewhat greater detail. Fourteen lifestyle and environmental factors were considered for each of 18 types of cancer. As expected, tobacco led the list, accounting for an estimated 19.4% of all cancer. Following, in rank order of importance, were diet, overweight and obesity, alcohol, occupation, exposure to the sun, infections, ionizing radiation, exercise, reproductive factors, and post-menopausal hormones. Estimates were provided of the contribution of each to the incidence of cancer. The overall conclusion was that fully one-third of all new cancer cases are preventable by modification of lifestyle. Considerably lower than Dr. Higginson's estimate from more than a half century ago but substantial nonetheless. More important, many of the same changes in lifestyle which protect against cancer are effective in reducing heart disease, stroke, a myriad of other afflictions, and, just possibly, dementia.

Based upon their massive review of the medical literature, Professor Parkin and his colleagues arrived at the following theoretical optimum exposure levels.

(1) tobacco smoke	none
(2) alcohol	none
(3) diet	
(a) fruit and vegetables	5 or more servings per day
(b) red and preserved meat	none
(c) fiber	23 or more grams per day
(d) salt (sodium chloride)	6 grams or less per day
(4) overweight and obesity	Body Mass Index of 25 or less
(5) exercise	30 minutes or more, 5 per week
(6) exogenous hormones	none
(7) infections	none
(8) ionizing radiation	none
(9) UV (solar) radiation	minimal
(10) occupational exposures	none
(11) reproductive factors	breastfeeding, min. of 6 months

In a perfect world we would be able to reach an ideal exposure to each identified risk factor. Alas, perfection will not be ours for several reasons. It is true that some of the goals are readily achieved, albeit with some discipline required. We can stop smoking, follow a DASH or Mediterranean diet, achieve a desirable body weight, and exercise regularly. Others are more problematic. For example, few who drink alcohol regularly are willing to eliminate it entirely and, as we will see in chapter 14, alcohol in moderation may have beneficial effects with respect to heart disease. (I will say more about alcohol and breast cancer in a moment.)

The risks inherent in items (6) through (10) can, at best, be minimized. Exogenous hormones for women come in two primary forms, oral contraceptives and post-menopausal hormone replacement therapy (HRT). It was concluded a decade ago that combined oral estrogen-progesterone contraceptives increase the risk of cancer of the breast, uterine cervix, and liver. However, equally convincing is the evidence that oral contraceptive use is protective against endometrial and ovarian cancer.

Balancing these effects is difficult but it was the conclusion of the Parkin group that use of oral contraceptives has a net positive effect, i.e., they reduce the total number of cancers. On the other hand, HRT, as I noted in the Preface, increases the risk of breast, endometrial, and ovarian cancer with no beneficial effect at other sites. The risks are relatively small, the greatest being a 3.2% increase for breast cancer. Clearly the decision by a post-menopausal woman to use HRT is a personal one based on multiple considerations.

The total contribution of infections to cancer is estimated to be about 8% of all cases. The infecting agents are hepatitis B and C, human immunodeficiency virus (HIV), human papillomaviruses (HPV), T-lymphotropic virus type-1, Epstein-Barr virus, human herpes virus 8, and *Helicobacter pylori*, a bacterium which is responsible for about one-third of all stomach cancer. Viral infection contributes to cancer of the oral cavity, liver, and colon. Of greatest current interest are the HPV's because, first, they are responsible for virtually all cervical cancer and, second, a highly effective vaccine is available.[17] This issue came to public attention during the 2012 Republican presidential debates when it was noted that Governor Rick Perry of Texas had supported the vaccination of girls in that state against HPV. To me the governor's decision appears perfectly rational in light of the fact that, in the United States, vaccination programs for both boys and girls have been recommended by the National Cancer Institute, the Food and Drug Administration, and the Centers for Disease Control and Prevention. Others view such vaccination as an unwarranted intrusion of government and, because HPV is a sexually transmitted disease, an invitation to sexual activity.

The discovery of X-rays at the end of the 19th century was followed quickly by their use in medical imaging. Also following quickly was the realization that they might cause skin cancer and leukemia. It is for this reason that dental and medical use of X-rays, especially CT scans, should be minimized. Another source of ionizing radiation is radon, a naturally occurring radioactive gas. Radon is the probable cause of most lung cancer in those who do not smoke and, for this reason, many communities require that homes be tested for radon before sale. As with X-rays, reaching a zero exposure level to radon is not practicable. The same might be said for solar radiation, the major cause of malignant melanoma which accounts for about three-quarters of all deaths from skin cancer. The dermatologists say it best: there is no such thing as a healthy tan whether from a tanning bed or from natural sunlight.

The Occupational Safety and Health Administration came into being in 1971 with the charge to ."..assure safe and healthful working conditions for working men and women... " During its stormy history, OSHA has been attacked from the left for doing too little and from the right for what are regarded as burdensome regulations. While occupational exposure to carcinogens cannot be totally avoided, Richard Doll provided us with an example of why constant vigilance is essential. He described a group of 19 men exposed to 2-naphthylamine, a solvent used in the dye industry. Eighteen died of bladder cancer and the last avoided that fate only by being killed in an accident.

Under reproductive factors in the table of theoretical optimum exposure levels, only breastfeeding is mentioned. This requires some explanation. The other elements considered were age at the onset of menstruation, age at menopause, number of children, and age at the birth of the first child. It is reasonably well established that the incidence of cancers of the uterus, ovary, and breast are reduced in woman who give birth at an early age, have multiple children, and who breastfeed. Conversely, the risk of these cancers is increased by an early onset of menstruation and by the total duration of menstruation. Because there are valid reasons not to give birth at an early age or to have multiple births, the Parkin group did not consider these as targets for prevention. With respect to an early onset of menstruation, it has long been known that good nutrition makes for bigger children and a younger age for sexual maturation. At this point in time, no one advocates the intentional underfeeding of our daughters as a means to reduce breast cancer. Preventing obesity is another matter entirely.

Because breast cancer is second only to smoking as a cause of cancer-related death in women, it deserves particular attention especially with respect to the role of nutrition and the drinking of alcohol. In the nearly four decades since Armstrong and Doll suggested a possible association between total fat consumption and breast cancer, much advice, often conflicting, has been offered to women. The origins of the notion that dietary fat and breast cancer might be linked can be traced to the discovery of a remarkable correlation between the amount of fat in women's diets and the incidence of breast cancer in 22 countries. Recall that I said that women in Japan eating a traditional diet have a low rate of breast cancer. Indeed, in 1964, when the data were published, Japan had both the lowest rate of breast cancer and the lowest fat consumption.[18] But, as I have said many times, correlation does not mean causation. Subsequent large epidemiological studies have found no consistent relationship. I mentioned earlier that an investigation called the Women's Health Initiative raised serious doubts about the wisdom of hormone replacement therapy for women. That same study found no association between total fat and the incidence of breast cancer. Walter Willett of the Harvard School of Public Health, is perhaps the most prominent naysayer. He suggests that the real culprits are childhood growth rates and midlife weight gain. Still more reassuring with respect to the fat content of the diet and breast cancer is the growing body of evidence that high-fat Mediterranean diets, relying as they do on vegetable sources of unsaturated fats and minimal animal fat, may actually be protective against cancers of all kinds including that of the breast.[19, 20]

In chapter 7 I talked at length about how obesity and the accompanying disordered function of adipose tissue might lead to a chronic state of inflammation. It is via this mechanism that I am inclined to account for the extensive epidemiological evidence that overweight and obesity increase the risk of cancer at multiple sites. For the obese, both men and women, there is an increased incidence of cancer of the esophagus, colon and rectum, pancreas, gall bladder, and kidney.[16] An additional hazard for women is an increase in cancer of the breast and uterus.[16]

Earlier in this chapter I noted that in 1982, the National Academy of Sciences report, Diet, Nutrition, and Cancer, recommended that alcoholic beverages be drunk only in moderation. The basis for this advice came from a study reported five years earlier in the *Journal of the National Cancer Institute* which found that smoking and drinking were associated with an increased risk of various cancers including that of the female breast. The report did not create much of a stir at that time partly because some of their other correlations appeared implausible. For example, a college education and high income were associated with a higher incidence of some cancers in men. However, since that time, numerous studies were conducted in this country and elsewhere and virtually all found an association between alcohol intake and breast cancer. The most recent and the most convincing evidence is found in what is called the Nurses' Health Study.

In 1980, 105,896 American nurses completed detailed questionnaires regarding, among other things, their drinking habits. They were then followed for twenty-eight years. During that period, a little over seven percent of them developed breast cancer. When the data were analyzed by Wendy Chen and her colleagues in 2011, there emerged what we called in chapter 1 a dose-effect relationship. The more alcohol drunk, the higher the risk of breast cancer. As little as 3-6 glasses of wine per week or their equivalent in beer or spirits had a perceptible effect. The authors estimated that around 10% of new cases of breast cancer could be avoided by abstention from alcohol. In the real world, what is a woman who enjoys modest amounts of alcohol to do? I quote the last sentence of Dr. Chen's report.

...an individual will need to weigh the modest risks of light to moderate alcohol use on breast cancer development against the beneficial effects on cardiovascular disease to make the best personal choice regarding alcohol consumption.[21]

However, a less sanguine conclusion was reached in 2013 by David E. Nelson of the National Cancer Institute and his colleagues.[22] In what they called "the first comprehensive study of alcohol-attributable cancer deaths in the United States in more than 30 years", they concluded that alcohol consumption causes 15% of breast cancer deaths and 3.5% of all cancer deaths. Furthermore, they discounted possible beneficial effects of alcohol on heart disease and suggested that alcohol cause ten times more deaths than it prevents. Finally, though they found that risk increased with the amount of alcohol consumed, they also could detect no lower level completely devoid of risk.

An article by Tara Parker-Pope in the *New York Times* for April 8, 2010 carried the headline "Eating Vegetables Doesn't Stop Cancer." That conclusion was based upon a study by Paolo Boffetta of the Mount Sinai School of Medicine and his colleagues of more than 478,000 Europeans for nine years.[23] The *Times* piece said that it was "the latest in a series of studies to debunk the potential of vegetables for lowering cancer risk." I rather hope that you didn't read the *Times* that day. As an anonymous writer in *The Lancet* put it, headlines like that could deflate even the most ardent healthy-eating campaigner.

I realize that the function of headlines is to gain our attention but that one did a disservice and, I would add, ignored what was said in the last paragraph of the report: "…our study supports the notion of a modest cancer preventative effect of high intake of fruits and vegetables…" However, despite that tepid endorsement of fruits and vegetable, a negative conclusion with respect to fruit and vegetable consumption and cancer was reached in 2014 by a group at the Harvard School of Public Health. The latter study brought together data from more than 800,000 people in sixteen separate studies. But, fearful as it may be, cancer is not the only reason we die and I would direct you to a further conclusion reached by the Harvard group in 2014: "…a higher consumption of fruit and vegetables is associated with a lower risk of all-cause mortality, particularly cardiovascular mortality."[24]

The recent comprehensive review by the Parkin group which I have already described to you, concluded that a deficiency in consumption of fruits and vegetables increases the risk of cancer of the oral cavity and pharynx, esophagus, stomach, larynx, and lung. Their fiber content contributes to a significantly lower risk of colorectal cancer. But any effect on cancer is a bonus. Fruits and vegetables displace less desirable components of the diet such as sugar and other refined carbohydrates and thus play an important role in the maintenance of a healthy weight. To the extent that they displace red and processed meat such as ham and bacon, they will reduce the risk, as does fiber, of colorectal cancer. Their beneficial effects related to heart disease and stroke will be noted in chapter 14. Eat your fruits and vegetables.

Before leaving the issue of diet and cancer, I want to say a few things about a particular nutrient, lycopene, and prostate cancer. Lycopene is a carotenoid such as those discussed in chapter 6.5 but, unlike *beta*-carotene, it is not converted into vitamin A. For the past twenty-five years, correlational studies have sometimes suggested that low levels of lycopene may be associated with an increased risk of prostate cancer but the question has remained unsettled. Presently the Food and Drug Administration does not permit claims to be made that lycopene prevents any form of cancer.

In chapter 10 it was pointed out that prostate cancer is the second leading cause of cancer death among American men and, as an elderly American man, I would most certainly like to avoid it. This is the reason, as stated in chapter 10, that I decline to artificially increase my levels of testosterone. On the other hand, I am an avid consumer of tomatoes and tomato products, the richest dietary sources of lycopene. I am influenced in this decision by a report from Ke Zu and his colleagues of the Harvard School of Public Health. Writing in 2014, they described an ongoing study begun in 1986 of more than 50,000 male American health professionals.[25] They examined the relationship between lycopene intake and total prostate cancer, lethal prostate cancer, and a marker for angiogenesis, an indicator of the aggressiveness of cancer. All three measures were reduced in those men with diets having the highest levels of dietary lycopene. Most impressive was that the risk of lethal prostate cancer was cut in half in those men in the highest quintile as compared with those in the lowest. Because processing of raw tomatoes increases the bioavailability of lycopene, items such as tomato soup, tomato paste, and ketchup are best. A good reason to eat, in moderation, pasta and pizza with red sauce. (I know, the food police often include pizza on their "never to eat" lists. Nonsense. Just go easy on the cheese and meat toppings.)

Cancer of all kinds is closely related to the aging process. Most attribute this to cumulative mutational damage to our DNA but, whatever the mechanism, it is a fact that more than 90% of all cancer arises in those beyond the age of 40. In 2014, the Centers for Disease Control estimated that cancer is 126 times more likely in those of us over age 75 than it was when we were teenagers.[2] All the more reason to do all that we can to avoid it. Although it inconceivable that cancer of all kinds will be eliminated in our lifetimes, and if it were would heart disease or dementia fill in the gap, each of us should take a close look at the theoretical optimum exposure levels presented by Dr. Parkin. Whatever age you may be at the moment, embark on a program of prevention. Not only will your risk of developing cancer be reduced but all other unwanted aspects of aging will be ameliorated as well.

CHAPTER 14

HEART DISEASE AND STROKE

The greatest killers

Nearly four centuries have passed since William Harvey described in detail the functioning of the heart and the circulation of the blood. Since that time, an enormous amount has been discovered about how our circulatory system works in health and in disease. Much that we have learned has been put to good use. The rate of death from heart and vascular disease in the United States has dropped by 70% from its peak in 1968. Nonetheless, more of us continue to die following a heart attack or stroke than from any other cause.[1] Cardiovascular disease is eight times more likely to kill a woman than is breast cancer. Deaths from prostate cancer number less than one-tenth those from heart disease. Fortunately, there is much that we can do to further reduce the likelihood of our suffering a stroke or heart attack.

In 1948, a study was begun in the town of Framingham, Massachusetts that would forever change the face of cardiovascular disease and, in the process, introduce the notion of risk factors.[2] A total of 5,209 residents of the town, aged 30-62, were recruited, given physical and laboratory examinations, questioned about their lifestyles, and then followed up every two years until they died. The Framingham study continues to this day and now includes the second and third generation descendants of the original participants.

As defined at Framingham, a risk factor is a characteristic which is associated with a greater than average probability of developing vascular disease. Eventually the number grew to include more than 250 but, as we have seen before, correlation does not equal causality. Those for which the evidence is strongest are just nine in number: family history, gender, age, high blood pressure, elevated serum cholesterol, obesity, diabetes, lack of exercise, and smoking. You already know that the smoking of nicotine-containing cigarettes is a deadly addiction to be condemned for multiple reasons and I'll say no more about it here.

Of the other factors listed, the first three, family history, gender, and age, are not under our control. However, we certainly can make use of them. In a way, it's the converse of "if it ain't broke, don't fix it." If you are male, you need to concern yourself more about heart disease than if you are a premenopausal woman. Likewise, all of us as we age need to pay ever greater attention to the state of our heart and blood vessels. But it is family history that provides the clearest picture of our possible future. We cannot change our genetic endowment but we can work to counter any disease to which that endowment predisposes us. Many a son whose father was taken at an early age by a heart attack has been inspired to follow a different path by altering the remaining risk factors.

The first principle of prevention is that neither risk factors nor preventive measures operate in isolation. Obesity and weight loss were considered at length in chapters 7 and 8. There I presented you with the hypothesis that the hormonal changes that occur in the presence of excess body fat are the primary cause of type 2 diabetes. Eighty percent of untreated diabetics are also hypertensive, i.e., they have high blood pressure. The adverse vascular effects of elevated blood sugar are exacerbated by high levels of serum cholesterol. On the preventive side, diet and exercise are recurring themes and should always be fully implemented before resorting to drugs. Altered patterns of eating as exemplified by the DASH and Mediterranean diets coupled with aerobic and anaerobic exercise can simultaneously alter obesity, hypertension, serum cholesterol, and diabetes. A massive study completed three decades ago concluded that men aged 35-57 who don't smoke and have appropriate levels of cholesterol and blood pressure will die from heart disease at a rate of 2.40 per 1,000. Hypertension increases the rate to 3.86; smoking to 5.62; elevated cholesterol to 6.12. But for the man who smokes, has high blood pressure, and has too much cholesterol in his blood, the rate of death increases to 17.49. In just five years, he is more than seven times as likely to die of heart disease.[3]

First, a word about guidelines. For fifty years and more, groups including the American Cancer Society, the United States Department of Agriculture, the American Heart Association, numerous branches of the National Institutes of Health, the National Kidney Foundation, the American Diabetes Foundation, and numerous professional societies have issued guidelines on a variety of issues related to our health. We have been given specific numbers to be achieved with respect to body weight, blood pressure, blood sugar, and serum cholesterol, details of screening for multiple diseases, and advice on all manner of dietary components such as vitamins, salt, and fats. The intentions have generally been good though the influence of Big Food, Big Pharma, and Big Agriculture has sometimes been evident. However, frustration on the part of the general public has arisen because of regular alterations in these guidelines. Should we reduce sodium in the diet? Should we screen for prostate cancer? At what level should we say you have hypertension and when should it be treated with drugs? At what age should women get mammograms? Absent is a guideline on guidelines. All such guidelines must be recognized as no more than informed opinion based on what is known, or thought to be known, at any given point in time. It is inevitable that advice in the form of guidelines will change with time. The great danger is that these changes will further undermine trust in the medical system and that well-founded advice will be ignored because of frustration with the uncertainty of it all.

At the root of heart disease and the majority of strokes is atherosclerosis, a condition in which blood vessels become blocked by deposits of cholesterol (atheroma) and hardened (sclerotic). Most often affected are the arteries, hence the related term arteriosclerosis, hardening of the arteries. For example, as atherosclerosis progresses, plaques forming in the arteries supplying blood to the heart can cause sudden attacks of chest pain in the condition called angina pectoris. If a plaque ruptures, coagulation occurs and a thrombus or clot is formed resulting in the complete block of blood flow in the artery. This is a myocardial infarction, a heart attack. If the clot breaks loose it is called an embolus which may travel to distant sites to block blood flow. A thrombus originating in a leg vein may be carried to the lung and block blood flow there. A clot that reaches the brain results in a stroke.

The current emphasis on the role of lifestyle in causing and preventing atherosclerosis might lead one to think that it is a new affliction. In fact, it is an ancient disease whose ultimate origins are still largely unknown. Modern imaging techniques applied to mummies dating to the second century B.C. in Egypt, Peru, and in Pueblo Indians of what is now the American Southwest have revealed the presence of atherosclerosis in nearly a third.[4] It is also a multifactorial disease, influenced by many different elements of our lives. Arguably the most important of these is hypertension. Like osteoporosis, it is a silent disorder; if our blood pressure is not checked regularly, we become aware of the disease only when bad things happen. The organs most often involved are heart, brain, eyes, and kidneys. The incidence of hypertension increases progressively with age. By age 65, more than 65% of Americans are affected.[5]

Blood pressure is nearly always given in terms of millimeters of mercury. Thus, 120/70 means that the peak pressure in the vascular tree, the systolic pressure, is equal to a column of mercury 120 millimeters high. The second number, the diastolic pressure, is a measure of the minimum pressure exerted by the blood on the walls.

No one doubts the damage done by hypertension but that is about the only thing that can be said without evoking controversy. In 1930, writing in the *Journal of the American Medical Association*, two prominent physicians defined hypertension as a reading of 160/95.[6] By 1990, the emphasis was on the diastolic pressure with mild hypertension defined as 90-104 mm. Ten years later, Peter Sever, a past president of the British Hypertension Society, said that we should abandon routine diastolic readings.[7] Until very recently, most guidelines suggested a diastolic pressure between 80 and 90 mm coupled with a systolic pressure of 140 mm. But Dr. Sever again: only a systolic pressure greater than 150 mm is cause for intervention and raise that to 160 mm for those without other risk factors or over age 65. He and others regard hypotension, too low a systolic pressure, and the falls associated with it, to be a particular hazard for the elderly.

In the United States, the latest guideline, published in February 2014, has done little to settle the issue.[8] The emphasis in the guideline is upon deciding at what blood pressure readings to begin medication. Three categories were created. If you are younger than 60: 140/90. For those of us 60 or older: 150/90. The third category is for those with diabetes or chronic kidney disease: 140/90.

Response to elevating the threshold for treatment to 150/90 for those age 60 and older was immediate. This was the first time that a recommended value had been increased in the nearly four decades over which American guidelines had been issued. Objections were raised by the American Heart Association, the American College of Cardiology, and the American Society for Hypertension. Participation by the National Heart Lung and Blood Institute in development of the guidelines was discontinued a year earlier and it was acknowledged by the authors of the guidelines that their report was neither sanctioned by the Institute nor did it "reflect the views of NHLBI."

What's a person to do? My own inclination is to listen to those who point out that primitive societies with systolic pressures less than 120 mm have remarkably little heart disease. That inclination is encouraged by the results of a study published in 2014 by Eleni Rapsomaniki and her colleagues of London's Farr Institute of Health Informatics Research.[9] They examined electronic health records of one and quarter million healthy adult patients. Over the five year course of the study, seven percent of the participants exhibited signs of heart or blood vessel disease. The investigators found that the risk was lowest in people with systolic readings of 90-114 and diastolic of 60-74; let's say 102/67. For some, such values can be reached by non-pharmacological means alone: smoking cessation, regular exercise, weight loss, low-sodium diet, etc. For most others, drug treatment will be necessary. However, only a knowledgeable physician, taking into account your personal history, can arrive at a prudent target. And, as always, the potential adverse effects of too aggressive treatment with drugs to reach an unrealistic and possibly unhelpful goal must be considered. As I already noted, this is of particular concern in the elderly for whom drug-induced low blood pressure may contribute to falls with all of their consequences.

The form of stroke I mentioned earlier, where blood vessels in the brain are blocked by an embolus, is more formally called cerebral ischemia-infarction. Brain tissue is deprived of essential oxygen and nutrients and quickly dies. A second type of stroke results when we have bleeding into the brain tissue when an artery bursts; this is called a hemorrhagic stroke and accounts for about 10% of all strokes. Control of blood pressure is the most important factor in reducing the risk of hemorrhagic stroke. Hypertension and hemorrhagic stroke become progressively more important as we age because of the weakening of the blood vessels of the brain by deposition of amyloid, the substance we talked about in chapter 12 as a possible cause of dementia.

The life and death of Franklin Delano Roosevelt, the 32nd President of the United States, illustrates both the consequences of the disease and how far we have come in its treatment. In early February, 1945, Roosevelt met with Winston Churchill and Joseph Stalin at Yalta to chart the course of World War II. His blood pressure at that time was 260/150 yet he appeared to function well. At that time, hypertension, while clearly hazardous, was deemed untreatable. On April 12, 1945, his personal physician, Commander Howard Bruenn, obtained a reading of 300/190.[10] A short time later, the President said "I have a terrific headache." Those were his last words. He quickly lost consciousness and was dead two hours later. Although no autopsy was performed, it is likely that he died of a massive hemorrhagic stroke. Writing in 1970, Dr. Bruenn commented "I have often wondered what the course of history might have been if the modern methods for the control of hypertension had been available then."[11] Roosevelt was 63 years of age.

The means to reduce blood pressure are varied and many of us will use multiple measures simultaneously. As I mentioned earlier, our first course of treatment takes the form of diet and exercise. In the late 1940's, J. N. Morris and his colleagues, under the auspices of the Medical Research Council of England, set out "to seek for relations between the kind of work men do and the incidence among them of coronary heart disease." The drivers of London's double-decker buses were compared to their conductors. In a day's work, the drivers sat while the conductors were in near-constant motion from front to back and from deck to deck of the bus.

In a pair of articles published in November of 1953, Morris reported that bus conductors suffered heart disease less often and in less severe form than did the drivers.[12, 13] Several years later Morris and Dr. Margaret Crawford speculated that "habitual physical activity is a general factor of cardiovascular health in middle-aged men" and that "regular physical exercise could be one of the 'ways of life' that promote health in middle age."[14]

It's hardly a practical approach to the prevention of heart disease simply to tell everyone to be a conductor rather than a driver. But if physical activity on the job is beneficial, might leisure-time exercise do as well? In earlier times, the nearly universal advice given to those with hypertension was to take it easy, to avoid strenuous exercise, so as not to strain the heart. In 1970, John Boyer and Fred Kasch of San Diego State University provided the first evidence that aerobic training, as we discussed in chapters 4 and 5, is useful in reversing hypertension.[15]

Drs. Boyer and Kasch chose for their study 45 sedentary men aged 35-61 who differed only in their blood pressure. The men they called normotensive had readings of 140/90 or less. The readings for the 23 men defined as having diastolic hypertension were 159/105. (At that time the emphasis was on the diastolic pressure.) The exercise program consisted of alternate walking and running for 30 minutes twice a week for six months. You may recall from chapter 5 that Waldo Harris and his colleagues at the University of Oregon had described jogging three years earlier.

At the end of 6 months, the normotensive group had an average drop of 6 mm in diastolic pressure. Still more impressive was what happened to the hypertensives. Diastolic pressure declined in all of the 23 and the average blood pressure reading fell to 146/93. In the years that followed, many have confirmed these findings and have concluded that aerobic exercise itself, independent of any weight loss that might occur, accounts for the drop in blood pressure. What is perhaps most surprising is that subsequent studies have found beneficial effects of strength training on blood pressure. This is still another reason to embark on a combined program of aerobic and anaerobic exercise as described in chapter 5.

Having read chapter 7, you already are aware that I regard obesity as I do the smoking of cigarettes; there is nothing good about it. All of us should strive to bring body fat to an acceptable level. That being said, there are some unknowns to be considered. What has been called the obesity paradox refers to the observation that those with pre-existing heart disease and hypertension seem not to be harmed by being over-weight. While there presently is no certain explanation of the obesity paradox or even agreement as to its existence, it has been pointed out that in nearly all studies in which it has been observed, obesity was defined in terms of body mass index (BMI).[16] We already have seen that many athletes in superb physical condition have BMI values which put them in the overweight or obese categories. BMI is a very rough tool for defining obesity. Indeed, if an alternative measure such as the waist to hip ratio is used, the obesity paradox largely disappears.

All are agreed that, with respect to hypertension and cardiovascular disease, exercise and avoidance of obesity are good ideas. But what about the specifics of what we eat? Here we come back to controversy in the form of what we might call the great salt debate.

Sodium is a soft silvery metal, liquid at 208 degrees, used as a coolant in some nuclear reactors. Drop it into water and an explosion beloved of every undergraduate chemistry major results. Chlorine is the poison gas of trench warfare in World War I. An odd couple, sodium and chlorine, but combine them and sodium chloride is formed. Its common name is table salt, essential for life and an item of commerce since antiquity. Dissolve salt in a watery environment such as the ocean, our digestive tract, or our blood, and its constituent sodium and chloride atoms are released. These charged forms, sodium and chloride ions, are essential for human life, not the least because each is required for the electrical activity of our hearts and our brains. Given their importance, the human body has elaborate mechanisms to maintain appropriate levels by balancing intake from the diet and excretion by the kidneys.

A connection has long been made between high blood pressure and dietary salt, usually expressed as milligrams of sodium. Beginning in the 1970's various national and international organizations have suggested that we reduce our salt intake in the interests of preventing or reducing hypertension and its cardiovascular consequences. The World Health Organization recommends no more than 2,500 mg per day. The 2010 Dietary Guidelines issued by the United States Department of Agriculture and endorsed by the American Heart Association go further: reduce daily sodium intake to less than 2,300 mg and further reduce intake to 1,500 mg among persons who are 51 and older and those of any age who are African American or have hypertension, diabetes, or chronic kidney disease.[17] To put 1,500 mg into perspective, it is estimated that a typical American adult today takes in somewhere between 3,500 and 5,000 mg of sodium. This is well above what the guidelines suggest and about ten times more than our minimal needs. Presently, about 90% of Americans exceed the 2,300 mg guideline and less than 1 in 100 is below 1,500 mg.

But where is the controversy? For decades, critics have argued that the calls for reduced sodium are misguided and that actual harm may be done by eating too little salt. Leading these critics, not surprisingly, has been the Salt Institute (which is not to be confused with the Salt Institute for Documentary Studies). The Institute describes itself as an "association of salt companies dedicated to helping consumers unlock the secrets of salt, sodium chloride." The medical establishment paid little attention to the Institute or its spokesman, Morton Satin (or as he is identified on the Institute's web site, the Salt Guru). The guidelines of groups such as the American Heart Association continued to be widely promoted to the general public and endorsed by such luminaries as Mayor Michael

Bloomberg and his health commissioner, Thomas A. Farley. In 2014, Dr. Farley called salt "the public health crisis hiding in our food."[18]

In 2011, the Cochrane Collaboration, a highly respected group in Oxford, England, reevaluated previous studies linking excessive sodium intake with hypertension and vascular disease.[19] The title of their article in the *American Journal of Hypertension* was Reduced Dietary Salt for the Prevention of Cardiovascular Disease. After writing that "Our findings are consistent with the belief that salt reduction is beneficial in normotensive and hypertensive people" they went on to express reservations. The data did not, in their opinion, prove that salt reduction reduces deaths from cardiovascular disease. Furthermore, they expressed concern that some might be harmed by drastically lowering sodium intake. Finally, doubt was raised as to whether dietary advice to the general public has had any effect on salt intake and speculated that it was the food processing industry that had to change.

Many rejected the Cochrane conclusions. In an editorial in *The Lancet*, a London-based medical journal, Graham MacGregor, a long-time foe of excess sodium, said flatly "These statements are incorrect."[20] On the other hand the media were quick to embrace them. A front page headline in the *Daily Express*, a British tabloid, read "Now salt is safe to eat – health fascists wrong after lecturing us all these years." The *New York Times* was more subdued: "Research questions the benefit of low-salt diet" and "Cutting salt has little effect on heart risk." In May 2013, more doubt was sprinkled on the low-salt campaign by a committee appointed by the Institute of Medicine at the request of the US Centers for Disease Control. Their conclusion, similar to that expressed earlier in the Cochrane review, was that reducing sodium is not as beneficial as was previously thought and, more alarming, that some might actually be harmed by intakes less than 2,300 mg.[21]

It remains to be seen what influence the conclusions of the Cochrane and Institute of Medicine reports will have the new US dietary guidelines to be issued in 2015. In the meantime, what are we to do while the opposing sides battle it out? First and foremost, be aware of your blood pressure. If, without medication, it is in the range of 120-130 mm systolic and less than 80 or so mm diastolic, you have little to worry about with respect to sodium. You may be one of those fortunate persons whose blood pressure is not influenced by dietary sodium. However, even the salt-insensitive should taste food before adding salt if only to flatter the chef whose seasoning is already, in her mind, perfect. On the other hand, if your blood pressure readings are higher than optimal, a modest reduction in salt intake may be helpful. Only regular monitoring of blood pressure can tell us if any given intervention is working. Home monitoring devices are reliable and relatively inexpensive.

A significant shaper of my feelings about sodium guidelines came from an editorial by Michael H. Alderman following release of the Cochrane report in 2011.[22] At the time, Dr. Altman was the editor-in-chief of the *American Journal of Hypertension* and professor of medicine and epidemiology at the Albert Einstein College of Medicine. In his article, he presented a figure showing a continuous decrease in blood pressure with lower levels of salt intake; just what the low-salt advocates emphasize. But the figure also showed a quite different relationship between dietary salt and cardiovascular events and those, after all, are what we really are interested in. The optimal point was at about 2,500 mg of sodium, the amount recommended by the World Health Organization. Above that value *and below that value*, disease increased in what has been called a J-shaped relationship. If there be truth in these data, they favor a reduction in sodium intake from current levels to about 2,500 mg but argue against more extreme reductions advocated by organizations such as the American Heart Association.

I will end this now rather long discussion of sodium with the thought that perhaps our emphasis has been misdirected. There is a second ion to be considered: potassium. It too is found in the foods we eat and its effects are generally opposite those of sodium. Current recommendations range from the World Health Organization's 3,000 mg per day to 4,700 mg per day in the United States. It has been estimated that fewer than 2% of the American population currently reach 4,700 mg.[23] As already noted, many studies have suggested a favorable effect on hypertension of reducing sodium. In contrast, an *increase* in dietary potassium lowers blood pressure. Most convincing of all are studies which examined the ratio of sodium to potassium. These indicate that a ratio of one to one may be optimal both with respect to hypertension and cardiovascular disease, stroke, and death.[24, 25]

There is a simple way to simultaneously decrease sodium and increase potassium. Eat more unprocessed fruits and vegetables. As a group these foods are low in sodium and rich in potassium. Particularly to be recommended are peas, beans and greens of all kinds, potatoes with the skin left on, bananas, whole grains, nuts, and fish: all of the foods so abundantly found in the Mediterranean and DASH diets. My favorite is the tomato and tomato products: virtually sodium-free and rich in potassium. Yogurt is a good choice in a processed food. Most brands have 2 to 5 times more potassium than sodium. Even a much-maligned sugar-sweetened cereal I eat most days of the week is sodium-free and a good source of potassium. Sodium content is now commonly listed for processed foods and soon it is hoped that potassium will be shown as well. As you have already read in chapters 2 and 6, I am generally opposed to the use of supplements and this is certainly true for potassium. Intake from unprocessed foods is perfectly safe but one can easily exceed a healthy level if supplements are used particularly in the presence of kidney disease.[26]

If hypertension is the leading risk factor for heart disease and stroke, type 2 diabetes is not far behind. Indeed, the two conditions are closely related.[27] Diabetes is a probable cause of much hypertension. As I noted earlier in this chapter, eighty percent of untreated diabetics are also hypertensive. The vascular damage that is done is a major factor in adult blindness, end-stage kidney disease, nerve damage leading to pain and loss of sensation, heart attack and stroke. The feet and legs are especially susceptible to ulcers, infection, and eventual amputation.

All forms of diabetes are defined in terms of blood glucose but it is important to distinguish between the two major types. What was previously called insulin-dependent or juvenile-onset diabetes is an autoimmune disorder that destroys the ability of the *beta* cells of the pancreas to produce insulin, the primary regulator of blood glucose levels. It is now designated type 1 diabetes. Presently we know of no way to prevent type 1 diabetes and its treatment remains imperfect despite the enormous contribution made by the discovery of insulin in the 1920's. In contrast, the majority of type 2 diabetes with all its terrible consequences is preventable by the avoidance or reversal of obesity. Returning to the comparisons made in chapter 7 of the states of Mississippi and Connecticut, I would point out that in Mississippi the rate of obesity is 58% higher and the incidence of diagnosed diabetes is greater by 75% than in Connecticut.

Cholesterol, the final risk factor to be considered, is the one perhaps best known to the general public. In chapter 6.2, I told you of the essential nature of cholesterol and the fact that we are able to manufacture our own thus freeing us of any need for a dietary source. In addition, I mentioned that a connection between saturated fat in our food and serum cholesterol was reported more than sixty years ago. The idea that high serum cholesterol has an effect on cardiovascular disease had been proposed in the 1850's but was not convincingly demonstrated until 1938 with the work of the Norwegian physician Carl Muller.[28] He described a group of patients with an inborn propensity to develop atherosclerosis. The name given to their disease, familial hypercholesterolemia, reflects its genetic basis and its primary sign, elevated levels of cholesterol in the blood. About one person in a million receives defective genes from both parents. These individuals are destined to suffer heart attacks as early as childhood. Despite its rarity, the study of familial hypercholesterolemia has provided insights likely to be of value to the majority of the world's population.

The primary site of cholesterol synthesis is the liver. But cholesterol is an oily, water-insoluble material, and the blood is a watery medium. Oil and water don't mix. How then are we to move cholesterol from the liver to all cells of the body? As any mister-mom knows, to disperse oil in water, you need a detergent. Nature's cholesterol-dispersing detergents are the lipoproteins. They are of various kinds and are usually addressed by their initials; best known are LDL, low density lipoprotein, and HDL, high density lipoprotein. LDL-cholesterol has come to be known as "bad cholesterol" because it is the form most often associated with cardiovascular disease. HDL-cholesterol, on the other hand, has been called "good cholesterol" because higher levels have long been thought to be beneficial. (This idea has recently been challenged.[29]) The Nobel Prize for Physiology or Medicine was awarded in 1985 to Drs. Michael Brown and Joseph Goldstein of the University of Texas for their discovery that those with familial hypercholesterolemia lack receptors for LDL-cholesterol with the result that normal entry of cholesterol into cells cannot occur.[30] The excess is deposited in arteries and atherosclerosis develops.

The Framingham Heart Study, begun in 1948, reported in 1965 that serum cholesterol is a major risk factor for coronary heart disease.[31] However, this conclusion was based purely on epidemiological data: higher cholesterol levels were correlated with an increased risk of atherosclerosis. There remained the uncomfortable facts, and they are still with us today, that a significant number of persons who suffer heart attacks have normal levels of cholesterol and nearly half of those with elevated cholesterol never have a heart attack. In 1973, the National Heart and Lung Institute began a study intended to buttress the case against high cholesterol. (With the addition of blood disease to its portfolio, the Institute is now called NHLBI.) It was decided not to do a simple diet/heart disease investigation in healthy people on the grounds that the expected effect would be too small to be identified except in an unreasonably large group of people. Instead they opted for a design in which persons at high risk would be treated with cholestyramine, a cholesterol-lowering drug popular at the time.

Nearly half a million men (no women) were screened to identify 3,806 whose total cholesterol put them in the top 5% in that regard. All subjects were placed on a diet expected to reduce serum cholesterol by 3-8%. Half received cholestyramine. The men were followed for an average of 7.4 years. The primary end point was death from coronary heart disease or a nonfatal heart attack.

The results of the LRCT were published in January 20, 1984 in the *Journal of the American Medical Association.*[32] Drug treatment reduced levels of cholesterol in the blood and that reduction was associated with fewer heart attacks and deaths from heart attacks. What followed may be described as an explosion of media attention. *Time* magazine had a cover story called "Hold the Eggs and Butter" with the subtitle "Cholesterol is proved deadly and our diets may never be the same." But, as we have seen before, the passage of information from the literature of science with all its reservations and caveats to the purity of the popular press is not always without distortion.

Let's first look at the numbers. Some 32 drug-treated men died of heart attacks versus 44 controls; 12 lives were saved, an impressive result. But there are other ways to die than by heart attack. Overall deaths in the cholestyramine group numbered 68 while 71 controls died. The difference is less impressive and, by the usual criteria of science, quite possibly the result only of chance. The thought crossed more than one mind that the drug treatment, though perhaps saving lives by reducing cholesterol, might be taking lives by some unknown toxic effect. To this day, no satisfactory explanation for the increase in non-heart disease deaths has been found; oddly enough, the excess deaths were caused by accident, suicide, and homicide.

The simple message carried by the media was "the more you reduce cholesterol and fat in your diet, the more you reduce your risk of heart disease." In fact, those were the words of Basil Rifkind, director of the LRCT, as quoted by *Time* magazine on March 26, 1984. But the LRCT wasn't a diet study. It was a drug study. And the LRCT didn't look at average people or even normal people. It was concerned with middle-aged white men with an average cholesterol level of 292 mg per deciliter of blood, nearly three times higher than what current guidelines recommend.

The LRCT coupled with an earlier study sponsored by the LHLBI now represented an investment which today would amount to nearly one billion tax payer dollars. The LHLBI had to do something with the results. On December 10, 1984, it convened a Consensus Development Conference to consider "lowering blood cholesterol to prevent heart disease." Drawing heavily upon the LRCT, the panel made a number of recommendations.[33] Among them was that all Americans aged 2 to 90 should reduce daily cholesterol intake to 250-300 mg or less. I have previously noted that two eggs alone will put you well over the limit.

Critics of that recommendation were quick to respond. M. F. Oliver, professor of medicine at Scotland's University of Edinburgh chose this title for his article in *The Lancet* : Consensus or Nonsensus Conferences on Coronary Heart Disease.[34] Professor Edward Ahrens of Rockefeller University said that recommendations "should be based, not on faith or zeal or alarm, but on hard scientific evidence" and added that "existing evidence is far from convincing."[35] Less restrained was Thomas Chalmers of the Mt. Sinai Medical School: "I think the panel made an unconscionable exaggeration of all the data."

In the years that followed, the NHLBI issued explicit total cholesterol goals for those at highest risk: smokers, diabetics, hypertensives, and the obese. The trend was ever downward, from 130 mg/dL in 1988 to less than 100 in 2002 to less than 70 in 2004. But what about healthy people, those without other risk factors? In mid-2013, advice from the Cleveland Clinic was this: "It is extremely important for everyone—men and women of every age, with or without known heart disease—to have a low LDL-cholesterol level...the optimal guideline level is less than 100 mg/dL."[36] The Mayo Clinic website was a little less demanding: 100-129 mg/dL.[37] And then came the publication, on November 12, 2013, of the American College of Cardiology-American Heart Association guidelines.[38]

In the first major revision since 2002, the ACC/AHA document was a dramatic departure from previous guidelines. Recommendations for drug therapy were no longer focused on cholesterol levels. Indeed, no routine assessment of LDL-cholesterol levels is advised. Instead, a "risk calculator" takes into account, in addition to cholesterol, multiple factors including gender, age, smoking status, family and personal history of heart disease, diabetes, height, weight, and waist size as an index of obesity, blood pressure, and level of triglycerides. For example, drug treatment would not be recommended for a person aged 40-75 years with a calculated risk of cardiovascular disease of less than 7.5% even with an LDL-cholesterol level as high as 189 mg/dL. At the other end of the scale, high-intensity drug therapy is recommended for all persons, independent of cholesterol levels, who have already suffered a stroke or heart attack or who have others signs of cardiovascular disease such as angina.

Before considering the reaction of the medical community to the new guidelines, a few words about the drugs to be used. They all belong to a family called statins. Their trade and generic names are familiar to many of us either because of personal experience or from their extensive advertising. They include Crestor (rosuvastatin), Lipitor (atorvastatin), Zocor (simvastatin), and Mevacor (lovastatin). All act to inhibit the enzyme in the liver responsible for cholesterol synthesis. Although initial sales were tepid, aggressive promotion and evidence from a series of clinical trials gradually convinced prescribers. From the time of its introduction in 1987 until its patent ran out on November 30, 2011, worldwide sales of Lipitor alone totaled $124 billion.

Reaction to the ACC/AHA guidelines was immediate and generally unfavorable. Much of the criticism centered on the risk calculator. Paul Ridker and Nancy Cook of Boston's Brigham and Women's Hospital argued that risk was overestimated by 75 to 150% thus exposing millions more to a lifetime of statin treatment.[39] They went on to say that virtually all men older than 66 years and women older than 70 years have a calculated risk factor greater than 7.5% even with optimal risk factors. Under the new guidelines, 13 million Americans would be added to the 43 million for whom statins were already recommended.

In articles in the *New York Times* by Gina Kolata, Steven Nissen, chief of cardiovascular medicine at the Cleveland Clinic was quoted as saying that "It's stunning...we need a pause to further evaluate this approach."[40] Peter Libby, chairman of cardiovascular medicine at Brigham and Women's

Hospital said "We're surrounded by a real disaster in terms of credibility."[41] John P.A. Ioannidis of the Stanford University School of Medicine wrote in the *Journal of the American Medical Association* that "It is uncertain whether this would be one of the greatest achievements or one of the worst disasters of medical history."[42] Dr. Ioannidis went on to point out that 8 of the 15 panelists writing the new guidelines have ties to the pharmaceutical industry. (It should be noted that this is an improvement over the guidelines of 2004 when all but one of the fifteen authors had ties to companies selling cholesterol-lowering drugs.[43]) Rita F. Redburg, editor of *JAMA Internal Medicine* offered the opinion that the guidelines "will benefit the pharmaceutical industry more than anyone else."[44]

What are you and I supposed to do? The answer of course is to "talk to your doctor" so that you may engage in "shared decision making." The statins are after all not without adverse effects including liver damage, muscle problems, and increased risk of diabetes and cataract. Perhaps of greatest concern in the elderly is the possibility of cognitive decline. In 2012, the Food and Drug Administration warned about memory loss, forgetfulness, amnesia, and confusion.[45] Clearly, as with all drugs, we need to balance benefit and risk. With respect to the statins, that balance must be reached on an individual basis.

To paraphrase an old maxim of clinical medicine, half of what we have been told about cholesterol is wrong and we don't know which half. The darker side of the current fascination with cholesterol is that we may lose site of the fact that atherosclerosis is a multifactorial disease. The sedentary hypertensive obese diabetic smoker who merely gives up eggs for breakfast is likely to be disappointed with the results. Before any drug treatment is considered, whether it be for reduction of cholesterol or an elevated blood pressure, non-pharmacological factors should be corrected: stop smoking, engage in regular aerobic and anaerobic exercise, achieve and maintain an appropriate body weight, and adopt a manner of eating in keeping with the principles of the DASH and Mediterranean diets.

CHAPTER 15

OSTEOPOROSIS

Of osteoclasts and osteoblasts

Like high blood pressure, bone loss due to osteoporosis is initially silent and symptom-free. Often we become aware of it only when an arm or a vertebra or a hip is fractured. Osteoporosis is not a new disease. The skeleton of an adult Egyptian female now housed in the Natural History Museum of the Smithsonian Institution is about 4,000 years old. It shows unequivocal evidence of osteoporosis and a hip fracture.

Because age is the primary risk factor for osteoporosis, it was little seen in ancient societies; few lived long enough for it to be manifest. This situation has changed dramatically as advances in medical science and public health have permitted more and more people to live to old and advanced old age. In 2013, it was estimated that 15 million persons living in the United States have the disease with the number of fractures approaching 2 million per year. Twenty-five percent of residents of nursing homes are victims. Treatment of the consequences of osteoporosis is a major contributor to steadily rising health care costs.[1]

More important than dollars, consider the cost of osteoporosis in human terms. One in five hip fracture victims is dead within one year. Only slightly less fortunate is that percentage of the hip-broken elderly who linger for years without ever again leaving their beds. (*Matratzengruft*, "mattress grave", is the expression Heinrich Heine used.) To this we must add the countless broken arms and the collapsed vertebrae of "dowager's hump" to begin to grasp the consequences of osteoporosis.

In chapter 6.15 on vitamin D we considered rickets and its adult form, osteomalacia. We saw that these conditions are characterized by soft bones because of inadequate calcification. Rickets and osteomalacia are almost always caused by vitamin D deficiency and the resultant inadequate absorption of calcium. Osteoporosis is a quite different disease. Bone appears to be normally calcified, but there is simply too little of it. In severe osteoporosis, the bones may be so thin that fractures occur with the slightest stress; a sneeze will sometimes suffice. The mechanisms by which these changes take place have been known for a long time but a means to prevent the disease and to cure it once established have remained elusive.

It is easy to imagine that bone once formed is solid and stable and unchanging. In fact, bone is one of the most active of tissues, constantly undergoing remodeling throughout our lives. The cells responsible are osteoblasts which build bone and osteoclasts which tear it down. Ideally these are in perfect balance, a balance influenced by multiple factors including testosterone, estrogen, and parathyroid hormone. When that equilibrium shifts, as for example when estrogen production is diminished at the time of menopause, osteoclasts predominate, bone is lost, and fractures may result.

Prior to World War II, those few who thought about osteoporosis were inclined to attribute it to a lack of dietary calcium. That is certainly the simplest explanation but even at that time its validity was challenged by some. However, in the May 31, 1941 issue of the *Journal of the American Medical Association*, a fresh idea made it appearance. The article by Drs. Fuller Albright, Patricia Smith, and Anna Richardson of the Massachusetts General Hospital was simply titled Postmenopausal Osteoporosis, Its Clinical Features.[2]

Dr. Albright and his colleagues "were inclined to minimize the effects of diet." They were aware of the work of A.R.P. Walker with the South African Bantu who, despite a calcium intake of only about one quarter of that presently recommended in the United States, have a very low incidence of osteoporosis and hip fracture.[3] Instead they focused on the fact that osteoporosis is more common in women than in men and that it occurs in women after the menopause or removal of the ovaries. Might then a relative or absolute lack of estrogen be the major causative factor in osteoporosis?

During the decades following World War II, the estrogen hypothesis became thoroughly imbedded in the thinking of American physicians. Osteoporosis came to be regarded as a rather simple disease caused by lack of estrogen; a disease equally simply prevented by providing estrogen to postmenopausal women. Furthermore, as I noted earlier, American physicians convinced themselves that the use of estrogen replacement therapy in menopause not only ameliorated the troublesome effects of this aspect of female aging and prevented osteoporosis but also reduced the incidence of heart disease. Then came the Women's Health Initiative and its finding, contrary to expectations, that estrogen replacement *increased* the risk of heart attack, of stroke, of blood clots, and of breast cancer.[4] Nonetheless, in a delicate balance between risk and benefit, estrogen replacement is still recommended for women at high risk for osteoporosis but in as low a dose and for as short a time as possible.

The diagnosis of osteoporosis is based on the measurement of bone mineral density (BMD) by something called dual X-ray absorptiometry (DXA). The National Osteoporosis Foundation recommends that all women have their BMD measured by age 65. Men can wait until age 70. However, measurement at earlier ages is in order if a fracture has already occurred, if there is a family history of the disease, or if one or more of a myriad of other risk factors are present. Most prominent among these factors are smoking (still another reason to quit), excessive alcohol use, and the use of corticosteroids in the treatment of inflammatory disorders including rheumatoid arthritis, chronic obstructive pulmonary disease (COPD), and inflammatory bowel disease. Our genes are important as well. It has long been known that persons of black African origin have more dense bones than do Caucasians. Though both races lose bone mass with age, blacks have a significantly lower risk of osteoporotic fractures. Indeed, a white woman is five times as likely to suffer a hip fracture as is a black man.

At this point in time there is no combination of measures that is guaranteed either to prevent or to cure osteoporosis. That having been said, there are a number of things we can do. It begins in childhood, adolescence, and young adulthood when bone growth is most vigorous and a skeleton is laid down which must serve us the rest of our lives. It is in our twenties that peak bone mass is achieved. Adequate but not excessive intake of vitamin D and calcium is especially desirable during these periods. And, as we have seen in so many other areas of health maintenance, exercise has a role to play. Frederik Detter and his colleagues, in a study done in Swedish school children and published in 2013, found significant increases in bone mineral density when exercise was increased from the Swedish standard of 60 minutes per week to 200 minutes. The boys and girls were 6 to 9 years of age at the start and were followed for five years.[5]

Although it remains to be proven that either calcium or vitamin D can prevent osteoporosis, current recommendations are to increase daily vitamin D intake by men and women over age 70 to 800 international units (IU) from the 600 IU suggested for younger adults. Also for women over 50, calcium from all sources, but preferably from the diet, should increase to 1,200 mg per day. For men, the increase in calcium can wait until age 70.[6] However, as I noted in chapters 6.15 and 6.18, both calcium and vitamin D can be hazardous in excess. Supplements of either, if they are to be used at all, should be taken with care. More is definitely not better. Smoking and alcohol in excess are never desirable. Every woman should discuss estrogen replacement with her physician at the time of menopause. For those with a strong family history of osteoporosis or other risk factors, the decision for estrogen replacement may well be a wise one.

In chapters 4 and 5, we saw how muscles respond to inactivity by shrinking and to stress by growing. Bones respond in a similar fashion. This remarkable property of bone is due to the fact that bone cells, osteocytes, are derived from the same precursor cells as are neurons and, just as do neurons, osteocytes send out long projections whose function it is to sense the stresses on bone imposed by muscle tension and gravity.

The term "post-traumatic osteoporosis'" first appeared in the medical literature more than a century ago. This is the phenomenon in which bone loss follows inactivity. Persons who suffer paralysis following an injury or a disease such as polio suffer bone loss along with atrophy of their muscles. Astronauts in space, freed of the forces of gravity, invariably excrete more calcium than they take in. As unnatural as we might wish to consider the weightlessness of space or muscle paralysis, the response of bone to these situations is entirely normal. Despite the presence of calcium in abundance, bone will not be formed in the absence of stress. It comes as no surprise then that loss of bone from inactivity cannot be prevented by calcium supplements. But, if lack of stress on bones causes them to become thinner than normal, might the imposition of greater stress cause them to become thicker? That reasonable question and its plausible answer are the basis for our hope that certain forms of exercise will prevent or even reverse osteoporosis.

A simple way to assess the effects of exercise on bone density is to compare athletes with non-athletes. An investigation by Drs. Bo Nilsson and Nils Westlin of the University of Lund in Sweden was the first of its kind and it has served as a model for many similar studies.[7] Their subjects were 64 athletes and, as controls, 39 "healthy men." The density of the thigh bone was measured in each subject. The athletes included weightlifters, runners, soccer players, and swimmers; nine had represented Sweden in international competition. The control subjects were divided into those who exercise regularly and those who did not.

The results obtained by Nilsson and Westlin certainly supported the idea that exercise increases bone density. As a group, the international-class athletes had a density half again as great as the non-exercising controls. However, a more important observation concerned the effects of exercise on the "non-athletic healthy men." Ordinary men who exercised had a 21% greater bone density than did those who did not and their densities were only 18% less than the most elite of the athletes, those who engaged in international competition. Indeed, there was no statistically significant difference between the exercising non-athletes and the national-class runners, soccer players, and swimmers.

Nilsson and Westlin reported their results in 1971. At that time, I was confident that the hypothesis that exercise prevents, perhaps even reverses, osteoporosis would be proven within a decade. Alas, more than forty years later, the matter is not yet settled to the satisfaction of all. Many studies have shown, as did Nilsson and Westlin, an increase in bone mineral density following regular exercise but BMD is only a surrogate endpoint. What we really want to know is whether the rate of fractures is reduced. In 2013, Professor Wolfgang Kemmler and his colleagues at the Institute of Medical Physics of the University of Erlangen in Germany, after assessing results of multiple studies over the past thirty years, came close to a definitive conclusion. Exercise was associated with a convincing decrease in all fractures and a nearly convincing reduction in vertebral fractures.[8]

I am going to ignore the present absence of absolute proof that exercise can reduce the number of fractures of the hip, assume that exercise is a very good idea, and say a few things about what kind of exercise we should choose. All that I have said in chapters 4 and 5 about aerobic and non-aerobic exercise is applicable. In particular I would emphasize strength training but in moderation and, at least when starting out, with formal guidance. The image of bulky men and women straining to lift enormous weights in competition is no more relevant to your strength training program than are masochistic ultra-marathoners to your aerobic conditioning. However, exercise of both kinds on a regular basis is important. For the compulsive, seven days a week for aerobics with strength training on alternate days. For the less dedicated, strength training plus aerobics at least twice a week.

If you are to adopt and maintain a program of exercise to increase bone density and decrease the probability of an osteoporotic fracture, it is essential that activities be chosen that you enjoy and can continue for many years. In terms of what is often called "high-impact weight bearing exercise", hiking, vigorous dancing, and tennis can be as valuable as more formal exercise such as jogging and high-impact aerobics. Something as simple as using the stairs instead of the elevator whenever possible can be helpful. Once again, however, the principles laid out in chapter 5 with respect to intensity and duration should be followed. A final element relates to balance. Strength training and aerobics will improve balance but something more formal is a good idea with advancing age. I earlier suggested regular use of a wobble board but the practice of yoga or Tai chi can be helpful as well.

If exercise is good for your bones, then the more exercise the less risk. Right? Wrong. The reasons for this are rather roundabout, but interesting. It seems that long ago evolution built into women a means to protect against pregnancy when times are hard. A million years ago nobody talked about unemployment rates or levels of poverty so Mother Nature used percentage of body fat as a barometer of hard times. When a woman's body fat falls below a certain level, circulating estrogen decreases and ovulation stops. No ovulation, no pregnancy; no ovulation, no menstruation.

For many women, absence of menstruation may sound like a good thing. Unfortunately, the low-fat fall in estrogen is the endocrinological equivalent of premature menopause which in turn is a powerful influence on accelerated loss of bone. If exercise increases bone density and excess loss of body fat indirectly leads to a decrease in bone density, where is the appropriate balance point? How does a woman know she's gone as far as she should go? The answer to these questions is not entirely clear. Perhaps the best indicator is irregularities in or cessation of menses. Most exercising, dieting women will never reach that point. On the other hand, the women's cross-country team at a West Coast university was said to be menstruation-free for a decade. In addition, loss of bone mass is well documented in a variety of eating disorders including anorexia. All women should carefully balance the benefits of high level training or the achievement of the thinness of a fashion model with possible harm to their bones. With respect to our bones, Bloomingdale's Law must be changed: you cannot be too rich but you can be too thin. (I say "our bones" because there is some evidence that similar low-fat bone loss occurs in men.)

A variety of chemical approaches to treating osteoporosis has been tried over the years and found wanting. However, at this time there are several drugs which are marginally effective in preventing fractures but which, like many drugs, carry with them some nasty adverse effects. A family of agents, the bisphosphonates, is exemplified by ibandronate. Many will know this drug by its trade name Boniva.

First approved in 2003, Boniva was popularized by Sally Field, two-time Academy Award winning actress, and self-described "post-meno-pausal woman with osteoporosis." She appeared in television and print advertisements extolling the virtues of Boniva. Its maker, Genentech, stated that "After one year on Boniva, 9 out of 10 women stopped and reversed their bone loss." Between 2005 and 2009, 150 million prescriptions were written for Boniva and similar drugs. However, beginning in 2010 the FDA forced Genentech to run advertisements carrying "An important correction: Boniva has *not* been shown to stop and reverse bone loss in 9 out of 10 women and is not a cure for postmenopausal osteoporosis…it is not known how long Boniva works."

Earlier, the FDA had warned of severe and sometimes incapacitating bone, joint, and muscle pain. When these FDA actions were coupled with widely publicized concerns about two rare effects of the bisphosphonates, deterioration of the jaw bone and thigh bone fractures, it was not surprising that sales of Boniva fell by 75% between 2008 and 2011. Nonetheless, the current consensus is that bisphosphonates have a role to play in the treatment of men and women at high risk of hip fracture.[9] In addition to Boniva, others in this group include Reclast, Fosamax, Zometa, and Actonel.

An alternative to Boniva-like drugs made its appearance in the United States in June 2010 with the FDA approval of Prolia (denosumab). Like Boniva, the drug has an actress promoting it, in this case Blythe Danner, who tells us that "My doctor and I chose Prolia" and suggests that you "Ask your doctor if Prolia is right for you." Prolia acts to alter the balance between the activity of osteoclasts and osteoblasts though by a somewhat different mechanism than do the bisphosphonates. Unfortunately, Prolia carries with it a multitude of possible adverse effects including suppression of the immune system with the possibility of life-threatening infections. Furthermore, thigh bone fractures and deterioration of the jaw bone as seen with the Boniva have also been reported following the use of Prolia. Nonetheless, with the adverse publicity which has attached itself to the bisphosphonates coupled with our attraction to anything new, it is expected that sales of Prolia will rise to $4 billion dollars by the year 2015. Whether it and similar drugs to follow will prove superior in their efficacy remains to be seen.

As we have earlier seen in our discussions of pain, dementia, cancer, and cardiovascular disease, osteoporosis is a condition which grows in incidence as we age. And, as is true of those conditions, total prevention is not presently within our grasp. However, we are able to diminish the risk of their occurrence. For osteoporosis, the list is both short and familiar: adequate nutrition especially with regard to dietary sources of vitamin D and calcium, appropriate body weight, no more than moderate use of alcohol, no smoking, and exercise of all kinds but with emphasis on those which stress the bones.

CHAPTER 16

THE FINAL CHAPTER

Death and dignity

*D*eath and Dignity was the title of an article published in the *New England Journal of Medicine* on March 7th, 1991.[1] Its author was Timothy Quill, an attending physician at the Genesee Hospital in Rochester, New York. In it Dr. Quill told how he had assisted the suicide by barbiturate overdose of Diane, a 45-year-old patient of his. Following her death, he informed the medical examiner that the cause was acute leukemia, a diagnosis Diane had received several months before. Dr. Quill's article was a remarkable admission not the least because in New York State a person convicted of aiding in a suicide is liable to 5-15 years imprisonment. (A grand jury in Rochester subsequently declined to indict him.)

Dr. Quill was certainly not the first to advocate or participate in the assisted death of a terminally ill patient. The deaths of Sigmund Freud and King George V of England give witness to that fact. However, as a respected physician and former director of a hospice program, he clearly was distinct from those such as Jack Kevorkian[2], a Michigan pathologist referred to by some as "Dr. Death", or Derek Humphry, a non-physician author of a best-selling book which listed lethal doses of 18 prescription drugs.[3] Mr. Humphry admits to assisting the deaths of three family members including his first wife. Instead, Dr. Quill represents those reasoned voices in the medical community who advocate assisted death for some. Writing 21 years after Diane's suicide, he put it this way: "...a small percentage of patients will suffer intolerably despite receiving state-of-the-art palliative care, and a few of these patients will request a physician-assisted death…physicians should search for the least harmful way to respond to intolerable end-of-life suffering in ways that are effective and also respect the values of the major participants…"[4]

First, we need to sort out some terms. Suicide is simplest: it is the act of taking one's life voluntarily and intentionally. Euthanasia, from the Greek *eu* plus *thanatos* meaning easy death, refers to the killing of a terminally ill person for humanitarian reasons. In the Netherlands, where euthanasia has been legal since 2002, the term has a more precise meaning: the administration of lethal drugs by a physician with the explicit intention to end a patient's life in accordance with a patient's request. The Dutch draw a distinction between euthanasia and physician-assisted suicide, also legal. In the latter, a patient administers a lethal medication that was prescribed intentionally by a physician. It is physician-assisted suicide (many advocates prefer to speak of physician-assisted dying) that is permitted in some parts of the United States, more about that in a moment.

I would ask you to consider two forms of suicide. One is an act, seemingly senseless and difficult for most of us to comprehend, the other the consequence of a rational decision. As a sometime chemist, I have known of Wallace Hume Carothers my whole adult life. His story has always served me as an example of suicide of the first kind. Dr. Caruthers was trained by some of the most eminent chemists in America and received his Ph.D. degree in 1924. After academic positions at the University of Illinois and Harvard University, he joined the Dupont Experimental Station. At DuPont, he and his team made the discoveries which would lead to the first synthetic rubber and to nylon, a truly revolutionary fiber. He was elected to the National Academy of Sciences in February 1936, a rare distinction at that time for an industrial scientist. Two months later he married a fellow DuPont chemist.

A year following his marriage, on April 29th, 1937, two days after his 41st birthday and seven months before the birth of his daughter Jane, Wallace Carothers took his own life in a Philadelphia hotel room by ingesting cyanide.[5] Ever the chemist, he washed it down with lemon juice knowing that an acidic environment would enhance the absorption of the poison. Looking back, it is clear that Dr. Carothers had struggled with endogenous depression, a form of the disease with no clear antecedents, for all of his short life. Drugs to treat the condition had not yet been discovered.

Despite today's confident talk of chemical imbalances, deranged neurotransmitters such as dopamine and serotonin, and the availability of several moderately effective drugs, endogenous depression of the kind suffered by Dr. Caruthers remains an enigmatic cause of suicide. Standing in contrast to suicide in the throes of endogenous depression is suicide as a rational act by a person unimpaired by cognitive or psychiatric disorders. There are many examples which might be given. I will limit myself to just four.

The education of every midshipman in the United States Navy begins with an introduction to the heroes of the service. Thus, in the mid-1950's, I learned of John Paul Jones, David Farragut, James Lawrence, and many others. From World War II there was Chester Nimitz, Jr., son of Fleet Admiral Chester Nimitz, Commander in Chief of our forces in the Pacific and architect of the naval victory over Japan. In August 1944, the younger Nimitz was commanding officer of the submarine *U.S.S. Haddo* which was on its seventh war patrol in the South China Sea. On that patrol, Nimitz gained lasting fame and the Navy Cross when his boat sank two Japanese destroyers, the nemesis of the submarine service.[6] For good measure, *Haddo* seriously damaged a third destroyer and sank 17,000 tons of shipping during that single patrol. Following his World War II and Korean War service, the now retired Rear Admiral Nimitz began a distinguished 23-year business career culminating in his being named chief executive officer of the PerkinElmer Corporation.

On January 2nd, 2002, Chester Nimitz, Jr. and Joan Nimitz, his wife of 63 years, took their own lives with an overdose of sleeping pills. At the time of their deaths they were 86 and 89 years of age, respectively. Ever in command, the admiral had waited until after the first of the year for tax reasons related to gifts to his children and grandchildren. In a note, he said this:

Our decision was made over a considerable period of time and was not carried out in acute desperation. Nor is it an expression of a mental illness. We have consciously, rationally, deliberately, and of our own free will taken measures to end our lives today because of the physical limitations on our quality of life placed upon us by age, failing vision, osteoporosis, back pain and painful orthopedic problems.[7]

A fear of many of us as we enter old age is loss of control over our lives. At the time of their deaths, Sara Rimer writing in the *New York Times* quoted Joan's sister: "They didn't want to think in any way that their final days would be controlled by some whippersnapper internist at the hospital." Ms. Rimer also quotes the admiral's sister, Mary Aquinas, a Catholic nun, who could not condone the act but added "If you cannot see any value to suffering for yourself or others, then maybe it does make sense to end your life."[7]

Morris E. Chafetz received his medical degree in 1948 and then trained in psychiatry at Harvard Medical School. Finishing his residency, the only position he could find was as the medical director of a newly established state-supported treatment center for alcoholics. Initially he was not enthused but soon recognized, as he put it, "my prejudices and the prejudices of others." Later he would be one of the first to advocate the creation of what would become the National Institute on Alcohol Abuse and Alcoholism. In 1970, he was named the first director of NIAAA.

Marion and Morris Chafetz were married in 1946. Sixty-five years later, at the age of 86, Marion died in an assisted living facility in Bethesda, Maryland. Early the next day, Dr. Chafetz called his three sons to inform them that he intended to take his own life. He was 87 years of age. In the words of Dennis Powell, a co-author of one of Dr. Chafetz' many books, "Living without Marion was not among the things he considered possible. So he was going to die now. Which he did."[8] Though the genders are reversed, the story of Marion and Morris Chafetz personifies for me the lines written more than three centuries ago by Sir Henry Wotton *Upon the Death of Sir Albert Morton's Wife*

> He first deceased; She for a little tried
> To live without him: liked it not, and died.

The last two instances of rational suicide that I want to tell you about both took place in Oregon. In that state there has been in effect since November 1997 something called the Death with Dignity Act. The act allows terminally-ill adult Oregonians to obtain from their physician a prescription for a lethal dose of a medication, usually a barbiturate. Through 2011, a total of 935 prescriptions were written and 596 deaths resulted. Most who availed themselves of the Act were white, well-educated, insured, had cancer, and were elderly; in 2011 the median age was 70. More than 95% were enrolled in hospice care and nearly 95% died at home.[9]

To enroll in the Oregon program, I need only complete a one-page form entitled the Request for Medication To End Life in a Humane and Dignified Manner. On the form I indicate that I am suffering from a specified terminal disease, whether I have informed my family of my decision, that I fully understand the consequences of my decision, that I have a right to rescind the request, and that I make the request voluntarily. My signature is witnessed by two persons, one of whom is neither a relative nor an heir to any part of my estate. The attending physician than completes a compliance form which attests, among other things, that I have made two requests separated by at least 15 days, that I have less than six months to live, that I am acting voluntarily, that I suffer from no psychiatric disorder, and that I am a resident of Oregon.

Forty years ago, Peter Goodwin, a physician in Oregon, helped a terminally ill patient to die. Just as was the case with Dr. Quill in Rochester, he risked imprisonment and loss of his career for his decision. Fortunately, his act was known only to the patient and his wife. Later, Dr. Goodwin became an advocate for what ultimately became the state's Death with Dignity Act. Ironically, it was that Act that allowed Dr. Goodwin on March 11, 2012 to take his own life. He did so in the company of his wife and his four children.

In a final interview with Belinda Luscombe of *Time* magazine, Dr. Goodwin described his affliction, a progressive degenerative neurological disease that left him with little voluntary muscular function, a disease that soon would kill him in a much more debilitated state.[10] Just as I have attempted to do, Dr. Goodwin distinguished his act from what he called a typical suicide: "...it's impulsive, it's often violent, and it's almost always in seclusion. (In contrast) this is a process done with the support of the family, after a great deal of consideration. And it's a gentle death." He added that "physicians are taught to treat and they often go on treating and treating...it's very difficult for physicians to give up... Physicians die in a different way from the majority of their patients, long before they've had a huge amount of chemotherapy. They know what's in store and they have an out." Oregon's Death with Dignity Act and similar measures in the states of Washington, Vermont, and Montana provide that "out" for non-physicians.

For those undecided about the wisdom of laws such as the Death with Dignity Act or who live in a state where such a measure will come up for a vote, I recommend seeing an HBO documentary called How to Die in Oregon. (I obtained my copy via NetFlix.) The film, directed by Peter Richardson, follows several persons as they make use of the Act.

A major part of How to Die in Oregon is devoted to the story of Cody Curtis, a 52 year old Oregonian who learns, two days after Christmas in 2007, that she has liver cancer. Surgery to reduce the tumor is performed but it soon is clear that the disease will kill her. Ms. Curtis recognizes that there will come a time when she will wish to "close my eyes and drift off." A prescription for secobarbital is filled and the drug is put aside for when it will be needed. Even as the disease progresses, this lovely, perceptive, and eloquent woman maintains her dignity and her optimism. But nature is cruel and, in November 2009, nearly two years after her diagnosis and with her episodes of pain increasing in frequency, she plans for the end. On the evening of December 7th, 2009, in the company of her husband, her two adult children, and her physician, Cody Curtis dies peacefully at home. I have not done justice to her story or the film. Please see it for yourself.

Christian doctrine holds suicide to be morally wrong. Indeed, St. Augustine pronounced that it is an unrepentable sin; a sin which surely damns one to hell. St. Thomas Aquinas later gave three reasons for this view: (1) suicide is contrary to natural self-love, whose aim is to preserve us, (2) it injures the community, and (3) it violates our duty to God because only He can determine the duration of our earthly existence. Clearly, neither Augustine nor Aquinas could have foreseen renal dialysis, feeding tubes, respirators, pacemakers or any of the other wonders of a 21st century Intensive Care Unit able to keep a body alive even in the absence of cognitive function. Furthermore, as a devote agnostic, I am not inclined to have another person's god dictate either my life or my death. However, as an American, I would not deny Christians or others whose religion marks suicide as a mortal sin the opportunity to avail themselves of any and all live-extending technologies so long as the community is not injured by diversion for this purpose of funds essential for medical services for others. In simpler terms, please don't put the bill on Medicare.

Daniel Greenberg said many years ago that planning for mortality has never been popular[11] and, I must confess that I have done less planning than I should. As to physician-assisted dying, Huibert Drion, a judge of the Dutch Supreme Court and a noted legal scholar, expressed my views nicely.

> It appears to me…that many old people would find great reassurance if they could have a means to end their lives in an acceptable way at the moment that to them…appears suitable…I do not know if I would use it, you know, because I am a coward…[12]

Judge Drion was spared that decision when he died thirteen years later in his sleep at home at age 87. Nonetheless, as did he, I look forward to the day when physician-assisted dying will be available to all who desire it.

NOTES

Abbreviations BMJ *British Medical Journal*
JAMA *Journal of the American Medical Association*
NEJM *New England Journal of Medicine*

Preface

1. Thomas D (1952) *The Collected Poems of Dylan Thomas.* P. 122. New York: New Directions.
2. Durant W (1953) *The Pleasures of Philosophy.* New York: Simon & Schuster.
3. Anonymous (2009) http://www.nobelprize.org/nobel_prizes/medicine/laureates/2009/blackburn-facts.html
4. Taylor HS, Manson JE (2011) Update on hormone therapy use in menopause. J Clin Endocrinol Metab 96(2):255-264.
5. Winter JC (1991) *True Nutrition, True Fitness.* Clifton, NJ: Humana.
6. Sepkowitz KA (2011) *New York Times*, April 26.
7. Anonymous (2000) Don't trust anyone over 30, unless it's Jack Weinberg. The *Berkeley Daily Planet,* April 4.

Chapter 1 Drugs *The Good, the Bad, and the Ugly*

1. Moynihan R (2011) Is your mum on drugs? BMJ 343:d5184.
2. Topol EJ (2004) Failing the public---Refocoxib, Merck, and the FDA. NEJM 35 (17):1707-1709.
3. Expert Panel, American Geriatrics Society (2012) Criteria for potentially inappropriate medication use in older adults. J Am Geriatr Soc 60:616-631.

4. Smith DE (2012) The process addictions and the new ASAM definition of addiction. J Psychoactive Drugs 44:1-4.
5. Davies D (1999) Please, not wrinkles. Lancet 354:264.
6. Lamas D, Rosenbaum L (2012) Painful inequities---Palliative care in developing countries. NEJM 366 (3):199-201.
7. Pizzo PA, Clark NM (2012) Alleviating suffering 101---Pain relief in the United States. NEJM 36 (3):197-199.
8. Garfinkel D, Mangin D (2010) Feasibility study of a systematic approach for discontinuation of multiple medications in older adults. Arch Int Med 170 (8):1648-1654.
9. Wolff T et al. (2009) Aspirin for the Primary Prevention of Cardiovascular Events: An Update of the Evidence for the U.S. Preventive Services Task Force (2009) Ann Intern Med 150:396-404.
10. Gordon B (1979) *I'm Dancing as Fast as I Can.* New York: Harper & Row.

Chapter 2 Dietary supplements *Who is watching out for us?*

1. Dietary Supplement Health and Education Act of 1994 (1994) Public Law No. 103-417.
2. Holmstedt B, Liljestrand G (1963) The sulfonamides. *Readings in Pharmacology*, New York: Pergamon.
3. Jackson CO (1970) Doctor Massengill's elixir. In: *Food and drug legislation in the New Deal. Pp, 151-174.* Princeton, NJ: Princeton University Press.
4. Public L. No. 75-717, 52 Stat. 1040 (1938).
5. Scheinlin, S (2011) The courage of one's convictions: The due diligence of Frances Oldham Kelsey at the FDA. Molecular Interventions 11:3-9.
6. Florence AL (1960) Is thalidomide to blame? BMJ December 31.
7. Lenz W, Knapp K. (1962) Thalidomide embryopathy. Arch Environ Health 5:100-105.

8. Kefauver-Harris Amendments (1961) Congressional Record, Washington, DC.

9. Cohen PA (2009) American roulette...Contaminated dietary supplements. NEJM 361:1523-1525.

10. Mencimer S (2001) Scorin' in Orrin. *Washington Monthly*, September.

11. Braico KT et al. (1979) Laetrile intoxication, Report of a fatal case. NEJM 300 (5):238-240.

12. News Highlights (1978) Appeals court backs Laetrile injunction. *FDA Consumer* 12:25.

13. Anonymous. (1977) Toxicity of Laetrile. FDA Drug Bulletin 7:25. For a detailed discussion of Laetrile and its use in cancer treatment see Herbert V (1979) Laetrile: the cult of cyanide. Promoting poison for profit. Am J Clin Nutr 32:1121-1158.

14. Moertel CG et al. (1982) A clinical trial of amygdalin (Laetrile) in the treatment of human cancer. NEJM 306:201-206.

15. Anonymous cited by Lattman P, Singer N (2012) *New York Times*, February 12.

16. Anderson JR (2011) *Army Times*, December 29.

17. Hutt PB quoted by Singer N, Lattman, P (2012) *New York Times*, April 28.

18. Di Lorenzo C et al. (2013) Could 1,3-dimethylamylamine (DMAA) in food supplements have a natural origin? Drug Test Anal 5(2):116-121.

19. Austin KG et al. (2014) Analysis of 1,3-dimethylamine concentrations in Geraniaceae, geranium oil, and dietary supplements. Drug Test Anal 6(7-8):797-804.

20. Offit PA (2012) Studying complementary and alternative therapies. JAMA 307:1803-1804.

21. Barker P (1991) *Regeneration*. London: Penguin.

Chapter 3 The aging brain. *The drug industry and the Battered Child of Medicine*

1. Gaboda D et al. (2011) No longer undertreated? Depression diagnosis and antidepressant therapy in elderly long-stay nursing home residents, 1999-2007. J Amer Geriatri Soc 59(4):673-680.
2. Park-Lee E et al. (2013) Dementia special care units in residential care communities: United States 2010. NCHS Data Brief Nov (134):1-8.
3. Molinar V (2010) Provision of psychopharmacological services in nursing homes. J Gerontol B Psychol Sci Soc Sci 65B(1):57-60.
4. Shorter (1997) *A History of Psychiatry, From the Era of the Asylum to the Age of Prozac.* Pp. 248-250, New York: Wiley.
5. Laborit H et al. (1952) Un nouveau stabilisateur vegetative (le 4560 RP). Press medicale 60:206-208.
6. Huybrechts KF (2012) Differential risk of death in older residents in nursing homes prescribed specific antipsychotic drugs: population based cohort study. BMJ 344:e977.
7. Anonymous (2014) Drug Sales Through March 2014. http://www.medscape.com
8. McCleery J, Fox R (2012) Antipsychotic prescribing in nursing homes. BMJ 344:e1093.
9. Schmidt MS, Thomas, K. (2012) Abbott settles marketing lawsuit. *New York Times* May 7.
10. Chedekel, L. (2013) High antipsychotic use in nursing homes stirs concerns. *The Day,* February 2.
11. Briesacher BA et al. (2013) Antipsychotic use among nursing home residents. JAMA 309(5):440-442.
12. Shorter (1997) *A History of Psychiatry, From the Era of the Asylum to the Age of Prozac.* Pp. 258-261, New York: Wiley.
13. Banerjee S et al. (2011) Sertraline or mirtazapine for depression in dementia (HTA-SADD): a randomized, multicentre, double-blind, placebo-controlled trial. Lancet. 378(9789):403-11.

14. Brodaty H (2011) Antidepressant treatment in Alzheimer's disease. Lancet 378(9789):375-376.

15. Coupland, C et al. (2011) Antidepressant use and risk of adverse outcomes in older people: population based cohort study. BMJ 343:d4551.

16. Rodda J et al. (2011) Depression in older adults. BMJ 343:d5219.

17. Greenblatt M. (1975) Psychiatry: the battered child of medicine. NEJM 292(5):246-250.

18. Cosgrove L et al. (2009) Conflicts of interest and disclosure in the American Psychiatric Association's Clinical Practice Guidelines. Psychother Psychosom 78(4):228-232.

19. Spence D (2012) Don't just blame big pharma. BMJ 345:e3825.

20. Harris G (2008) Top psychiatrist didn't report drug makers' pay. *New York Times*, October 4.

21. Ibid.

22. Rosenthall MB, Mello MM (2013) Sunlight as disinfectant---New rules for disclosure of industry payments to physicians. NEJM 368 (22):20151-2052.

23. Bass E et al. (2007) Risk-adjusted mortality rates of elderly veterans with hip fractures. Ann Epidemiol 17 (7):514-519.

24. Rebensdorf, A (2001) Sarafem: The Pimping of Prozac for PMS. www.AlterNet.org.

25. Obiora E et al. (2013) The impact of benzodiazepines on occurrence of pneumonia: a nested case-control and survival analysis in a population-based cohort. Thorax 68:163-170.

Chapter 4 A training effect *The Alvin Roy revolution*

1. Quinn TJ (2009) Pumped-up pioneers: the '63 Chargers. http:// sports.espn.go.com/espn/otl/news/story?id=3866837

2. Ibid.

3. Sherrington C et al. (2008) Effective exercise for the prevention of falls: a systematic review and meta-analysis. J Am Geriatric Soc 56:2234-2243.

Chapter 5 A program of exercise *The good addiction*

1. Anonymous. (2008) Physical Activity Guidelines for Americans. *www.health.gov/PAGuidelines/*

2. Nes BM et al. (2013) Age-predicted maximal heart rate in healthy subjects: The HUNT fitness study. Scand J Med Sci Sports 23(6):697-704.

3. U.S. Department of Health and Human Services (2008) Physical Activity Guidelines for Americans. http://www.nhlbi.nih.gov/health/health-topics/topics/phys/recommend.html

4. Hegsted DM (2004) Frederick John Stare (1910-2002). J Nutr 134:1007-1009.

5. Harris WE et al. (1967) Jogging, An adult exercise program. JAMA 201(10):133-135.

6. Brody JE (2012) Changing our tune on exercise. *New York Times*, August 27.

Chapter 6 Nutrition
6.1 Introduction

1. Lietch I (1942) The evolution of dietary standards. Nutr Abs rev 11:509-521.

2. Roberts LJ (1958) Beginnings of the Recommended Dietary Allowances. J Am Diet Assoc 34:903-908.

3. Anonymous (2010) *Dietary Guidelines for Americans*, 7th ed., US GPO, www.cnpp.gov/dietaryguidelines.htm

4. Anonymous (2013) *Guidance for Industry: A Food Labeling Guide* (14. Appendix F: Calculate the Percent Daily Value for the Appropriate Nutrients) U.S. Food and Drug Administration. *www.fda.gov/food/.../ucm064928.htm*

6.2 Fat *Lessons from sheep sex*

1. Anitschkow N. (1913) Uber die veranderungen der kaninchenaorta bei experimenteller cholesterinsteatose. Beitr Pathol Anat 56:379–404.

2. Lichtenstein AH et al. (2006) Diet and lifestyle recommendations revision 2006: a scientific statement from the American Heart Association Nutrition Committee. Circulation 114(1):82-96.

3. Eckel RH et al. (2014) 2013 AHA/ACC Guideline on Lifestyle Management to Reduce Cardiovascular Risk: A Report of the American College of Cardiology/American Heart Association Task Force on Practice Guidelines. J Amer Coll Cardiol 63 (25 pt. B):2960-2984.

4. Kinsell LW et al. (1952) Dietary modification of serum cholesterol and phospholipid levels. J Clin Endocrinol Metab. 12(7):909-13.

5. Pugliese MT et al. (1983) Fear of obesity. A cause of short stature and delayed puberty. NEJM 309 (9):513-518.

6. Burr GO, Burr MM (1929) A new deficiency disease produced by the rigid exclusion of fat from the diet. J Biological Chem 82:345-367.

7. Hansen AE et al. (1963) Role of linoleic acid in infant nutrition. Pediatrics 31:171-192.

8. Holman RT et al. (1982) A case of linolenic acid deficiency involving neurological abnormalities. Amer J Clin Nutr 35:617-623.

9. von Euler US (1973) Some aspects of the actions of prostaglandins. Arch int Pharmacodyn Ther 202 (S):295-307.

10. Bergström S, Samuelsson B. (1968) The prostaglandins. Endeavour 27102:109-113.

11. Vane JR (1976) The mode of action of aspirin and similar compounds. J Allergy Clin Immunol. 58(6):691-712.

12. Hamberg M et al. (1975) Thromboxanes: a new group of biologically active compounds derived from prostaglandin endoperoxides. Proc Natl Acad Sci U S A. 72(8):2994-2998.

13. Anonymous. (2009) Aspirin for the prevention of cardiovascular disease. U.S. Preventative Services Taskforce. http://www.uspreventiveservicestaskforce.org/index.html

14. Dyerberg J, Bang HO (1979) Haemostatic function and platelet polyunsaturated fatty acids in Eskimos. Lancet 314 (8140):433-435.

15. Whittaker N et al. (1976) The chemical structure of prostaglandin X (prostacyclin). Prostaglandins. 12(6):915-928.

16. Bang HO et al. (1971) Plasma lipid and lipoprotein pattern in Greenlandic west coast Eskimos. Lancet 297 (7710):1143-1145.

17. Fodor JG et al. (2014) "Fishing" for the origins of the Eskimos and heart disease story: facts or wishful thinking? Can J Cardiol 30:864-868.

18. Bertelsen A (1940) Medical statistics and nosography in Greenland: the usual disease pattern in Greenland. Meddelelser om Gronland 117(3).

19. Bjerregaard P et al. (2003) Low incidence of cardiovascular disease among the Inuit—what is the evidence? Atherosclerosis 166:351-357.

20. Smith SC et al. (2011) AHA/ACCF secondary prevention and risk reduction for patients with coronary and other atherosclerotic vascular disease: 2011 update. Circulation 124:2458-2473.

21. Bosch J et al. (2012) n-3 fatty acids and cardiovascular outcomes in patients with dysglycemia. NEJM 367(4):309-318.

22. Rizos EC et al. (2012) Association between *omega*-3 fatty acid supplementation and risk of major cardiovascular disease events: a systematic review and meta-analysis. JAMA 308(10):1024-1033.

23. Manson JE et al. (2012) The VITamin D and OmegA-3 TriaL (VITAL): Rationale and design of a large randomized controlled trial of vitamin D and marine *omega*-3 fatty acid supplements for the primary prevention of cancer and cardiovascular disease. Cotemp Clinical Trials 33:159-171.

24. Harris WS et al. (2009) *Omega*-6 fatty acids and risk for cardiovascular disease: A science advisory from the American Heart Association. Circulation 119(6):902-907.

25. Brasky TM et al. (2013) Plasma phospholipid fatty acids and prostate cancer risk in the SELECT trial. J Natl Cancer Inst 105(15):1132-1141.

26. Willett WC et al. (1993) Intake of trans fatty acids and risk of coronary heart disease among women. Lancet 341(8845):581-585.

27. Chowdhury R et al. (2014) Association of dietary, circulating, and supplement fatty acids with coronary risk. Ann Internal Med 160:398-406.

28. Sanders A (2014) Plant compared with marine n-3 fatty acid effects on cardiovascular risk factors and outcomes: what is the verdict? Am J Clin Nutr 100 (S1):453S-458S.

6.3 Protein *Too much of a good thing?*

1. Otten JJ et al. (2006) Dietary Reference Intakes: The Essential Guide to Nutrient Requirements. http://www.nap.edu/11537.html

2. Pasiakos SM et al. (2013) Efficacy and safety of protein supplements for U.S. Armed Forces personnel: consensus statement. J Nutr 143:1811S-1814S.

3. Luscombe B (2012) Ultramarathoner Scott Jurek on 100-mile races, craving tempeh and why hallucinations are no big deal. *Time*, July 23.

4. Scrimshaw N (1961) Plant mixtures as a source of protein in human nutrition. Rev Col Med Guatem 12:1-3.

5. Shinwell ED, Gorodischer R (1982) Totally vegetarian diets and infant nutrition. Pediatrics 70(4):582-586.

6. Crim MC, Munro HN (1977) *Defined Formula Diets for Medical Purposes*. Chicago: American Medical Association.

7. Anonymous (2008) Nutrition Recommendations and Interventions for Diabetes. A position statement of the American Diabetes Association. Diabetes Care 31(S1):S67-S78.

8. Eisenberg ME et al. (2012) Muscle-enhancing behaviors among adolescent girls and boys. Pediatrics 130(6):1019-1026.

6.4 Carbohydrates *Sugar is not a poison.*

1. Banting FG et al. (1922) Pancreatic Extracts in the Treatment of Diabetes Mellitus. Can Med Assoc 12(3):141-146.

2. Yudkin J, Roddy J (1964) Levels of dietary sucrose in patients with occlusive atherosclerotic disease. Lancet 2:6.

3. Yudkin J (1972) *Pure, White, and Deadly: The Problem of Sugar.* London: Davis-Poynter.
4. Cleave TL (1974) *The Saccharine Disease.* Bristol: John Wright & Sons.
5. Dufty W (1975) *Sugar Blues.* Radnor, PA: Chilton.
6. Lustig RH et al. (2012) Public health: The toxic truth about sugar. Nature 482(7383):27-29.
7. Katz D (2011) Sugar isn't evil: a rebuttal. www.huffingtonpost.com/david-katz/ April 19.
8. Tappy L (2012) 'Toxic' effects of sugar: Should we be afraid of fructose? BMC Biology 10:42-53.
9. Walker AR (1956) Some aspects of nutritional research in South Africa. Nutr Rev 14(11):321-324.
10. Trowell HC (1960) Non-infective disease in Africa: the peculiarities of medical non-infective diseases in the indigenous inhabitants of Africa south of the Sahara. London: Arnold.
11. Burkitt DP (1961) Observations on the geography of malignant lymphoma. East Afr Med J 38:511-514.
12. Burkitt DP et al. (1974) Dietary fiber and disease. JAMA 229(8):1068-1074.
13. Wrick KL et al. (1983) The influence of dietary fiber on human intestinal transit and stool output. J Nutr 113(8):1464-1479.
14. Anonymous (1913) Sugar as food. JAMA 61(7):492-493.

6.5 Vitamin A and *beta*-carotene *Of polar bears and flamingos*

1. Wald G (1967) The Molecular Basis of Visual Excitation. Nobel lecture, December 12. The Nobel Foundation.
2. Bloch CE (1924) Blindness and other diseases in children arising in consequence of deficient nutrition (lack of fat soluble A factor). J Dairy Sci 7(1):1-10.
3. McCollum E, Davis M (1913) The necessity of certain lipids in the diet during growth. J Biol Chem 15:167-175.

4. Osborne TB, Mendel LB (1913) The influence of butter fat on growth. J Biol Chem 16:423-437.

5. McCollum EV (1918) *The Newer Knowledge of Nutrition. The Use of Food for the Preservation of Vitality and Health.* New York: MacMillan.

6. Steenbock H (1919) White corn vs. yellow corn and a probable relation between the fat-soluble vitamin and yellow plant pigments. Science 50:352-353.

7. Moore T (1929) Vitamin A and carotene: The association of vitamin A activity with carotene in the carrot root. Biochem J 23(4):803-11.

8. McLaren DS, Zekian D (1971) Failure of enzymic cleavage of *beta*-carotene. The cause of vitamin A deficiency in a child. Am J Dis Child. 121(4):278-80.

9. Hume EM, Krebs HA (1949) Med Res Counc (Gt Brit) Spec Rep Ser 264.

10. Rodahl K, Moore T. (1943) The vitamin A content and toxicity of bear and seal liver. Biochem J 37:166-168.

11. Gerber A et al. (1954) Vitamin A poisoning in adults; with description of a case. Am J Med 16(5):729-745.

12. White PL (1977) The lid is off. JAMA 238(6):1761-1762.

13. Cohlan SC (1953) Excessive intake of vitamin A as a cause of congenital anomalies in the rat. Science 117:535-536.

14. Miller RK et al. (1987) Position paper by the Teratology Society: Vitamin A during pregnancy. Teratology 35:267-268.

15. Otten JJ et al. (2006) Dietary Reference Intakes: The Essential Guide to Nutrient Requirements. http://www.nap.edu/11537.html

16. Mata-Granados JM et al. (2013) Vitamin D insufficiency together with high serum levels of vitamin A increases the risk of osteoporosis in postmenopausal women. Arch Osteoporos 8(1-2):124-129.

17. Peto R et al. (1981) Can dietary *beta*-carotene materially reduce human cancer rates? Nature 290:201-208.

18. The Alpha-Tocopherol *Beta*-Carotene Cancer Prevention Study Group. (1994) The effect of vitamin E and *beta*-carotene on the incidence of lung cancer in male smokers. NEJM 330:1031-1035.

19. Omenn GS et al. (1996) Effects of a combination of *beta* carotene and vitamin A on lung cancer and cardiovascular disease. NEJM 334(18):1150-1155.

6.6 Thiamine (vitamin B₁) *Polished rice and beriberi*

1. Gerrard PN (1906) Beri-Beri: Its Symptoms and Symptomatic Treatment. Kessenger Legacy Reprints www.kessenger.net/

2. Takaki K (1905) Three lectures on the preservation of health amongst the personnel of the Japanese Navy and Army. Lancet 167(4316):1369-1374; 167(4317):1451-1455; 167(4318):1520-1523.

3. Sugiyama Y, Seita A (2013) Kanehiro Takaki and the control of beri-beri in the Japanese Navy. J Roy Soc Med 106(8):332-334.

4. Carpenter KJ, Sutherland B (1995) Eijkman's contribution to the discovery of vitamins. J Nutr 125:155-163.

5. Eijkman C (1929) Nobel Prize for Physiology or Medicine. http://www.nobelprize.org/nobel_prizes/medicine/laureates/1929/eijkman-lecture.html

6. Grijns G (1935). Researches on vitamins, 1910-1911. J Noorduyn en Zoon, Gorinchem, Holland. http://www.worldneurologyonline.com/article/gerrit-grijns-in-java-beriberi-and-the-concept-of-partial-starvation/#sthash.u4yL8KKr.dpuf

7. Jansen BCP, Donath WF (1926) The isolation of the anti beri beri vitamin. Med J Dutch East Indies 66:1-2.

8. Otten JJ et al. (2006) Dietary Reference Intakes: The Essential Guide to Nutrient Requirements. http://www.nap.edu/11537.html

9. Luxemburger C (2003) Beri-beri: The major cause of infant mortality in Karen refugees. Trans Roy Soc Trop Med Hyg 97:251-255.

10. Nardone R et al. (2013) Thiamine deficiency induced neurochemical, neuroanatomical, and neuropsychological alterations: a reappraisal. Scientific World Journal. Oct 21:309143.

6.7 Niacin (vitamin B$_3$) *Pellagra and madness*

1. Casal G (1932) *The natural and medical history of the principality of the Asturias.* In *Classic Descriptions of Disease.* Springfield IL: CC Thomas.
2. Searcy GH (1907) An epidemic of acute pellagra. JAMA 49:37.
3. Goldberger JG (1914) The cause and prevention of pellagra. Public Health Rep 29:2354-2357.
4. Siler JF et al. (1914) Further studies of the Thompson-McFadden pellagra commission. JAMA 63:1090-1093
5. Goldberger JG et al. (1915) The prevention of pellagra. A test diet among institutionalized inmates. Public Health Rep 30:3117-3131
6. Goldberger JG et al. (1923) Pellagra prevention by diet among institutionalized inmates. Public Health Rep 38:2361-2368.
7. Goldberger JG, Wheeler GA (1915) Experimental pellagra in the human subject brought about by a restricted diet. Public Health Rep 30:3336-3339
8. Goldberger JG, Wheeler GA (1920) The experimental production of pellagra in human subjects by means of diet. Hygienic Laboratory Bulletin 120:7-116.
9. Goldberger JG (1916) The transmissibility of pellagra. Experimental attempts at transmission to the human subject. Public Health Rep 31:3159-3173.
10. Sebrell WH (1981) History of pellagra. Fed Proc 40(5):1520-1522.
11. Elvehjem CA et al. (1937) Relation of nicotinic acid and nicotinic acid amide to canine black tongue. Am Chem Soc J 59:1767-1768.
12. Fouts PJ et al. (1937) Treatment of human pellagra with nicotinic acid. PSEBM 37:405-407.
13. Krehl WA et al. (1945) Growth retarding effect of corn in nicotinic acid-low rations and its counteraction by tryptophane. Science 101:489-490.
14. Vilter et al. (1949) The therapeutic effect of tryptophane in human pellagra. J Lab Clin Med 34:409-413.

15. Otten JJ et al. (2006) Dietary Reference Intakes: The Essential Guide to Nutrient Requirements. http://www.nap.edu/11537.html
16. Altschul R, Hoffer A (1960) The effect of nicotinic acid on hypercholesterolemia. Canada M.A.J. 82:783-785.
17. The AIM-HIGH Investigators (2011) Niacin in patients with low HDL cholesterol levels receiving intensive statin therapy. NEJM 365:2255-2267.
18. HPS2-THRIVE Collaborative Group (2014) Effects of extended release niacin with laropiprant in high-risk patients. NEJM 371:203-212.
19. Lloyd-Jones DM (2014) Niacin and HDL cholesterol—Time to face facts. NEJM 371:271-273.

6.8 Riboflavin (vitamin B$_2$) *A vitamin for depression?*

1. Booher LE (1933) The concentration and probable chemical nature of vitamin G. J Biol Chem 102:39-46.
2. Sterner RT, Price WR (1973) Restricted riboflavin: within-subject behavioral effects in humans. Am J Clin Nutr 26(2):150-160.
3. Miller BJ et al. (2013) Dietary supplements for preventing postnatal depression. Cochrane Database Syst Rev 10:CD009104.
4. Otten JJ et al. (2006) Dietary Reference Intakes: The Essential Guide to Nutrient Requirements. http://www.nap.edu/11537.html

6.9 Pyridoxine (vitamin B$_6$) *Not just for morning sickness*

1. Gyorgy P (1934) Vitamin B2 and the pellagra-like dermatitis in rats. Nature 133:498-499.
2. Harris SA, Folkers K (1939) Synthetic vitamin B$_6$. Science 89:347.
3. Spies T et al. (1939) A note on the use of vitamin B$_6$ in human nutrition. JAMA 112:2414-2415.
4. Hawkins WW, Barsky J (1948) An experiment on human vitamin B6 deprivation. Science 108(2802):284-6.
5. Snyderman SE et al. (1953) Pyridoxine deficiency in the human infant. J Clin Nutr. 1(3):200-7.

6. Molony CJ, Parmalee AH (1954) Convulsions in young infants as a result of pyridoxine (vitamin B6) deficiency. JAMA 154(5):405-406.
7. Coursin DB (1954) Convulsive seizures in infants with pyridoxine-deficient diet. JAMA 154(5):406-407.
8. Otten JJ et al. (2006) Dietary Reference Intakes: The Essential Guide to Nutrient Requirements. http://www.nap.edu/11537.html
9. Baumgart et al. (2014) Atypical vitamin B6 deficiency: a rare cause of unexplained neonatal and infantile epilepsies. J Child Neurol 29(5):704-707.
10. Malouf R et al. (2003) The effect of vitamin B6 on cognition. Cochrane Database Syst Rev (4):CD004393.
11. Bendich A (2000) The potential for dietary supplements to reduce premenstrual syndrome (PMS) symptoms. J Am Coll Nutr 19(1):3-12.
12. Aufiero E et al. (2004) Pyridoxine hydrochloride treatment of carpal tunnel syndrome: a review. Nutr Rev 62(3):96-104.
13. Schaumburg H (1983) Sensory neuropathy from pyridoxine abuse. A new megavitamin syndrome. NEJM 309(8):445-448.
14. Institute of Medicine (2006) Dietary Reference Intakes. Washington, DC: The National Academies Press.
15. Milliken R (1993) Thalidomide doctor found guilty of medical fraud. *The Daily Telegraph*, February 20, Sydney, Australia.
16. Slaughter SR et al. (2014) FDA approval of doxylamine-pyridoxine therapy for use in pregnancy. NEJM 370:1081-1083.

6.10 Pantothenic acid *Burning feet and gray hair*

1. Lunde G, Kringstad H (1940) The anti grey hair vitamin, a new factor in the vitamin B complex. J Nutr 19:321-331.
2. Simpson J (1946) Burning feet in British prisoners-of-war in the Far East. Lancet.1(6409):959-61.
3. Denny-Brown D (1947) Neurological conditions resulting from prolonged and severe dietary restriction; case reports in prisoners-of-war, and general review. Medicine 26(1):41-113.

4. Gopalan C (1946) The burning feet syndrome. Ind Med Gaz 81:22-26.
5. Bean WB, Hodges RE (1954) Pantothenic acid deficiency induced in human subjects. Proc Soc Exp Biol Med 86(4):693-8.
6. Otten JJ et al. (2006) Dietary Reference Intakes: The Essential Guide to Nutrient Requirements. http://www.nap.edu/11537.html
7. Allbutt TC (1904) *Notes on the Composition of Scientific Papers.* London: Keynes Press.

6.11 Biotin *Did Rocky know about Avidin?*

1. Boas MA (1927) The Effect of desiccation upon the nutritive properties of egg-white. Biochem J 21(3):712-724.
2. du Vigneaud V et al. (1940) On the identity of vitamin H with biotin. Science 92:62-63.
3. du Vigneaud V (1942) The structure of biotin. Science 96(2499).
4. Eakin RE et al. (1940) Egg-white injury in chicks and its relationship to a deficiency of vitamin H (biotin). Science 92:224-225.
5. Williams RH (1943) Clinical biotin deficiency. NEJM 228:247-252.
6. Sydenstrycker VP (1942) Preliminary observations on "egg white injury" in man and its cure with biotin concentrate. Science 95(2459):176-177.
7. Jay AM et al. (2014) Outcomes of individuals with profound and partial biotinidase deficiency ascertained by newborn screening in Michigan over 25 years. Genet Med Aug 21. doi: 10.1038/gim.2014.104.
8. O'Keefe SJ et al. (2009) Products of the colonic microbiota mediate the effects of diet on colon cancer risk. J Nutr 139(11):2044-2048.
9. Otten JJ et al. (2006) Dietary Reference Intakes: The Essential Guide to Nutrient Requirements. http://www.nap.edu/11537.html

6.12 Vitamin B$_{12}$ *Dr. Castle's pre-digested hamburger*

1. Addison T (1855) *On the constitutional and local effects of disease of the suprarenal capsules.* London: Highly.

2. Herbert V (1984) An 'extrinsic factor' and pernicious anemia. JAMA 251(4):522-523.

3. Minot GR, Murphy WP (1926) Treatment of pernicious anemia by a special diet. JAMA 87(7):470-476.

4. Whipple GH, Robscheit-Robbins FS (1925) Favorable influence of liver, heart, and skeletal muscle in diet on regeneration in anemia. Am J Physiol 72:408-418.

5. Whipple GH, Minot GR, Murphy WP (1934) www.nobelprize.org/ nobel_prizes/medicine/laureates/1934/

6. Castle WB (1929) Observations on the etiologic relationship of achylia gastrica to pernicious anemia: I. The effect of administration to patients with pernicious anemia of the contents of the normal human stomach recovered after the ingestion of beef muscle. Am J Med Sci 178(6):748-763

7. Shorb MS (1947) Unidentified essential growth factors for *Lactobacillus lactis* found in refined liver extracts and in certain natural materials. J Bacteriol 53(5):669.

8. Rickes EL et al. (1948) Crystalline vitamin B_{12} Science 107:396-397.

9. West R (1948) Activity of Vitamin B_{12} in Addisonian Pernicious Anemia. Science 107(2781):398.

10. Castle WB (1953) Development of knowledge concerning the gastric intrinsic factor and its relation to pernicious anemia. NEJM 249(15):603-613.

11. Berlin H et al. (1968) Oral treatment of pernicious anemia with high doses of vitamin B_{12} without intrinsic factor. Acta Med Scand. 184(4):247-58.

12. Otten JJ et al. (2006) Dietary Reference Intakes: The Essential Guide to Nutrient Requirements. http://www.nap.edu/11537.html

13. Lam JR et al. (2013) Proton pump inhibitor and histamine 2 receptor antagonist use and vitamin B_{12} deficiency. JAMA 310(22):2435-2442.

14. de Jager J et al. (2010) Long term treatment with metformin in patients with type 2 diabetes and risk of vitamin B-12 deficiency: a randomized placebo controlled trial. BMJ 340:c2181doi:10.1136/bmj.c2181
15. Stabler S (2013) Vitamin B_{12} deficiency. NEJM 368(2):149-161.
16. Higginbottom MC et al. (1978) A syndrome of methylmalonic aciduria, homocystinuria, megaloblastic anemia and neurologic abnormalities in a vitamin B_{12}-deficient breast-fed infant of a strict vegetarian. NEJM 299(7):317-323.
17. The Vegetarian Society of the United Kingdom (2014] Fact sheet: vitamin B_{12}. www.vegsoc.org/b12
18. Blanco G, Peters HA (1983) Myeloneuropathy and macrocytosis associated with nitrous oxide abuse. Arch Neurol 40:416-418.

6.13 Folic acid *Lucy Wills in the slums of Bombay*

1. Tylden E (1986) Tropical macrocytic anaemia. Lancet 327(8472):94-95.
2. Wills L, Evans BDF (1938) Tropical macrocytic anemia: Its relation to pernicious anemia. Lancet 232(5999):416-421.
3. Mitchell HK et al. (1941) The concentration of "folic acid." JACS 63:2284.
4. Heinle RW, Welch AD (1947) Folic acid in pernicious anemia. Failure to prevent neurological relapse. JAMA 133:739-741.
5. Herbert V (1962) Experimental nutritional folate deficiency in man. Trans Assoc Amer Phys 75:307-320.
6. Greenberg M, Driscoll HG (1968) Failure of multivitamin preparations to prevent folic acid deficiency in pregnancy. Am J Obstet Gynecol. 100(6):879-81.
7. Farber S et al. (1948) Temporary remissions in acute leukemia in children produced by folic acid antagonist, 4-aminopteroyl-glutamic acid (Aminopterin). NEJM 238:787-793.

8. Smithells RW et al. (1980) Possible prevention of neural-tube defects by periconceptional vitamin supplementation. Lancet 1(8164):339-340.
9. Otten JJ et al. (2006) Dietary Reference Intakes: The Essential Guide to Nutrient Requirements. http://www.nap.edu/11537.html
10. Schmidt RJ (2012) Maternal periconceptional folic acid intake and risk of autism spectrum disorders and developmental delay in the CHARGE (CHildhood Autism Risks from Genetics and Environment) case-control study. Am J Clin Nutr 96(1):80-9.

6.14 Vitamin C *Scurvy, Dr. Pauling, cancer, and colds*

1. Lind JA (1753) *Treatise on Scurvy*. Edinburgh: Sands, Murray, and Cochrane.
2. Cook J (1776) James Cook to Sir John Pringle. Phil Trans Roy Soc London 66:402-406.
3. Holst A, Frolich T (1907) Experimental Studies Relating to "Ship-beri-beri" and Scurvy. J Hyg (Lond) 7(5):634-71.
4. Jukes TH (1988) The identification of vitamin C, an historical summary. J Nutr 118(11):1290-1293.
5. Otten JJ et al. (2006) Dietary Reference Intakes: The Essential Guide to Nutrient Requirements. http://www.nap.edu/11537.html
6. Crandon JH et al. (1940) Experimental human scurvy. NEJM 223(10):353-368.
7. Abt AF, Farmer CJ (1938) Vitamin C: pharmacology and therapeutics. JAMA 111(17):1555-1565.
8. Stone I (1972) *The Healing Factor: Vitamin C Against Disease*. New York: Grosset and Dunlap.
9. Pauling L (1970) *Vitamin C and the Common Cold*. San Francisco: Freeman.
10. Anderson TW et al. (1972) Vitamin C and the common cold: a double-blind trial. C.M.A. Journal 107:503-508.

11. Hemila H, Chal E (2013) Vitamin C for preventing and treating the common cold. Cochrane Database Syst Rev 1:CD000980.
12. Cameron E, Campbell A (1974) The orthomolecular treatment of cancer. II. Clinical trial of high-dose ascorbic acid supplements in advanced human cancer. Chem Biol Interact 9(4):285-315.
13. Cameron E, Pauling L (1976) Supplemental ascorbate in the supportive treatment of cancer: Prolongation of survival times in terminal human cancer. Proc Natl Acad Sci U S A. 73(10):3685-9.
14. Cameron E, Pauling L (1978) Supplemental ascorbate in the supportive treatment of cancer: reevaluation of prolongation of survival times in terminal human cancer. Proc Natl Acad Sci U S A. 75(9):4538-42.
15. Cameron E, Pauling L (1978) Experimental studies designed to evaluate the management of patients with incurable cancer. Proc Natl Acad Sci U S A 75(12):6252.
16. Creagan ET et al. (1979) Failure of high-dose vitamin C (ascorbic acid) therapy to benefit patients with advanced cancer. A controlled trial. NEJM 301:687-690.
17. Cameron E, Pauling L (1993) *Cancer and Vitamin C.* Philadelphia: Camino Books.
18. Moertel CG et al. (1985) High-dose vitamin C versus placebo in the treatment of patients with advanced cancer who have received no prior chemotherapy. NEJM 312(3):137-141.
19. Padayatty SJ et al. (2004) Vitamin C pharmacokinetics: implications for oral and intravenous routes. Ann Intern Med 140:533-537.

6.15 Vitamin D *Hormone or vitamin?*

1. Mayer J (1957) Armand Trousseau and the arrow of time. Nutr Rev 15:321-323.
2. Palm TA (1890) The geographic distribution and etiology of rickets. Practitioner 45:270-279.
3. Bland-Sutton J (1889) Rickets in monkeys, lions, bears, and birds. J Comp Med Surg Phila 10:1-29.

4. Findlay L, Ferguson M (1918) *A study of social and economic factors in the causation of rickets, with an introductory historical survey.* Medical Research Council Special Report #20. London, H.M.S.O.
5. Mellanby E (1919) An experimental investigation on rickets. Two lectures delivered at the Royal College of Surgeons of England. Lancet 193(4985):407-412.
6. Huldschinsky K (1919) Heilung von Rachitis durch kunssliche Hohensonne. Dtsch Med Wochenschr 45:712.
7. Chick H (1974) Study of rickets in Vienna 1919-1922. The 1974 Prize Lecture of the British Nutrition Foundation. Medical History 20:41-51 (1976).
8. McCollum EV et al. (1922) Studies on experimental rickets. XXI. An experimental demonstration of the existence of a vitamin which promotes calcium deposition. J Biol Chem 53(2):293-313.
9. Institute of Medicine (2010) Dietary reference intakes for calcium and vitamin D. www.iom.edu/vitamind
10. Dawson-Hughes B et al. (2010) IOF position statement: vitamin D recommendations for older adults. Osteoporos Int 21:1151-1154.
11. Holick MF et al. (2011) Evaluation, treatment, and prevention of vitamin D deficiency: an Endocrine Society clinical practice guideline. J Clin Endocrinol Metab 96(7):1911-30.
12. Heaney RP (2013) Health is better at serum 25(OH)D above 30 ng/ml. J Steroid Biochem Mol Biol 136:224-228.
13. Sattar N et al. (2012) Increasing requests for vitamin D measurement: costly, confusing, and without credibility. Lancet 379(9811):95-96.
14. Stolezenburg-Solomon R et al. (2006) A prospective nested case-controlled study of vitamin D status and pancreatic cancer risk in male smokers. Cancer Res 66(20):10213-10219.
15. Stolzenberg-Solomon R et al. (2010) Circulating 25-hydroxyvitamin D and risk of pancreatic cancer. Am J Epidemiol 172:81-93.
16. Manson JE et al. (2012) The VITamin D and OmegA-3 TriaL (VITAL): Rationale and design of a large randomized controlled trial of vitamin D and marine *omega*-3 fatty acid supplements for the

primary prevention of cancer and cardiovascular disease. Contemp Clinical Trials 33:159-171.

6.16 Vitamin E *A vitamin in search of a disease*

1. Evans HM, Bishop KS. (1922) On the existence of a hitherto unrecognized dietary factor essential for reproduction. Science 56 (1458):650-651.
2. Evans HM (1962) The pioneer history of vitamin E. Vitam Horm 20:389-387.
3. Evans HM et al. (1936) The isolation from wheat germ oil of an alcohol, alpha-tocopherol, having the properties of vitamin E. J Biol Chem 113:319-332.
4. Horwitt MK (1960) Vitamin E and lipid metabolism in man. Am J Clin Nutr 8:451-461.
5. Otten JJ et al. (2006) Dietary Reference Intakes: The Essential Guide to Nutrient Requirements. http://www.nap.edu/11537.html.
6. Horwitt MK (2001) Critique of the requirement for vitamin E. Am J Clin Nutr 73(6):1003-1005.
7. Horwitt MK (1980) Therapeutic uses of vitamin E in medicine. Nutr Rev 38(3):105-113.
8. The HOPE and HOPE-TOO Trial Investigators (2005) Effects of long-term vitamin E supplementation on cardiovascular events and cancer. A randomized controlled trial. JAMA 293(11):1338-1347.
9. Miller ER et al. (2005) Meta-analysis: High-dosage vitamin E supplementation may increase all-cause mortality. Ann Intern Med 142:1-11.
10. Klein EA et al. (2011) Vitamin E and the risk of prostate cancer. The selenium and vitamin E cancer prevention trial (SELECT). JAMA 306(14:1549-1556.
11. Albanes D et al. (2014) Plasma tocopherols and risk of prostate cancer in the Selenium and Vitamin E Cancer Prevention Trial (SELECT). Cancer Prev Res 7(9):886-895.
12. Garnick M (2014) Harvard Health Letter, Feb. 28.

6.17 **Vitamin K** *A balancing act*

1. Woods CW et al. (2013) Vitamin K deficiency bleeding, a case study. Adv Neonatal Care 13(6):402-407.

2. Committee statement on nutrition (1961) Vitamin K compounds and the water-soluble analogues: use in therapy and prophylaxis in pediatrics. Am Acad Pediatr 28:501-507.

3. Townsend C (1894) The hemorrhagic disease of the newborn. Arch Pediatr 11:559.

4. Golding J et al. (1992) Childhood cancer, intramuscular vitamin K, and pethidine given during labour. Brit Med J 305:341-346.

5. Anonymous (2014) Why do parents decline vitamin K for their newborns? JAMA 311(4):351.

6. Dam H (1934) A deficiency disease in chicks resembling scurvy. Biochem J. 28(4):1355-9.

7. Dam H (1935) The antihemorrhagic vitamin of the chicken: occurrence and chemical nature. Nature 135:652-653.

8. DAM H (1946) The discovery of vitamin K, its biological functions and therapeutical application. *Nobel Lecture, December 12, 1946. http://www.nobelprize.org/nobel_prizes/medicine/laureates/1943/dam-lecture.pdf*

9. Doisy EA et al. (1940) Vitamin K. Science 91(2351):58-62.

10. Schofield FW ((1922) A brief account of a disease in cattle simulating hemorrhagic septicemia due to feeding sweet clover. Can Vet Record 3:74-78.

11. Shaw K (2014) Vitamin K and bone health in older adults. J Nutr Gerontol Geriatr 33(1):10-22.

12. Otten JJ et al. (2006) Dietary Reference Intakes: The Essential Guide to Nutrient Requirements. http://www.nap.edu/11537.html

13. Ruff CT et al. (2014) Comparison of the efficacy and safety of new oral anticoagulants with warfarin in patients with atrial fibrillation: a meta-analysis of randomized trials. Lancet 383(9921):955-962.

14. Thomas K (2014) $650 million to settle blood thinner lawsuits. *New York Times*, May 28.

6.18 Calcium *A fallen star*
1. Sherman HC (1920) Calcium requirement for maintenance in man. J Biol Chem 44:21-27.
2. Institute of Medicine (2010) Dietary reference intakes for calcium and vitamin D. www.iom.edu/vitamind
3. Hegsted DM et al. (1952) A study of the minimum calcium requirements of adult men. J Nutr 46:1810201.
4. Hegsted DM (2002) Diet, calcium and hip fractures. Minerva Gastroenterol Dietol 48(3):211-213.
5. Walker ARP (1972) The human requirement of calcium: should low intakes be supplemented? Am J Clin Nutr 25:518-530.
6. Larsson CL, Johansson GK (2002) Dietary intake and nutritional status of young vegans and omnivores in Sweden. Amer J Clin Nutr 76:100-106.
7. Bolland MJ et al. (2008) Vascular events in healthy older women receiving calcium supplementation: randomised controlled trial. BMJ336(7638):262-266.
8. Larsson SC (2013) Are calcium supplements harmful to cardiovascular disease? JAMA Intern Med 173(8):647-648.

6.19 Iron *Tonic or toxin?*
1. Burnum J (1986) Medical vampires. NEJM 314(19):1250-1251.
2. Weinberg ED (2010) The hazards of iron loading. Metallomics 2(11):732-740.
3. Fonseca-Nunes A et al. (2014) Iron and cancer risk: a systemic review and meta-analysis of the epidemiological evidence. Cancer Epidemiol Biomarkers Prev 23(1):12-31.
4. NIH Office of Dietary Supplements [2014] http://ods.od.nih.gov/factsheet/iron-healthprofessional

5. Deriemaeker P et al. (2010) Nutritional status of Flemish vegetarians compared with non-vegetarians: a matched samples study. Nutrients 2(7):770-780.

6. Walker AR (1953) Iron overload in the South African Bantu. Trans R Soc Trop Med Hyg 47(6):536-548.

7. Herbert V ((1988) Recommended dietary allowances for vitamins. JAMA 260(9):1243.

8. Crosby WH (1986) Hemochromatosis: the missed diagnosis. Arch Intern Med 146(6):1209-1210.

9. Mursu J et al. (2011) Dietary supplements and mortality rate in older women. Arch Intern Med 171(18):1625-1632.

Chapter 7 Obesity *I know it when I see it.*

1. 1 Ogden CL et al. (2014) Prevalence of childhood and adult obesity in the United States, 2011-2012. JAMA 311(8):806-814.

2. Winter J et al. (2014) BMI and all-cause mortality in older adults: a meta-analysis. Am J Clin Nutr 99(4):875-890.

3. Durant W (1953) *The Pleasures of Philosophy*. New York: Simon & Schuster.

4. Schulz LO et al. (2006) Effects of traditional and eastern environments on prevalence of type 2 diabetes in Pima Indians in Mexico and the U.S. Diabetes Care 29(8):1866-1871.

5. Anonymous (2009) MMWR Weekly 58(27):740-744.

6. Miller WR et al. (1996) What predicts relapse? Prospective testing of antecedent models. Addiction 91S:S155-172.

7. Manolescu B et al. (2008) Review article: The role of adipose tissue in ureamia-related insulin resistance. Nephrology 13(7):622-628.

8. King D (2011) The future challenge of obesity. Lancet 378:743-744.

9. Swinburn BA (2011) The global obesity pandemic: shaped by global drivers and local environments. Lancet 378:804-814.

10. Satran J (2012) Soda taxes shot down by voters in two California towns. *The Huffington Post*, November 8.

Chapter 8 Weight loss and maintenance *Never say diet.*

1. Taller H (1961) *Calories don't count.* New York: Simon & Schuster.
2. Bouchard C et al. (1990) The response to long-term overfeeding in identical twins. NEJM 322(21):1477-1482.
3. de Boer JO et al. (1986) Adaptation of energy metabolism of over-weight women to low-energy intake, studied with whole-body calorimeters. Am J Clin Nutr 44(5):585-595.
4. Allbaugh LG (1953) *Crete: a case study of an underdeveloped area.* Princeton, NJ: Princeton University Press.
5. Keys A, Keys M (1959) *Eat Well and Stay Well.* New York: Doubleday.
6. Tangney CC et al. (2014) Relation of DASH- and Mediterranean-like dietary patterns to cognitive decline in older persons. Neurology 83(16):1410-1416.
7. Scarmeas N et al. (2006) Mediterranean diet and risk for Alzheimer's disease. Ann Neurol 59:912-921.
8. Sacks F et al. (1995) Rationale and design of the Dietary Approaches to Stop Hypertension (DASH). A multicenter controlled-feeding study of dietary patterns to lower blood pressure. Ann Epidemiol 5(2):108-118.
9. Appel LJ et al. (1997) A clinical trial of the effects of dietary patterns on blood pressure. DASH Collaborative Research Group. NEJM 336(16):1117-1124.
10. Jebb SA et al. (2011) Primary care referral to a commercial provider for weight loss treatment versus standard care: a randomized controlled trial. Lancet 378:1485-1492.
11. Willett WC (2011) The great fat debate: total fat and health. J Am Dietetic Assoc 111(5):660-661.

Chapter 9 Enhancement of performance *Athletic, cognitive, sexual*

1. Papagelopoulos PJ (2004) Doping in ancient and modern Olympic Games. Orthopedics 27(12):1226-1231.

2. Rasmussen N (2011) Medical science and the military: the Allies use of amphetamine during World War II. J Interdis History 42:205-233.

3. Smith GM, Beecher HK (1959) Amphetamine sulfate and athletic performance. I. Objective effects. JAMA 170(5):542-557.

4. Smith GM et al. (1963) Effects of amphetamine and secobarbital on coding and mathematical performance. J Pharmacol Exp Ther 141:100-104.

5. Bradley, C (1937) Behavior of children receiving Benzedrine. Am J Psychiat 94:577-582.

6. Volkow ND, Swanson, JM (2013) Adult attention deficit-hyperactivity disorder. NEJM 369(20):1935-1944.

7. Stolberg VB (2011) The use of coca: history, prehistory, and ethnography. J Ethn Subst Abuse 10(2):126-146.

8. Sheff N (2008) *New York Times* February 26.

9. Bastuji H, Jouvet M (1988) Successful treatment of idiopathic hypersomnia and narcolepsy with modafinil. Prog Nueropsychopharmacol Biol Psychiatry 12(5):695-700.

10. Volkow ND et al. (2009) Effects of modafinil on dopamine and dopamine transporters in the male human brain: clinical implications. JAMA 301(11):1148-1154.

11. Fox M (2013) Richard Ben Cramer, writer of big ambitions, dies at 62. *New York Times, January 8.*

12. Anonymous (1912) The influence of caffein (sic) on mental and motor efficiency and on the circulation. Reprinted JAMA 307(11):1118-1119.

13. Meier B (2012) Monster Energy drink cited in deaths. *New York Times*, October 22.

14. Freedman N et al. (2012) Association of coffee drinking with total and cause-specific mortality. NEJM 366(20):1891-1904.

15. Kruse P et al. (1986) *beta*-Blockade used in precision sports: effect on pistol shooting performance. J Appl Physiol 61(2):417-420.

16. Brantigan CO et al. (1982) Effect of *beta* blockade and *beta* stimulation on stage fright. Am J Med 72(1):88-94.
17. Herculano-Houzel S (2012) The remarkable, yet not extraordinary, human brain as a scaled-up primate brain and its associated cost. PNAS USA 109(S1) 10661-10668.
18. Jaeggi SM et al. (2008), Improving fluid intelligence with training on working memory. Proc Natl Acad Sci U S A. 105(19):6829-33.
19. Rebok GW et al. (2014) Ten-year effects of the Advanced Cognitive Training for Independent and Vital Elderly Cognitive Training Trial on cognition and everyday functioning in older adults. J Am Geriatr Soc 62:16-24.
20. Yoest H (2014) *Plants with Benefits.* Pittsburgh: St. Lynn's Press.
21. Furchgott RF (1999) Endothelium-derived relaxing factor: discovery, early studies, and identification as nitric oxide. Biosci Rep 19(4):235-251.
22. Karlovsky M et al. (2004) Increasing incidence and importance of HIV/AIDS and gonorrhea among men aged >/= 50 years in the US in the era of erectile dysfunction therapy. Scand J Urol Nephrol 38(3):247-252.

Chapter 10 Steroids *From dog testicles to "Is it low T?"*

1. Brown-Sequard CE (1889) The effects produced on man by subcutaneous injections of liquid obtained from the testicles of animals. Lancet 2:105-107.
2. Berthold A (1849) Transplantation der hoden. Arch Anat Physiol Wissenschr 42-47
3. Kendall EC (1915) The isolation in crystalline form of the compound containing iodin (sic), which occurs in the thyroid. Its chemical nature and physiologic activity. JAMA 64:2042-2049
4. David KG et al. (1935) Über krystallinisches mannliches Hormon aus Hoden (Testosteron) wirksamer als aus harn oder aus Cholesterin bereitetes Androsteron. Hoppe Seylers Z Physiol Chem 233 (5–6): 281-288.

5. Kenyon AT et al. (1937) The urinary excretion of androgenic and estrogenic substances in certain endocrine states. Studies in hypogonadism, gynecomastia, and virilism. J Clin Invest 16(5):705-17.

6. Macur J (2011) Former girlfriend details changes in Bonds. *New York Times*, March 29.

7. Bauer M et al. (1994) Psychological and endocrine abnormalities in refugees from East Germany: Part II. Serum levels of cortisol, prolactin, luteinizing hormone, follicle stimulating hormone, and testosterone. Psychiatry Res 51(1):75-85.

8. Handelsman DJ (2013) Mechanisms of action of testosterone— Unraveling a Gordian knot. NEJM 369:1058-1059.

9. Harman SM et al. (2001) Longitudinal effects of aging on serum total and free testosterone levels in healthy men. J Clin Endocrinol Metab 86(2):724-731.

10. Mayer C (2011) Amortality. Why acting your age is a thing of the past. *Time*, April 25.

11. Nieschlag E et al. (2005) Investigation, treatment, and monitoring of late-onset hypogonadism in males: ISA, ISSAM, and EAU recommendations. Int J Andrology 28:125-127.

12. DeSantis CE et al. (2014) Cancer treatment and survivorship statistics. CA Cancer J Clin 64(4):252-271.

13. Powell IJ (2010) Evidence supports a faster growth rate and/or earlier transformation to clinically significant prostate cancer in Black than in White American men, and influences racial progression and mortality disparity. J Urol 183:1792-1797.

14. Basaria S et al. (2010) Adverse events associated with testosterone administration. NEJM 363(2):109-122.

15. Vigen R (2013) Association of testosterone therapy with mortality, myocardial infarction, and stroke in men with low testosterone levels. JAMA 310(17):1829-1836.

16. Multiple authors (2014) Deaths and cardiovascular events in men receiving testosterone. JAMA 311(9):961-965.

17. Xu L et al. (2013) Testosterone therapy and cardiovascular events among men: a systematic review and meta-analysis of placebo-controlled randomized trials. BMC Medicine 11:108-120.
18. Finkle WD (2014) Increased risk of non-fatal myocardial infarction following testosterone therapy prescription in men. PLOS ONE 9(1):1-7.
19. Saiontz & Kirk, P.A. (2014) www.youhavealawyer.com
20. Schwartz LM, Woloshin S (2013) Low "T" as in "template": how to sell disease. JAMA Intern Med 173(15):1460-1462.

Chapter 11 Pain *A more terrible lord of mankind than even death*

1. Editorial (2011) Managing pain effectively. Lancet 377:2151.
2. Brand P, Yancey P (1997) *The Gift of Pain.* Grand Rapids, MI: Zondervan.
3. Vogelsang ThM (1978) Gerhard Henrik Armauer Hansen 1841–1912. The discoverer of the leprosy bacillus. His life and his work. Int J Lepr Other Mycobact Dis 46: 257–332.
4. Burney F (1812) Henry W. and Albert A. Berg Collection of English and American Literature. New York Public Library.
5. Bigelow HJ (1846) Insensibility during surgical operations produced by inhalation. Boston Med Surg J 35(16):309-317.
6. Richardson R (2013) The art of medicine. Joseph Lister's domestic science. BMJ 382:e8-e9.
7. Davy H (1800) *Researches, Chemical and Philosophical.* London: Biggs and Cottle.
8. Long CW (1849) An account of the first use of sulphuric ether by inhalation as an anaesthetic in surgical operations. In Cole F (1965) *Milestones in Anesthesia.* Omaha: University of Nebraska Press.
9. Holmstedt B, Liljestrand G (1963) *Readings in Pharmacology,* pp. 117-121, New York: MacMillan.
10. Niemann A (1860) Ueber eine neue organische Base in den Cocablattern. Inaug. diss. Gottingen

11. Koller C (1884) Ueber die Verwendung des Cocain zur Anasthesirung am Auge. Wein med wschr 34:1276-1228, 1309-1311.
12. Murray AT (1919) *Homer The Odyssey*. The Loeb Classical Library, Cambridge, MA.
13. Schmiedeberg O (1918) Uber die Pharmaka in der Ilias und Odyssee. Schriften d. wiss. Gesellsch Strassburg 36: 37-42.
14. Berridge V (1999) *Opium and the People*. New York: Free Association Books LTD.
15. Taylor N (1965) *Plant Drugs That Changed the World*, p. 212. New York: Dodd, Mead &Co.
16. Serturner FWA (1817) Ueber das Morphium, eine neue salzfahige Grundlage, und die Mekonsaure, als Hauptbestandtheile des Opiums. Gilbert's Ann d Physik Leipsig 25:56-89.
17. Jones CM et al. (2013) Pharmaceutical overdose deaths, United States, 2010. JAMA 309(7):657-659.
18. Moore A et al. (2013) Expect analgesic failure; pursue analgesic success. BMJ 346:f2690.
19. Phillip DM (2000) JCAHO Pain management standards are unveiled. JAMA 284:428–429.
20. Deandrea S et al. (2008) Prevalence of under-treatment in cancer pain. Ann Oncol 19:1985-1991.
21. Atasoy S (2009) Statement to the United Nations Economic and Social Council. www.incb.org/documents/President-statements-09/2009 4404.
22. Moszynski P (2009) Lack of palliative care causes unnecessary suffering for India's terminally ill people. BMJ 339:b4404.
23. Vargas-Schaffer G (2010) Is the WHO analgesic ladder still valid? Twenty-four years of experience. Can Fam Physician 56(6):514-517.
24. Saunders C (2000) The evolution of palliative care. Patient Educ Couns 41(1):7-13.
25. Turk DC et al. (2011) Treatment of chronic non-cancer pain. Lancet 377(9784):2226-2235.

26. Morgan JP (1985) American opiophobia: customary underutilization of opioid analgesics. Adv Alcohol Subst Abuse 5(1-2):163-173.
27. Jeal T (2013) *Livingstone: Revised and Expanded Edition.* New Haven: Yale University Press.

Chapter 12 Dementia *Augusta Deter and Dr. Alzheimer*
  1. Maurer K et al. (1997) Auguste D and Alzheimer's disease. Lancet 349:1546-1549.
  2. Alzheimer A (1906) Uber einen eigenartigen schweren Erkrankungsprozes der Hirnrind. Neurologisches Centralblatt 23:1129-1136.
  3. Alzheimer's Association (2014) Alzheimer's Disease Facts and Figures. www.alz.org/facts
  4. Jacoby S (2011) *Never Say Die. The Myth and Marketing of the New Old Age,* P. 111. New York: Pantheon Books.
  5. Chinthapalli K (2014) Alzheimer's disease: still a perplexing problem. BMJ 349:g4433.
  6. Jonsson T et al. (2012) A mutation in *APP* protects against Alzheimer's disease and age-related cognitive decline. Nature 488:96-99.
  7. Doody RS et al. (2013) A phase 3 trial of semagacestat for treatment of Alzheimer's disease. NEJM 369(4):341-350.
  8. Doody RS et al. (2014) Phase 3 trials of solanezumab for mid-to-moderate Alzheimer's disease. NEJM 370(4):311-321.
  9. Salloway S et al. (2014) Two phase 3 trials of bapineuzumab in mild-to-moderate Alzheimer's disease. NEJM 370:322-333.
  10. Bateman RJ et al. (2012) Clinical and biomarker changes in dominantly inherited Alzheimer's disease. NEJM 367:795-804.
  11. Friedrich MJ (2014) Researchers test strategies to prevent Alzheimer's disease. JAMA 311(16):1596-1598.
  12. Aisen PS et al. (2008) High-dose B vitamin supplementation and cognitive decline in Alzheimer disease. A randomized controlled trial. JAMA 300(15):1774-1783.

13. Clarke R et al. (2014) Effects of homocysteine lowering with B vitamins on cognitive aging: meta-analysis of 11 trials with cognitive data on 22,000 individuals. Am J Clin Nutr 100(2):657-666.
14. Franke K et al. (2014) Gender-specific impact of personal health parameters on individual brain aging in cognitively unimpaired elderly subjects. Front Aging Neurosci 6:94-111.
15. Pitkala KH (2013) Effects of the Finnish Alzheimer disease exercise trial (FINALEX). A randomized controlled trial. JAMA Intern Med 173(10):894-901.
16. Ohman H et al. (2014) Effect of physical exercise on cognitive performance in older adults with mild cognitive impairment or dementia: A systematic review. Dement Geriatr Cogn Disord 38(5-6):347-365.

13 Cancer *The optimal lifestyle for prevention*

1. Anonymous (2014) Getting close and personal. *The Economist*, P. 61, January 4.
2. Henley SJ et al. (2014) Invasive cancer incidence - United States, 2010. MMWR Morb Mortal Wkly Rep 63(12):253-259.
3. Hurria A et al. (2013) Improving the quality of cancer care in an aging population. JAMA 310(17):1795-1796.
4. Del Vecchio M et al. (2014) Efficacy and safety of ipilimumab 3 mg/kg in pretreated, metastatic, mucosal melanoma. Eur J Cancer 50(1):121-127.
5. Leaf C (2013) *The Truth in Small Doses: Why We're Losing the War on Cancer---and How to Win It.* New York: Simon & Schuster.
6. Saika K, Sobue T (2009) Epidemiology of breast cancer in Japan and the US. JMAJ 52(1):39-44.
7. Inoue M, Tsugane S (2005) Epidemiology of gastric cancer in Japan. Postgrad Med J 81:419-424.
8. Higginson J, Oettle AG (1960) Cancer incidence in the Bantu and 'Cape Colored' races of South Africa: report of cancer survey in Transvaal (1953-1955). J Natl Cancer Inst 24:589-671.

9. Doll R, Hill AB (1952) A study of the aetiology of carcinoma of the lung. BMJ 2(4797):1271-86.

10. Anonymous (2012) Tobacco in the USA: smoke and mirrors. Lancet 379:288.

11. Armstrong B, Doll R (1975) Environmental factors and cancer incidence and mortality in different countries, with special reference to dietary practices. Int J Cancer 15(4):617-31.

12. Anonymous (1982) National Research Council (US) Committee on Diet, Nutrition, and Cancer. Washington, DC: National Academies Press.

13. Kushi M (1983) *The Cancer-Prevention Diet*. New York: St. Martins.

14. Gorbach S, Zimmerman DR (1984) *The Doctors' Anti-Breast Cancer Diet: How the Right Foods Can Reduce Your Risk of Breast Cancer*. New York: Simon & Schuster.

15. Boeke CE et al. (2014) Dietary fat intake in relation to lethal breast cancer in two large prospective studies. Breast Cancer Res Treat 146(2):383-392.

16. Parkin DM et al. (2011) The fraction of cancer attributable to lifestyle and environmental factors in the UK in 2010. Br J Cancer 105:S77-S81.

17. Prue G (2014) Vaccinate boys as well as girls against HPV: it works, and it may be cost effective. BMJ 349:g4834.

18. Segi M et al. (1964) Geographical and epidemiological considerations on cancer with special reference to the status of cancer in Japan as compared with other nations. Naika 13:1031-1041.

19. Schwingshackl L, Hoffmann G (2014) Adherence to Mediterranean diet and risk of cancer: a systematic review and meta-analysis of observational studies. Int J Cancer 135(8):1884.

20. Mourouti N et al. (2014) Adherence to the Mediterranean diet is associated with lower likelihood of breast cancer: a case-control study. Nutr Cancer 66(5):810-817.

21. Chen WY et al. (2011) Moderate alcohol consumption during adult life, drinking patterns, and breast cancer risk. JAMA 306(17):1884-1890.

22. Nelson DE et al. (2013) Alcohol-attributable cancer deaths and years of potential life lost in the United States. AJPH 103(4):641-648.

23. Bofetta P et al. (2010) Fruit and vegetable intake and overall cancer risk in the European Prospective Investigation into Cancer and Nutrition (EPIC). J Natl Cancer Inst 102:529-537.

24. Wang X et al. (2014) Fruit and vegetable consumption and mortality from all causes, cardiovascular disease, and cancer: systematic review and dose-response meta-analysis of prospective cohort studies. BMJ 349:g4490. 349:g4834.

25. Zu K et al. (2014) Dietary lycopene, angiogenesis, and prostate cancer: A prospective study in the prostate-specific antigen era. J Natl Cancer Inst 106(2):djt11430.

Chapter 14 Heart disease and stroke *Still the greatest killers*

1. Go AS et al. (2014) Heart disease and stroke statistics---2014 update: a report from the American Heart Association. Circulation 129(3):e28-e292.

2. Mahmood SS et al. (2014) The Framingham Heart Study and the epidemiology of cardiovascular disease: a historical perspective. Lancet 383:999-1008.

3. Epstein FH (1968) Multiple risk factors and the prediction of coronary heart disease. Bull N Y Acad Med 44(8):916-35.

4. Thompson RC et al. (2013) Atherosclerosis across 4000 years of human history: the Horus study of four ancient populations. Lancet 381:1211-1222.

5. Centers for Disease Control and Prevention (2012) Vital signs: awareness and treatment of uncontrolled hypertension among adults—United States, 2003–2010. *MMWR* 61(35):703–9.

6. Weiss S, Ellis LB (1930) The rational treatment of arterial hypertension. JAMA 311(21):2238.

7. Sever P (1999) Abandoning diastole. BMJ318:1773.

8. James PA et al. (2014) Evidence-based guideline for the management of high blood pressure in adults: report from the panel members appointed to the Eighth National Committee (JNC 8). JAMA 311(5):507-520.

9. Rapsomaniki E et al . (2014) Blood pressure and incidence of twelve cardiovascular diseases: lifetime risks, healthy life-years lost, and age-specific associations in 1.25 million people. Lancet 383:1899-1911.

10. Susmano A (2012) Franklin Roosevelt's last illness. Hektoen Int 4(1).

11. Bruenn HG (1970) Clinical notes on the illness and death of President Franklin D. Roosevelt. Ann Intern Med 72(4):579-91.

12. Morris JN et al (1953a) Coronary heart disease and physical activity of work. Lancet 262(6795):1053-1057.

13. Morris JN et al (1953b) Coronary heart disease and physical activity of work. Lancet 262(6796):1111-1120.

14. Morris JN, Crawford M (1958) Coronary heart disease and physical activity of work; evidence of a national necropsy survey. BMJ 2(5111):1485-1496.

15. Boyer JL, Kasch FW (1970) Exercise therapy in hypertensive men. JAMA 211(10):1668-1671.

16. Chrysant SG, Chrysant GS (2013) New insights into the true nature of the obesity paradox and the lower cardiovascular risk. J Am Soc Hypertens 7(1):85-94..0

17. Department of Agriculture, DHHS (2010) Dietary guidelines for Americans. Washington, DC: Government Printing Office.

18. Farley TA (2014) The public health crisis hiding in our food. *New York Times*, April 20.

19. Taylor RS et al. (2011) Reduced dietary salt for the prevention of cardiovascular disease: a meta-analysis of randomized controlled trials (Cochrane Review) Am J Hyperten 24(8):843-853.

20. He FJ, MacGregor GA (2011) Salt reduction lowers cardiovascular risk: meta-analysis of outcome trials. Lancet 378:380-382.

21. Institute of Medicine (2013) Sodium intake of populations: Assessment of evidence. Washington DC: National Academies Press.

22. Alderman MH (2011) The Cochrane review of sodium and health. Am J Hyperten 24(8):354-356.

23. Cogswell ME et al. (2012) Sodium and potassium intakes among US adults. Am J Clin Nutr 96(3):647-657.

24. O'Donnell M (2014) Urinary sodium and potassium excretion, mortality, and cardiovascular effects. NEJM 371:612-623.

25. Yang Q et al. (2011) Sodium and potassium intake and mortality among US adults. Arch Intern Med 171(13):1183-1191.

26. John SK et al. (2011) Life-threatening hyperkalemia from nutritional supplements: uncommon or undiagnosed? Am J Emerg Med 29(9):1237.e1-2.

27. Ferrannini E, Cushman WC (2012) Diabetes and hypertension: the bad companions. Lancet 380:601-610.

28. Müller C (1938) Xanthoma, hypercholesterolemia, angina pectoris. Acta Med Scandinav 95(S89): 75-84.

29. Rader DJ, Hovingh GK (2014) HDL and cardiovascular disease. Lancet 384(9943):618-625.

30. The Nobel Prizes (1986) Editor William Odeberg. Stockholm: Nobel Foundation.

31. Kannell WB et al. (1961) Comparison of serum lipids in the prediction of coronary heart disease. RI Med J 48:243-250.

32. Lipid Research Clinics Program (1984) The Lipid Research Clinics primary prevention trial results. JAMA 251:351-364.

33. Anonymous (1985) Lowering blood cholesterol to reduce heart disease. JAMA 253(14):2080-2086.

34. Oliver MF (1985) Consensus or nonsensus conferences on coronary heart disease. Lancet 1(8437):1087-1089.

35. Ahrens EH (1985) The diet-heart question in 1985: has it really been settled? Lancet 1(8437):1085-1087.

36. Cholesterol Guidelines (2013) my.clevelandclinic.org/services/heart/prevention/risk-factors/cholesterol

37. Mayo Clinic Staff (2013) Cholesterol levels: What numbers should you aim for? http://www.mayoclinic.com/health/cholesterol-levels/CL00001

38. Stone NJ et al. (2013) ACC/AHA guideline on the treatment of blood cholesterol to reduce atherosclerotic cardiovascular risk in adults. Circulation 129(25 S2):S1-45.

39. Ridker P, Cook N (2013) Statins: new American guidelines for prevention of cardiovascular disease. Lancet 382:1762-1765.

40. Kolata G (2013) Heart and stroke study hit by wave of criticism. *New York Times*, November 26.

41. Kolata G (2013) Risk calculator for cholesterol appears flawed. *New York Times*, November 17.

42. Ioannidis JPA (2014) More than a billion people taking statins? Potential implications of the new cardiovascular guidelines. JAMA 311(5):463-464.

43. Abramson JE et al. (2204) Petition to the National Institutes of Health seeking an independent review panel to re-evaluate the national cholesterol education project guidelines. http://cspinet.org/new/pdf/finalnihltr.pdf

44. Abramson JD, Redburg RF (2013) Don't give more patients statins. *New York Times*, November 13.

45. United States Food and Drug Administration (2012) FDA drug safety communication: important safety label changes to cholesterol-lowering statin drugs. Silver Spring, MD. www.fda.gov/Drugs/DrugSafety/ucm293101.htm

Chapter 15 Osteoporosis *Of osteoclasts and osteoblasts*

1. International Osteoporosis Foundation (2014) Incidence and economic burden of osteoporosis. http://www.iofbonehealth.org/facts-statistics

2. Albright F et al. (1941) Postmenopausal osteoporosis: its clinical features. JAMA 116(22):2465-2474.

3. Walker ARP, Walker BF (1981) Recommended dietary allowances and third world populations. Am J Clin Nutr 34:2319-2321.

4. Nabel EG (2013) The Women's Health Initiative---A victory for women and their health. JAMA 310(13):1349-1350.

5. Detter FTL et al. (2013) A 5-year exercise program in pre- and peripubertal children improves bone mass and bone size without affecting fracture risk. Calcif Tissue Int 92:385-393.

6. Institute of Medicine. Dietary reference intakes for calcium and vitamin D. Washington, DC: National Academies Press, 2011.

7. Nilsson BE, Westlin NE (1971) Bone density in athletes. Clin Orthoped Rel Res 77:179-182.

8. Kemmler W et al. (2013) Effects of exercise on fracture reduction in older adults: a systematic review and meta-analysis. Osteoporos Int 24(7):1937-1950.

9. Park-Wyllie LY et al. (2011) Bisphosphonate use and the risk of sub-trochantric or femoral shaft fractures in older women. JAMA 305(8):783-789.

Chapter 16 The final chapter *Death and dignity*

1. Quill T (1991) Death and dignity, a case of individualized decision making. NEJM 324(10):691-694.

2. Stafford N (2011) Jack Kevorkian, former pathologist and controversial assisted suicide activist. BMJ 342:d4100.

3. Humphry D (2002) *Final Exit*, 3rd ed. Delta Trade. *https://openlibrary.org/publishers/Delta_Trade_Paperbacks*

4. Quill T (2012) Physicians should "assist in suicide" when it is appropriate. J Law Med Ethics 40(1):57-65.

5. Knight S (2008) The tragic story of Wallace Hume Carothers. *Financial Times*, November 29, www.ft.com › Life&Arts

6. General Orders, Commander 7th Fleet: serial 03563 (1944) Navy Cross, Chester William Nimitz, Jr.

7. Rimer S (2002) With suicide, an admiral keeps command until the end. *New York Times*, January 12.
8. Powell D (2011) Dr. Chafetz and Marion---a love story. *The View from Mudsock Heights*. www.athensnews.com
9. Anonymous (2012) Oregon's Death with Dignity Act—2011. http://public.health.oregon.giv/ProviderPartnerResources/ EvaluationResearch.DeathwithDignityAct/Documents/year14.pdf
10. Luscombe B (2012) The doctor who pushed for Oregon's right-to-die law, Peter Goodwin, on brain disease and facing the hereafter. *Time*, March 16, p. 62.
11. Greenberg DS (1991) Dying, doctors, and politics. Lancet 338:1446-1447.
12. Anonymous (2004) Huibert Drion, Dutch Supreme Court judge who became a leading advocate of euthanasia. BMJ328:1204.

ABOUT THE AUTHOR

Jerrold Winter, Ph.D., is Professor of Pharmacology and Toxicology in the School of Medicine and Biomedical Sciences of the University at Buffalo. For nearly five decades he has taught the principles of pharmacology, the elements of addiction, and the drug treatment of anxiety, depression, and psychosis to graduate and medical students. Research in his laboratory has centered on hallucinogens and other drugs of abuse. He is the author of more than one hundred scientific publications. His previous book for the general public, *True Nutrition True Fitness*, was published in 1991.

INDEX

Made in the USA
Lexington, KY
06 May 2016